ESSENTIALS OF CRANIO-SACRAL OSTEOPATHY

Ronald R. McCatty

Ph.D., D.O., M.Cr.O.A.,
M.G.O.(Lon.), M.B.E.O.A., M.N.T.O.S., L.C.S.P.(Phys.)

ASHGROVE PRESS, BATH

First published in Great Britain by
ASHGROVE PRESS LTD
4 Brassmill Centre, Brassmill Lane
Bath BA1 3JN

© Ronald R. McCatty 1988

First published 1988

McCatty, Ronald R.
    Essentials of cranio-sacral osteopathy
    1. Medicine. Cranial osteopathy
    I. Title
    615.5'33
    ISBN 0-906798-90-6

Photoset in 11/12½ Palatino by
Ann Buchan (Typesetters), Middlesex
Printed in Great Britain by
Dotesios Printers
Bradford on Avon, Wiltshire

Essentials of Craniosacral Osteopathy

ERRATA

page 50 *Top caption, for* Thoracic Pump *read* Thoracic Inlet
Bottom caption, for Thoracic Inlet *read* Thoracic Pump

page 208 *Figure 67, delete* page *after figure number*

Contents

FOREWORD		ix
PREFACE		xi
	PART I	1
CHAPTER 1	The Cranio-Sacral Concept	3
2	The Cranio-Sacral Mechanism & Cranial Rhythmic Impulses	15
3	The Primary Respiratory Mechanism & Cerebro Spinal Fluid	30
4	Body Fluids	45
5	Cranio-Sacral Balance & Fluid Mechanics	56
6	The Significance of the Sphenoid in the Cranial Concept	64
7	The Endocrine Umbrella	75
8	Fourth Ventricle Compression	106
9	Diagnosis & Evaluation	116
10	Lesions – Vault & Base	128
11	The Facial Complex	145
12	Special Techniques	158
13	Gynaecology	177
14	Extracranial Considerations	190
15	The Minimal Lesion	199
16	More Case Histories	204
	PART II	215
CHAPTER 17	Cranial Landmarks & other Charts	217
18	The Vault	232
19	The Base	248
20	The Face	261
21	Ancillary Bones of the Skull	288
22	The Foetal Skull	295
23	The Sacrum & Coccyx	298
GLOSSARY		308
INDEX		319

List of Illustrations

	PART I	Page
1	The Skull. Articular Relationships	4
2 & 3	Pioneers. A.T. Still & W.G. Sutherland	6
4	Pioneer J.M. Littlejohn	8
5	The Human Skull I & II	10
6	The Human Skull III & IV	11
7	The Human Skull V & VI	12
8	Diagnostic Indications	16
9	Dural Attachments of the Spine	18
10	Palpation & Evaluation	20
11	Attachments of Dural Membranes (Poles of Attachment)	24
12	Sacro-Occipital Relationship	26
13	The Straight Sinus & Its Neighbours	31
14	Cranial Embryological Development	32
TABLE A	Cranial Embryological Development	34
15	Ventricles of the Brain and C.S.F. distribution	36, 37
16	The Dural Meninges	40
17	Cranial Venous Sinuses & Arterial Supply	42, 43
18	Lymphatic System	47
TABLE B	Distribution of Fluids. Body Constituents	48
19	Lymphatic Drainage	50
TABLE C	Body Fluids	52
20	Dural Meninges	57
21	Sphenobasilar Symphysis I & II	58
22	III & IV	59
23	Cranial Palpation	60
24	Sphenoidal Muscles	66
TABLE D	Sphenoidal Muscles, Ligaments & Foramina	67, 68
25	Sphenobasilar Torsion	69
26	Sphenobasilar Symphysis. Superior & Lateral Aspects	70
27	Sphenobasilar Symphysis. Anterior Aspect	72

	28	The Endocrine System	76
	29	Lemniscate Action	77
	30	Bi-Temporal Rolling	80
	31	The Endocrine Glands. Pineal & Pituitary	82
	32	Cranial Procedures. Thyroid & Sacral Flexion	88
	33	The Endocrine Glands. Thyroid, Parathyroid & Thymus	90
	34	The Endocrine Glands. Pancreas & Adrenals	95
35 & 36		The Endocrine Glands. Ovary and Testis	101 & 102
	37	Hand Position for 4VC	107
	38	Fourth Ventricle Compression	108
	39	Sacro-Occipital Balancing	109
	40	Cranial Techniques with Two Operators. Flexion & Extension I & II	110
	41	Cranial Techniques with Two Operators. Sacral Flexion	112
		Cranial Techniques with Two Operators. Contralateral Flexion III IV & V	113
TABLE E		Fourth Ventricle Compression — Summary	114
	42	Diagnosis & Evaluation. Observation	117
	43	Pedic Angles	118
	44	Facial Foramina	120
	45	Concavities	124
	46	Sagittal Spread	126
	47	The Foetal Skull & Birth	129
	48	Body Attitudes	130
TABLE F		Cranio-sacral Lesions & Body Attitudes	132
	49	Cranial Base Techniques. Decongestion, Decompression	136
	50	Vault Lifts	138
	51	Quadrant Analysis	142
	52	Flaring the Maxillae	146
	53	Vomer & Zygoma	148
	54	Increasing the Diameter of the Orbit	150
	55	Nasals & Lacrimals	152
	56	E.T.T. Four Finger Technique	159
	57	Energy Transference Techniques. Four Finger Technique	160
	58	Special Techniques. Ear Pull & Falx Cerebri	166
	59	Special Techniques. Coccygeal Adjustment	169
	60	Moulding	172
	61	Gynaecology. Female Reproductive Organs	180
	62	Gynaecology. Lateral View of Pelvic Bowl	182
	63	Fascial Planes	184
	64	Iliopsoas & Piriformis Muscles	192
	65	Draining the Psoas	194
	66	Crossover Point L2/3	196

TABLE G	Adaptation of Martindale's Postulation. Minimal Lesion	200
67 & 68	Mrs Bray's Sketches	208
69	Cranial Hypothesis	212

PART II

70	Cranial Landmarks	216, 217
TABLE H	Main Osseous Components of the Cranio-sacral Concept	218
TABLE I	Articulations	219–222
TABLE J	Key Vertebrae	223–226
TABLE K	Key Vertebrae. Key Pairs	226
TABLE L	Physiological Movement	227–230
71	Vault Sutural Bevels	233
72	Frontal Bone	235, 236
73	Frontal Bone	237
74	Parietal Bone	240, 241
75	Occipital Bone	244, 245
76	Basal Relationships	249, 250
77	Sphenoid Bone	252, 253
78	Temporal Bone	258, 259
79	Facial Relationships	262
80	Facial Relationships. Nasal, Orbital	263
81	The Mandible	266, 267
82	Anterior (External) Facial Bones. Zygoma, Maxilla	274, 275
83	Anterior (External) Facial Bones. Lacrimal & Nasal	276
84	Posterior (Internal) Facial Bones. Ethmoid	278, 279
85	Posterior (Internal) Facial Bones. Palatine, Vomer, & Inf. Nasal Choncha	284, 285
TABLE M	Hyoidal Muscles & Ligaments	289, 290
86	Ancillary Bones of the Skull	293
87	Full Term Foetal Skull	295, 296
88	The Sacrum	300, 301
89	The Coccyx	304

Foreword

It is a privilege to be requested to write a foreword to this book on advanced Osteopathic methods of treating disorders. *Essentials of Cranio-Sacral Osteopathy* by Dr Ronald R. McCatty is a landmark of progress in Osteopathic medicine. This book is the outcome of the practical experience of many years gained in this field. Osteopathy as a form of therapy is still an expanding science and its application in treatment of disease is widening.

In his book *Essentials of Cranio-Sacral Osteopathy* Dr McCatty has indeed succeeded in bringing to life a form of healing that many people are not familiar with. Dr McCatty primarily having treated patients using osteopathy has found that by observing the patient and merely adjusting the cranium and sacrum, many disorders can be successfully treated. He clearly and concisely describes the diagnosis and treatment which would otherwise evade the healer.

Cranial irregularities and dysfunctions are, we discover, responsible for many disorders including migraine, sinusitis, backache, etc. Using his experience in a busy practice, the author illustrates this treatment with patients under his care.

I commend this book to the student and practitioner for study. The practical application of the scientific knowledge expounded in this valuable work will be another milestone in the progress of alternative medicine.

Professor Dr Anton Jayasuriya
M.B.B.S. (Cey.), D.Phys.Med. R.C.P. (Lond.),
R.C.S. (Eng.), M.Ac.F. (Sri Lanka), Ph.D.,
F.Ac.F. (India), D.Litt.

THE BIBLE

'... the whole body fitly joined together and compacted by that which every joint supplieth, according to the effectual working in the measure of every part...'
Ephesians 4:16

'... and not holding the head, from which all the body by joints and bands having nourishment ministered, and knit together increaseth...'
Colossians 2:19

'... heal me, for my bones are vexed...'
Psalm 6:2

Preface

This book is intended to be a guide and working companion for practitioners and students on many different levels – Doctors, Chiropractors, Osteopaths, Dentists, Naturopaths, and allied professions. It is meant to be practical, illustrative, and devoid of obscure jargon.

Much of the nomenclature of Cranial Osteopathy owes its origin to the late Dr William Garner Sutherland, the pioneer of Cranio-Sacral Osteopathy. Certain words were either 'coined' or adapted by him and subsequent devotees to demonstrate the difference between the traditional allopathic concepts, and the body's self-regulating systems. They help to explain the various rhythms and cycles which are often hidden from normal observation because they are not anticipated – not taught. They do not accord with the more usual anatomic and physiological jargon.

There are two basic concepts peculiar to Cranial Osteopathy. Dr Sutherland spoke of these as being 'cranial sutural motion' and 'a distinct series of rhythmic impulses within the cranium:' and this book is mostly concerned with the practical application of this premise and all that follows from it.

It is not my idea, however, to present the last word on an almost inexhaustible subject. Nothing could be farther from my mind. But I have yielded to pressure from colleagues, students, and friends to write this book. Therefore, after two years, almost to the day, I am breathing a sigh of relief as the last few words are being added to the M.S.

It has been a stimulating exercise – certainly not merely a collecting or collating of facts and ideas, but a devotion to the cause of promoting health and well-being.

Particular attention is directed to the presentation of the body's physiological systems. Accordingly much space is given to the functional unity of the entire human organism, and the sketches and diagrams are aimed at minimising complexity.

Since Sutherland's 'The Cranial Bowl' and Magoun's 'Osteopathy in the Cranial Field' osteopathy has greatly benefited from a profusion of literary contribution. Some of these are indeed milestones which have marked the place for educational development and practical therapeutic excellence for which we can only be grateful. Many may never be surpassed in style and simplicity of application; and why should they be? There is no competition after all! Each contributor to the scholastic and heuristic pool deserves the highest accolade for adding fresh and enduring lustre to this ever unfolding concept which will outlast many that are 'here today and gone tomorrow.'

Essentials of Craniosacral Osteopathy is not presented as a substitute for any other book, but simply to amplify the spread of information that might prove a life-line to the 'drowning' practitioner!

We read so much these days of Cranial techniques being a mere adjunct to the osteopathic armoury; and it is true that many of these individual techniques can be used on a purely mechanical level – as another way to achieve this or that result.

But 'real' Cranial Osteopathy is a thing apart. It may take you two years to perceive even the basic rhythms; then when you have even that small beginning, you will wonder how you ever managed without it. It can take seven, eight, or ten years to become fully aware of what is happening under your fingers – to know what you are feeling, experiencing, affecting, and, just as you think 'that's it! I've got it now!' you are immediately aware that it's just another small part of the vast jig-saw of human physiology slotting into place.

Denis Brookes said a little while before he died 'I've worked over forty years with this, and I'm just beginning to learn what it is all about.' So don't be discouraged by those who say 'there's nothing to it' – after five minutes acquaintance with the subject, or by the fact that you will never come to terms with the human body and its workings entirely – it is so inexplicable at times, never the same, always changing in the one person from one time to another; and, of course, from person to person. Be encouraged by the thrill that you get when you suddenly find that you can sit at the head of a couch with a patient's head in your hands and, say, move his feet and legs; or remove a pain from his back, and begin to accomplish that balanced state you've desired to achieve.

Or experience the excitement of seeing a man walk into your practice crippled, with a long standing back problem, and by the merest feather-like touch on occiput and sphenoid, etc. see that man walk out better than he has been for years, because you have unlocked a restriction acquired a long time ago. The body is only too eager to restore homeostasis if it is given the right helping hand.

So, if I have merely given you a new set of techniques to add to your osteopathic armamentarium; or if you look on this book to give exact instructions to be used in certain circumstances, then I've failed.

But if you take hold of the idea – the concept – and make it your own, always studying to know more of the underlying stresses, strains, fluid patterns, etc. that are the real pre-cursors to pathology; and then learn to harness these to effect the well-being of the patient, then I will know that what I have tried to convey has been a success.

As far as possible study the pioneers, Sutherland, Magoun, Brookes, and not forgetting Still, whose original thought laid the foundations – they are still valid despite all our modern technological expertise, and you will be rewarded – as I have been – with a knowledge that far outreaches anything else you might learn about the human body.

Years ago my own thirst for knowledge was satisfied by contact with one of the greatest cranial osteopaths on the continent of Europe.

His name was Denis Brookes, and further mention will inevitably be made of him in the following text. It seems fitting for me to pay the highest possible tribute to that great man who became my teacher and revered mentor. I esteem it a great honour and privilege to have in my possession a Diploma bearing his signature.

He gave more than forty years to the profession and his knowledge of anatomy, physiology, and endogenous endocrinotherapy, etc. was profound, equalled only by his ability to impart that knowledge to his students. In a word he was brilliant.

If for no more than these reasons, I believe, that many of my colleagues and friends who came under his tutelage will join with me in acknowledging that his name is indelibly written not only in our minds but in the annals of Cranial Osteopathic history, as one of the Greats.

I am also indebted to the writings of Still, Magoun, Arbuckle, Burns, Stretch, the Lippincotts, and many others for the contribution they have made to Osteopathy as a whole, and Cranial Osteopathy in particular. Some of these innovators are quoted in this book.

A great many people have either consciously or unconsciously contributed to this volume, some by their helpful comments, and others by providing the requisite ambience for research and perceptive analysis.

My thanks are particularly extended to :- a graphic artist, Brian J. Brown who has been responsible for many of the illustrations: my assistant Joan Gazeley, for her long hours of hard work helping with the research, preparation, and compilation of the manuscript; and last – but certainly not least – to my wife, Nancy, without whose patience and encouragement through the years of study, research, and writing, none of this would have been possible.

I will end with this quotation from Dr Schooley (in relation to our concern with holistic medicine) 'Our corrective procedures should be to move or carry the articulation in the direction in which it moves most freely, at a point where the tissues feel under no stress, and fluids between the cells exert themselves and return the tissue spaces to their normal space relationships or shapes.'

HIPPOCRATES

'And each (disease) has its own peculiar nature and power, and none is of an ambiguous nature, or irremediable. And the most of them are curable by the same means as those by which they were produced. For any one thing is food to one, and injurious to another. Thus, then, the physician should understand and distinguish the season of each, so that at one time he may attend to the nourishment and increase, and at another to abstraction and diminution.'

'Men's heads are by no means all like to one another, nor are the sutures of the head of all men constructed in the same form . . .'

'. . . knowledge of the body depends upon the knowledge of the whole man.'

PART I

CHAPTER ONE

The Cranio-Sacral Concept

Any inquiry into the Cranial (or cranio-sacral) Concept must be preceded by a good understanding of osteopathic principles. This concept does not replace traditional Osteopathy, it enhances it.

The body is relentlessly self-protecting and resists the imposition of force. Hence, therapeutically the most profound results are arrived at by gentleness. No wonder William Garner Sutherland, the founder of Cranial Osteopathy, spoke of thinking, feeling, seeing, knowing fingers. He had great respect for the human body, his fingers dexterously perfecting balance of tissue tension when making corrections.

Regarding Osteopathy as a 'non-incisive surgical art' he never used force in his practice. He believed rather that the body possesses the inherent mechanism for self-correction over and above any considered external force that might be applied to it.

The reasoning behind Sutherland's thinking is yet another pointer to the fact that homeostatically the body is dependent on the integrity of its fluid systems – blood, lymph, C.S.F., etc.

Contrary to some schools of thought, all circumstances being normal, the cranial sutures (or joints of the head) do not fuse – regardless of age, race, sex, or geographical location. They are perpetually motile, influencing the dynamics of fluid exchange and membraneous tension within the cranio-sacral mechanism.

Beginning with a simple review of the cranium it will soon become obvious how these principles may be applied. Convenience is best served by dividing and sub-dividing the cranium into areas. For instance, Gray lists the various aspects as Norma Verticalis, Basalis, Occipitalis, Frontalis, Lateralis; and these are then sub-divided into smaller sections – orbit, fossae, etc.

Denis Brookes favours Cranial, Facial, Ossicle, Cervical groupings, along with a detailed list of the various features of each region. But for the purpose of this book it is probably easiest to follow Sutherland. In his treatise 'The Cranial Bowl' he has omitted the tedium of a lengthy discourse on anatomy and has devoted his text more to explaining the sutural mobility and function of the

1 THE SKULL
ARTICULAR RELATIONSHIPS

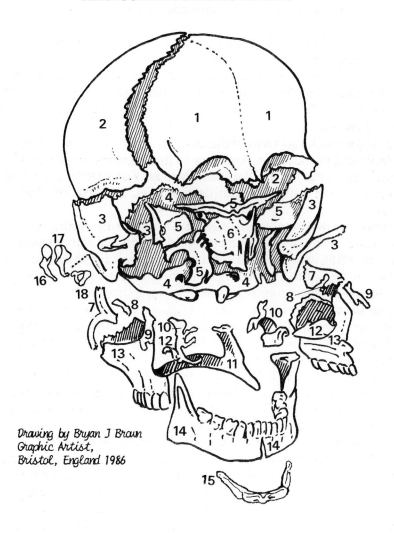

Drawing by Bryan J Brown
Graphic Artist,
Bristol, England 1986

1	Frontal	10	Palatine
2	Parietal	11	Vomer
3	Temporal	12	Inferior concha (turbinates)
4	Occipital	13	Maxilla
5	Sphenoid	14	Mandible
6	Ethmoid	15	Hyoid
7	Zygoma (Malar)	16	Malleus
8	Lacrimal	17	Incus
9	Nasal	18	Stapes

skull, its lesion possibilities and cranial technique. In so doing he originated and presented the profession with a new and most important concept that was, and still is, a tremendous contribution to the world of medicine.

That the medical profession did not, and still does not, pay homage to Dr Sutherland's findings is not our concern within these pages. Suffice it to say his discoveries have given rise to a whole new dimension in osteopathic thought and practice. He has outlined the phenomenon of the cranio-sacral mechanism, its functional unity and harmonious integration with the rest of the body's systems.

The motile (or working) areas of the cranium as he saw it, may be regarded as Basilar, Vault and Facial areas. Ancillary to these are the stapes, incus, malleus and hyoid. It is worth noting that the latter are not specifically related to the cranio-sacral concept, but cannot be omitted because of their position anatomically.

Sutherland was laying down the foundation for understanding some of the most basic functions of the human body. It must be remembered that his ideas originated in 1899, whilst but a student at Kirksville, Missouri, School of Osteopathy, in the United States of America – studying a skull belonging to the founding Father of Osteopathy, Andrew Taylor Still.

There had been no previous investigation regarding what we now know as the cranio-sacral system, and no-one else even remotely had any idea of such a concept. It was for this reason that for some twenty years Sutherland refrained from making his findings public.

Rather than being branded a divergent so early in his career, which would obviously have ruined his potential as a practitioner and subsequently as the originator of the Cranial concept, he kept it and devised many means of practicing on himself for furthering his knowledge.

His experiments were conducted with crude home-made mechanical devices such as straps, and a type of football helmet. Applying these to his skull he created the required pressures at the right places, often startling his wife, Adah, with his resulting personality changes. But, because of his prodigious knowledge of anatomy he was always able to correct the anomalies produced, and in the process of time began to apply his newly learned principles of diagnosis and treatment to his patients.

The most profound aspect of Sutherland's findings was that the structure of the cranial articular surfaces was significant. He could see that the design indicated mobility. Later he was to prove conclusively that the bones of the skull do in fact move, albeit slightly, also the brain, intracranial membranes, spinal cord, and intraspinal membranes; whilst the enclosed cerebrospinal fluid fluctuates rather than circulates. Perceiving the constancy of the motile behaviour peculiar to this system, Sutherland called it the Primary Respiratory Mechanism and stated that this includes the mobility of the sacrum between

2 & 3 PIONEERS

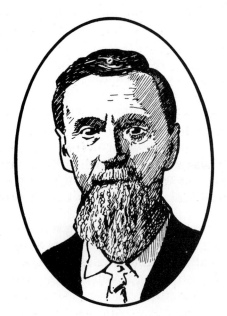

Andrew Taylor Still
Founding Father of Osteopathy

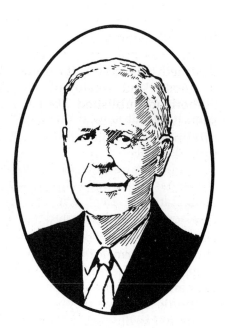

William Garner Sutherland
Pioneer of Cranial Osteopathy

the ilia. This he also stated is distinct from the diaphragmatic respiration, which is secondary.

Sutherland's career must be reviewed in the context of the then dominant trend of osteopathic thought. It was R.B. Taylor, biochemist, who saw the body as a thermodynamic system, subject to the laws of energy interchange and conservation. He said 'a system and its surroundings are in equilibrium in such a way that any change in the energy of the system will lead to change also in the energy of the surroundings.'

When there is a chronic disturbance of this state of equilibrium there is bound to be an increase or loss of energy. In the human body this is how disease occurs, and, for the osteopath as well as any other therapist, restoration and maintenance of homeostasis must be the goal.

It was through Sutherland that the osteopathic lesion was best understood as either membraneous or ligamentous strain. If joints are positioned so that the reciprocal tension in the whole body-mechanism can operate to change the relationship of these particular parts, the requisite ease is produced, thereby effectively releasing any strain that might be present.

It is by virtue of this induced balance that the ligaments and membranes are allowed to move the bones of the joints. In this way the body itself does the correction. Through diligent research Sutherland made these discoveries and simultaneously his sensory perception and dexterity developed. Claiming no fame for his ingenuity he maintained the stance that his findings originated from within the science of osteopathy as taught by Still.

This was not very convincing, but Cranial Osteopathy was nevertheless destined to succeed. Its tremendous benefit to humanity was obvious. In diagnosis and treatment its virtues were unsurpassed. When in 1939 Sutherland published *The Cranial Bowl* it was met with much ridicule and suspicion. The world of medicine, as it then stood, was unprepared for such profundity of original thought. This epoch making volume was soon followed by Harold Ives Magoun's *Osteopathy in the Cranial Field*, and within a year the concept was more generally accepted.

By 1946 the resistance had manifestly declined whereupon the birth of the Osteopathic Cranial Association took place. This was later to become the Cranial Academy (in 1960) which regularized the pattern of cranial osteopathic education and established research programmes. Dr Magoun's book was a shot in the arm for the progress of Cranial education. He was at pains to amplify the concept, stressing in particular that this therapeutic modality was primarily concerned with the motion found in the cranial sutures and the rhythmic impulses palpable within the cranium.

There was obviously then, no competition between the pioneer of Cranial Osteopathy, and the author of *Osteopathy in the Cranial Field*. The former began by studying the bones of the cranium, their reciprocal bevelling for gliding movement, and their postural accommodative motility. His scientific reasoning is a fact of history, and is only surpassed by his genius, much of which was particularly concerned with the fact that the bones of the skull originate in cartilage at the base, whilst those of the vault originate in membrane – membrane for articular expansile mobility, which then accommodates movement at the basal articular cartilage.

As touched on before, Sutherland tested his own reasoning upon himself. This provided him with a distinct advantage over his peers because he was aware of physiological changes that no one else had ever experienced. It was as a result of all this that he was able to postulate after some thirty years the mobility of the cranial bones, together with the function of the reciprocal tension membranes, the integrated unit mechanism of the cranio-sacral complex, the role of the C.S.F., and the synchrony of the whole, as related to the movable fulcrum at the straight sinus.

It is worthy of note that neither Sutherland nor any of the subsequent devotees of the cranial concept ever claimed that this was a panacea 'that

4 PIONEER

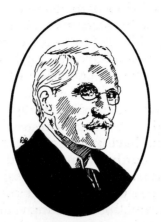

John Martin Littlejohn
Father of Osteopathy in Britain

dysfunctions present in the cranio-sacral system would only respond to cranial osteopathy.' The over-riding emphasis was always that the aetiology of many disturbed conditions was traceable to the cranio-sacral mechanism, which had no longer to be disregarded.

On the other hand, it became more and more obvious that many of these conditions could best be investigated, verified, and treated within this concept.

Furthermore research revealed that many dysfunctions that earlier were classified as incurable by conventional means responded admirably to cranial osteopathy; birth trauma, for instance, certain allergies, asthma, and Bell's palsy.

Through developing a new kind of sensory perception in his hands Sutherland was famous in discerning the patterns of motion occuring within the skull and brain. By his efforts he gained further valuable information that really fired his imagination for even deeper research.

By this time he was discovering cranial rhythms in people of all ages, which he soon found to be in correspondence with a palpable motion at the sacrum. This he reasoned, occurred by virtue of the spinal dural connection between the occiput and the sacrum.

Where there is motion at the dural link between the squamous part of the occiput and the foramen magnum, there must be the same motion occurring at the sacrum, he hypothesised. The only plausible reason he could see for there being any difference was if pathology were present. On this basis of reasoning he invented a model representing the cranium with the sphenoid as the centre of the cranial osseous activity. It was as a result of his tremendous success that many of his contemparies capitulated to the practice of Cranial Osteopathy.

However, it is true that many conventional osteopaths still do not easily embrace this concept, and there are sound though not good reasons for this.

Basically lack of application is to blame. I remember my cranial tutor saying 'two-thirds of those who train in this particular therapy do not practise it!' He was always careful to explain to his students that the cranial concept is not in any way a manipulative modality. He further said 'the lack of application was due to the fact that those osteopaths have never got over being mechanistic in their approach to treatment, whereas cranially this is both uncalled for and unhelpful.'

Much more shall be said in the succeeding text against even the least idea of manipulation in the cranial field, but in this preamble I take this opportunity of making this early comment, having special regard for what Denis Brookes used to say 'you simply put your hand on the head and wait. Wait until the head tells you what to do. If it tells you to do nothing, you do nothing. You do not manipulate the cranium, else you could be courting disaster.'

What he was really saying, and this only became obvious to me after a long time of patiently listening and learning, was that you must wait on the rhythms, impulses, and sutural resilience under your hands to begin to manifest themselves. You will discern whether they are thready, weak, strong, rapid, slow, sluggish, oscillating, A.P. (anteroposterior) or whatever, and with trained tactile capacity direct and use these therapeutically.

The concept is concerned with this physiological system of rhythms, pulsations, impulses and sutural mobility. Functionally it is wholly related to the central nervous system, musculoskeletal system, autonomic nervous system, endocrine system, and ultimately the entire human organism. Specifically it is bounded by the meningeal membranes and more particularly the dura mater.

Most conventional osteopaths will argue that their daily work is mostly concerned with manipulation. That is what they have been taught, and this is how they think. No-one should despise this because at some time or other we were all taught that way. This volume is not intended either to raise or inflame an argument, but simply to point out that the cranial concept, although embracing Still's teaching, is chiefly concerned with facilitating the dynamism of fluid pressure circulation and fluctuation.

It perhaps needs reiteration that, contrary to what some well-meaning but unsuspecting practitioners think, there is really no conflict between conventional and cranial osteopathy. Cranial osteopaths who are being successful in their efforts to help the sick and suffering are usually as humble as Sutherland used to be in acknowledging that the conventional and the cranial go hand in hand; neither is the solution to every condition, and the one is not complete without the other.

Listen to what Still wrote, 'the structure of the body is reciprocally related to its function. The body's musculoskeletal system, bones, ligaments, muscles, fascia (connective tissue) etc, forms a structure which when disordered may effect changes in the function of other parts of the body. This effect may be

5 THE HUMAN SKULL

I

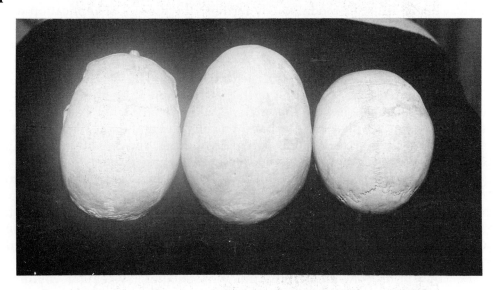

Note the variations in shape and sutural details
The sutures of the middle skull are almost obliterated

II

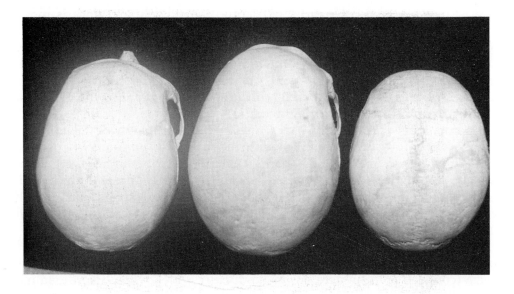

THE CRANIO-SACRAL CONCEPT

6 THE HUMAN SKULL

III

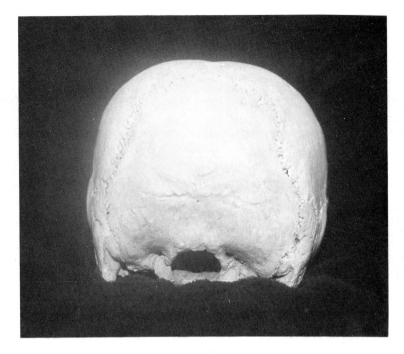

OCCIPUT & FORAMEN MAGNUM

IV

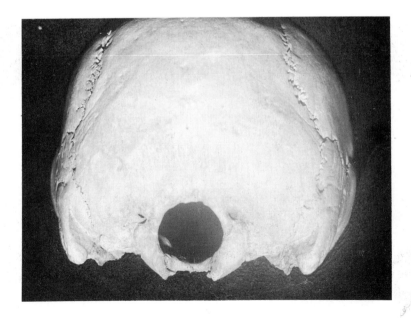

ESSENTIALS OF CRANIO-SACRAL OSTEOPATHY

7 THE HUMAN SKULL

V

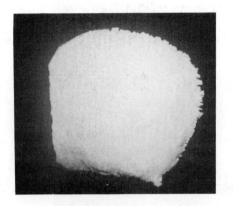 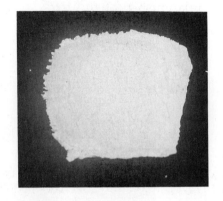

PARIETAL
External Surface

PARIETAL
Internal Surface

VI

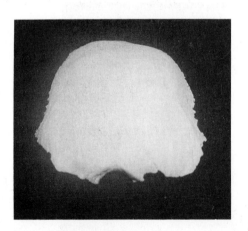 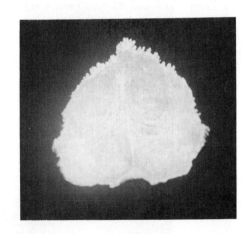

OCCIPITAL
External Surface

OCCIPITAL
Internal Surface

THE CRANIO-SACRAL CONCEPT

created through irritation and abnormal response of the nerve and blood supply to other organs of the body.'

The cranial concept embraces all this under the guiding principle of the restoration of free fluid circulation within the body, including the cranium and face. The aim is the positioning of joints and other structural parts so that reciprocal tension in the mechanism can operate to change the relationship of the parts, and produce ease, followed by active release of strain. The body is capable of doing its own work. This is why Sutherland emphasised that this concept came from within the science of osteopathy as expressed by Still. Nevertheless, he urged that cranial osteopathy should never become a specialization in itself as it has tended to do.

You may ask what then is the first practical step for the budding cranial osteopath to take. He must start with sensing the motion. There is no difference between perceiving cranial motion and palpating the arm, abdomen, back, or leg for tone. It is taken for granted here that he is already aware of the difference between a tense, rigid, fibrous tissue, and one that is normal. The osteopath needs only put his hand lightly on the patient's head and wait. By virtue of his previous experience in the profession he will soon begin to gather useful tactile information whether or not he has ever known anything of the cranial concept before.

Some heads are less pliant than others. There is a vast range – from hard to soft, pliable or normal tissues. The practitioner is not looking for structural irregularities, deformaties, or any bony malposition although there will be such. He is simply acquainting himself with cranial motion and intracranial rhythms. They will indicate the condition of the patient. They will tell the osteopath all he needs to know. Of course, this will be gone into at greater depth in the following chapters.

WILLIAM GARNER SUTHERLAND

'The idea (of Cranial articular mobility) originated while I was viewing the disarticulated bones of a skull . . . the articular surfaces seemed to me to indicate that they were designed for articular mobility.'

'A Master Mechanic designed and made the human skull in membrane for accommodative flexion in the vault, and in cartilage for mobility at the basilar area.'

'There are various types of cranial membraneous articular strains, or lesions; including the traumatic, reflex, mental strain and shellshock.'

CHAPTER TWO

The Cranio-Sacral Mechanism & Cranial Rhythmic Impulses

It was Sutherland who postulated 'a membraneous articular mechanism manifesting motion in the articulations of the skull and sacrum' (the bevelling of the bones of the skull and face allowing a certain amount of articular interaction and mobility) and who made this sophisticated, complex, physiological system into a concept that has, ever since, been available to be utilized diagnostically and therapeutically.

Most of the patients visiting our clinics with lesions of one kind or another are helped, but how much? If they have a pain their favourite osteopath might heroically do wonders for them. Relieved of their pain and suffering the patients go away feeling really satisfied only to come back later with similar troubles. Why?

In the light of cranial knowledge this is not mysterious. Often all these patients have received was first aid. They might have been helped to a better state of health had their practitioner's knowledge been equal to the situation. When we examine our patients cranially we find many more lesions than we were accustomed to noticing. Even if we had seen these before we might not have thought them diagnostically significant.

In the ordinary sense, examining the spine from the occiput to the sacrum we may find ten or even fifteen major lesions. These are usually recognisable without any real depth of investigation. Let this examination be a little more extensive. Taking a clinical look at the patient's face we are sure to have a revelation. (Of course, clinical investigation, and often treatment should be undertaken with the patient in the supine position). The obvious lesions here, and their patterns, many of which correspond to those of the sacrum and occiput, are legion.

What are we seeing? Changes in the facial symmetry. Having a clear mental picture of what the norm should be there is no difficulty in discerning the anomalous. For example, one eye may be higher than the other, one frontal promontary higher than the other. The superciliary ridge could also be more elevated on the one side – probably significant of myopia. And what about the naso-labial folds? The depth of these could be very revealing. So also might be

8 DIAGNOSTIC INDICATIONS

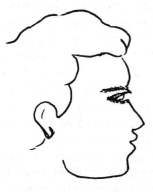

PROMINENT FRONTAL
Bilateral Extension

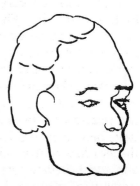

RECEDING FRONTAL
Bilateral Flexion

Unilateral finding indicates torsion or side-bending rotation

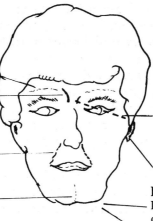

SUPERCILIARY FOLDS
Deeper when frontal is impacted anteriorly

SUPRANASAL FOLDS
These lateralize when the fronto-zygomatic border moves posteriorly

NASOLABIAL FOLDS
Deeper on side of externally rotated maxilla

MENTAL CREASE
Lateralizes to side of externally rotated Temporal

OBLIQUE DIAMETER OF EYE
Increased on side of high great wing (Eyeball will also appear larger)

LEVEL OF EARS
Lateral flare indicates external rotation of Temporal

RETRUSION OF JAW
Indicates bilateral external rotation of Temporal

PROTRUSION OF JAW
Indicates bilateral internal rotation of Temporal

the ears, one higher or closer to the head than the other. Then there is the malar prominence – this too might possess certain irregularities.

This could be a very daunting conglomeration of lesions. What are we going to do about them? Firstly, we need to consider what might have given rise to any or all of these lesions. Birth trauma is a cardinal offender. Genetic mutative deficiency cannot be ruled out. Sudden shock on trauma resulting from pelvic lesions due to cerebro-spinal-fluid bombardment . . . the list is endless.

In pelvic lesions no better authority can be quoted than Dr Still who wrote 'the osteopath has great demands for his powers of reason when he considers the relation of diseases generally to the pelvis and this knowledge he must have before his work can be attended with success. I want you to camp out on the borders of the pelvis and stay there with your microscopes both in hand and head. I have found the ischia too close together in all cases of enlarged prostate glands that I have examined and treated in the last 30 years.'

Dr Charles Owen also takes up this point in his book on Chapman's Reflexes 'an innominate lesion always indicates an endocrine disturbance.' Later in his work he shows how the endocrine secretions of the pelvic organs influence the thyroid, induce acidosis, affect the urine, and set up digestive disturbances.

Understanding the cranio-sacral mechanism therefore, requires a specialized survey of anatomy and physiology, coupled with a lively appreciation of the body as an integrated unit of function.

The cranio-sacral mechanism is in measured motile activity throughout life – a rhythm that does not vary with physical exertion, rest, or weather conditions, as does the cardio-vascular system; nor does it depend on our active co-operation as does (at least in part) the musculo-skeletal system. Therefore this mechanism is clinically dependable in evaluating pathology.

Cranial Rhythmic Impulse (C.R.I.) is to the cranio-sacral mechanism/motion what the measured apical beat is to the systemic circulation. Both are a method of monitoring what is happening in the particular system. We generally evaluate C.R.I. at the temporal squama where it is best detected with the hypothenar eminence of the practitioners hand, under which a slight pulsation occurs at a rate of 10–14 per minute in normal adults, and 12–16 per minute in children.

A word of caution – under certain conditions this rate varies. In the case of fear, up to 20 seconds may elapse without a pulsation. Fever produces a heightening influence and so does the presence of oxygen; while in the presence of carbon dioxide, or insomnia, the opposite reaction occurs.

In many mentally disturbed people it has been found that this rate is decreased by as much as half and this appears unaffected by sedatory drugs, tranquilizers, etc.

Aetiological factors which used to defy thorough or useful clinical investigation, are not only traceable through this system, but can be positively solved. Many patients who were written off by their doctors or specialists as

9 DURAL ATTACHMENTS OF THE SPINE

FORAMEN MAGNUM (POSTERIOR RING)
2nd & 3rd Cervical Vertebrae
First firm attachments

LIGAMENTUM DENTICULATUM
21 'toothed' segments either side of spinal cord, between Anterior & posterior nerve roots – ending between D12 & L1. Medially connect with Pia Mater, laterally with Dura Mater.

2ND SACRAL VERTEBRAE
Last firm contact of dura (now combined with other meningeal layers).

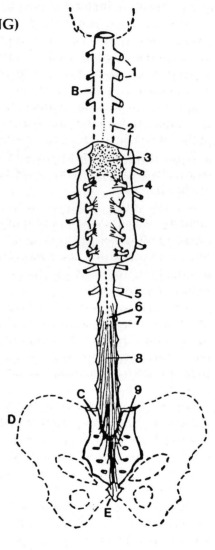

- A Occiput
- B Spinal cord
- C Sacrum
- D Ilium
- E Coccyx

1. Spinal nerve roots
2. Dura Mater
3. Arachnoid Mater
4. Pia Mater
5. Level of D12
6. Conus Medullaris
7. Level of L1
8. Cauda Equina
9. Filum Terminale

incurable are now being helped by those who practice cranio-sacral therapy. The label 'aetiology unknown' has lost its popularity.

Obscure causative factors are traceable through the musculoskeletal system and eradicated, instead of the continual dependance on palliatives.

Palpated most easily at the temples, cranio-sacral motion has two distinct phases of activity – flexion and extension – and in health this gentle pulsating pendulum measures out the hours, days, months, and years in perfect cadence, as seen in the harmonious workings of the grandfather clock.

This steady 'tick' is felt rather than heard by the Cranial Osteopath, but here we need to dig a little deeper – Still's words were 'dig deep.' Palpably there is a relaxation phase – a slight pause which takes place at the point of full excursion of the one cycle just prior to the commencement of the other – the phenomenon of long bones rotating internally, and the whole body lessening in girth, coincides with the extension phase (cranio-sacrally) and the opposite happens during flexion.

Let us for a moment consider the cranium itself. Here you cannot mechanically adjust or manipulate anything. You may try, but the consequences can be disastrous. You dare not manipulate a mal-positioned bone – should there be such. The most you can do (and then only with the utmost gentleness) is incline or encourage the bone in the direction where it would normally go.

The cranium is very delicate and particularly vulnerable in wrong or untrained hands, so intelligence and lightness of touch must reign over force or ignorance. Heavy-handedness will only make matters worse. Any alteration, however slight, will affect the rest of the body, so it is the practitioner's finesse that is on trial. It is his expertise which will bring results for good or ill.

Hence it is important that his palpating hand be not only warm, but dry, when handling the patient's head, behind which he should be comfortably sitting. Very gentle coaxing is all that is required. Remember also that the twenty nine cranial bones in the adult skull are bevelled for articular motion. Any aberrant suture injudiciously handled can be the 'launching of a battleship'.

Dr Sutherland's method of treatment is worth bearing in mind. He depended on the inherent corrective forces of the membranes for influencing motion and mobilizing therapeutic physiological forces. He regarded the dura mater of the cranium and spinal cord as a regulatory component of the articular mobility, not only of the basilar area of the cranium, but of the sacrum between the ilia during respiration.

The lesions are named in favour of the mobile side of the articulation. When a correction is intended the point chosen for applying the pressure should be at the farthest possible convenient area contralaterally. Normally the pressure should last no more than a minute or two, decreasing to

ESSENTIALS OF CRANIO-SACRAL OSTEOPATHY
10 PALPATION & EVALUATION

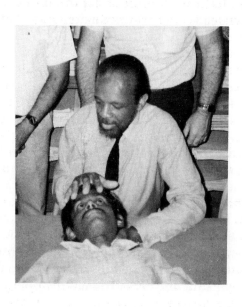

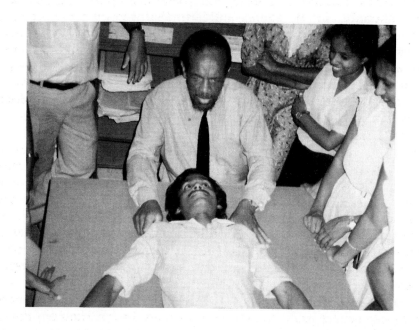

being as the touch of a feather. During this time rhythmic impulses will be felt by the practitioner under the hand or finger applying the pressure. Also there will be a slight indication of expansion of the underlying bones together with a sense of the corrective energy having arrived at its intended destination.

Physiologically, the strong dural meninges extending from the occiput to the sacrum are a positive connection which not only facilitate but regulate and maintain co-ordinated movement. This is the spinal reciprocal membraneous tension, distinct from any local mobility in the area.

The sacrum swings in an arc represented by the combined sweep of both auricular arms, with little or no change in the tension of the sacroiliac ligaments. This action is comparable with the combined fulcrum-pivot mechanism of the jugular process in the skull for temporal movement on the occiput.

It is important that we recognise there are no muscles connecting the sacrum with the ilia. Nor are there any muscles in the cranium (between the sutures) connecting the osseous structures to facilitate cranial articulation. Both the sacral and the cranial mobility are involuntary. Curved and wedge-shaped forming the base of the vertebral column, the sacrum is located between the ilia, completing the dorsal boundary of the pelvis.

Of its three important surfaces, two lateral are for its articulation with the ilia, while the third positioned superiorly, is the base of support for the spine.

During sphenobasilar flexion (inhalation) that anterosuperior elevation of the foramen magnum lifts the dural tube slightly and so moves the sacrum, its base going posterosuperiorly along the cephalad arm of the sacroiliac articulation, while its apex moves anteriorly towards the pubic symphysis along the auricular arm. In the extension phase (exhalation) the opposite occurs. The Pituitary gland in the sella turcica is therefore affected, it's activity being enhanced.

If the sacrum is maladjusted, so will the occiput be, and vice-versa.

To prove this we have only to observe what happens when the sacrum is tipped so that one side is posterior and inferior. The cranium will invariably go into torsion with the occiput low on the same side. Similarly, if the occiput moves inferiorly with the torsion at the symphysis, then the sacral base will be low on the same side, and somewhat posterior.

Therefore it is a truism that the spine will always conform to the direction of the curve beginning at either the occiput or the sacrum in line with the tilt. Rotation of the occiput on its anteroposterior axis, as in torsion or sidebending rotation, is suggested by the tilt of the head on the atlas, as well as the corresponding inclination of the occiput from side to side. The ramifications of a malpositioned sacrum may be manifold through the ganglion of Impar, for instance, which lies just in front of the sacrum, and has influence over the hypogastric plexus.

An understanding of this sacro-occipital relationship may provide the answer to haemorrhoids in this sense involving the liver and venous back pressure.

In sacro-occipital lesions it is well to remember that some are ascending and others descending. It is worth amplifying this. In the first instance some lesions ascend from the sacrum to the occiput. Others descend from the cranium through the cervical, dorsal and lumbar regions. Differential diagnosis is therefore of the utmost importance, and should include careful analysis of the effects on the spine below, from sphenobasilar torsion and sphenobasilar sidebending rotation.

In the event of sphenobasilar torsion it is usual for C1/2 to displace towards the low Great Wing side, and the rest of the Cervical spine 3, 4, 5, 6, & 7, curve to the high side. The Dorsal spine all rotate or displace to the low side while Lumbar's 1, 2, 3, & 4 displace to the high side. Accommodated to the sacrum, L5 alone displaces to the low side with the Ilium usually relatively anterior to the Sacrum on the low side.

Here then is the positive link between the cranium and the sacrum – the very reason why we cannot intelligibly talk about the one without the other. If the sacral base is tipped anteriorly and inferiorly, then we look for sidebending rotation cranial lesions. If the sacrum goes into torsion, so will the sphenoid.

Talking about the sphenoid we would benefit from noting that, together with the occiput – these are the two cranial bones which are always responsible, in one way or another, for any resistant lesioning whenever this occurs among the cranial osseous structures. This, of course, doesn't include peripheral traumatically induced lesions. These can sometimes lock the entire mechanism, and require local correction before the integrity of the sphenobasilar symphysis may be restored.

Occipital malposition and especially the masto-occipital suture, as far as these are likely to effect adverse changes in the jugular foramen, can produce far reaching consequences whereby through the dura the whole of the cranial mechanism might be unbalanced. Unlike dysfunctions occasioned by flexion, extension, side-bending and torsion lesions, which are for the most part rarely seriously incapacitating or debilitating, lesions of the cranial base, and impaction (compression) lesions, will often recur unless somatic imbalance has been treated first.

It is, however, of some comfort to relate that careful analysis of the gross unphysiological patterns of the sphenobasilar symphysis will always reveal the necessary corrective measure.

Now a word about diagnosis. In examining the cranium we might see what was described by Denis Brookes as the 'banana' (or dolicephalic) head. What's the first thing that comes to mind when we see this? We think of sphenobasilar side-bending. Then we can begin to look elsewhere for the correlating lesions and their ramifications.

The moment you even attempt to test a head, if there is a kink in the straight sinus you are likely to liberate it – and in so doing you will release chronic toxic states into the circulation. Furthermore, you will liberate endorphine – you will open up the infundibulum, you will open up the locus coeruleus – you will give the tissue the chance to flow straight through, from front to back, and instantly the whole of those cerebral structures are nourished and neutralized.

Then we have this fascinating question of psychosomatic release. When you alter the behaviour of the straight sinus you may expect anything. You achieve memory release – you release a neuro-hormone transmitter – you liberate endorphines and change behavioural patterns.

So when you put a patient on the couch and very gently undo a kink, you have started a chain of events, launched out into the deep, and the patient will know that something has happened.

It is all important that fluid stasis does not occur in any area. Life demands this. That kink in the straight sinus can be, and often is, one of the primary causes of epilepsy and internal hydrocephalus; a kink creates a blockage, the aqueduct is blocked. The Foramen of Munro is blocked. Cellular fluids cannot get back into circulation. They build up back pressure – fluid retention.

And again, change of direction of C.S.F. from anterior–posterior to lateral is of paramount importance in the sleep-wake phenomenon. When you are standing there is parallel action of C.S.F. flow. When you lie down with your head on a pillow this alters, you impinge on one or other temporal bone, you decelerate C.S.F. activity. You, as it were, slow down the pendulum. You inhibit parallel action.

By inhibiting this pendulum you automatically produce an anteroposterior swing which is parasympathetic; that is to say, the parts of the autonomic nervous system that slow down the action of the heart when the body is not under stress, in order to conserve bodily energy.

It is the cerebrospinal fluid under the auspices of the primary respiratory mechanism that does the correction. It will carry that bone right back to its correct sphere of operation.

Inside the skull the dura mater forms support for the brain. This is vital. The brain must be protected; but, what I really want to highlight just now, is the dura-fascial relationship at the various foramina, at the cranial base. Here we find the dura is linked with the extracranial fascia, and it is for this reason tensions occuring outside the cranium in muscles, may often be traced to cranial anomalies.

Traction upon intracranial structures then, may be influenced by the position of the head in flexion and extension. And, although the anatomy of the cranium varies so considerably from that of the spinal areas, physiologically lesions affecting either area appear to be very much alike.

It is pertinent to relate membranes to fascia. Fascial bands direct lymph flow; and the dura is continuous with fascial bands throughout the body, thus

11 ATTACHMENTS OF DURAL MEMBRANES
(POLES OF ATTACHMENT)

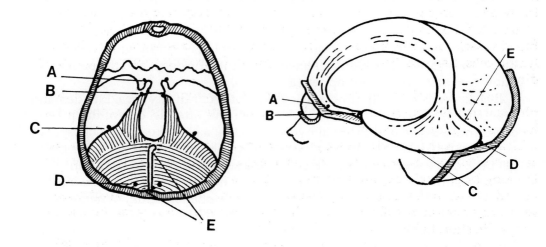

SUPERIOR VIEW   **LATERAL VIEW**

- **A** Anterior Superior Pole – at Crista Galli & Ethmoidal Notch
- **B** Anterior Inferior Pole – at Clinoid Process
- **C** Lateral Pole – at Petrous portion of Temporal
- **D** Posterior Poles – at Internal Occipital Protuberance & Straight Sinus
- **E** Straight Sinus

integrating the cranium, not only with the sacrum, but with the entire organism.

It was Dr Still who used to say of fascia 'in you I exist, through you I express myself, by you I live or die.' For some of us though, fascia doesn't usually occupy any significant place in our osteopathic reasoning. Yet, homeostasis is largely dependant on the fascia being in good working condition. This is to say, a steady state of health will not be experienced by the person whose fascia is interrupted in its course, as it envelops and caresses the various structures of the body . . . organs, muscles, ligaments, bones, tendons, nerves, and so on.

In a word, it is concerned with intervisceral support. It is the resting place for blood vessels, and the manufacturing site for intercellular substances, blood, lymph cells, heparin, histamine, and seratonin. It also transports prostaglandins.

Normally, fascial integrity doesn't vary, but trauma or shock, whether physical or psychological, will result in its distortion, which can, of course, have far-reaching consequences.

The phenomenon of breathing provides us with a perfect example of some aspects of fascia's activity under normal conditions. At the end of inspiration the long bones roll outwards, occasioning a stretch reflex, and this is fascia bound. Stretch reflex liberates prostaglandins. This is the all-important reason why long bones must roll outwards. This is an automatic prostaglandin release trigger, in short bursts of 90 seconds in tissue.

Our breathing in and breathing out, also provides just the right example of techniques for which some of our patients ought to have the opportunity of thanking us. This is to say, you can put your patient's arm into long axial rotation – coinciding with his inspiration or expiration. Let him hold his breath and in the light of your knowledge of the stretch reflex, and prostaglandin release, you can reverse physiology, by having your patient to do the respiratory opposite and achieve that painless desirable adjustment.

This is immediately effective on the Pineal body – the starting point of the endocrine system and the still point for cranial mobility, osseous, membraneous, ligamentous. These have a central point around which they work – the straight sinus to the fourth ventricle, directly in line with the Pineal body.

A look at the primary respiratory mechanism supports this. During inspiration convexity of the sphenobasilar junction appears to increase, the occiput is lowered, the Greater Wing of the Sphenoid flares outward and downwards, the temporals rotate so that the tip of the mastoid moves posteromedially.

The squama of the temporals flare away from the head and its petrous portion moves anteriorly and laterally. During exhalation these movements are reversed.

We have already said that the cranial bones determine the physiological

12 SACRAL-OCCIPITAL RELATIONSHIP

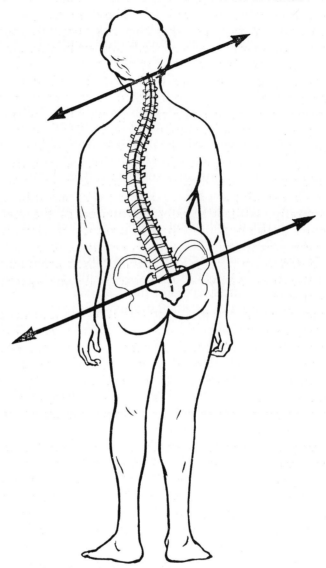

The sacrum mirrors the action of the Occiput

behaviour of the entire human organism. You may ask what these bones do. They do not of themselves do anything. It is what happens by their behaviour during sphenobasilar flexion and extension that is of particular interest to us. In sphenobasilar flexion the facet heads change position. The frontals move into flexion. They recede.

Visualize the frontals as two bones. Embryologically they are two bones with a central metopic suture which in 9% of skulls does not fuse or become obliterated but remains into adult life. They move as two, there can be one frontal in internal rotation, and the other in external rotation. As they recede the vomer rolls outwards, the malar rolls outwards, changing its position; the diameter of the orbit also changes. It rolls outwards in an oblique fashion. Speaking of eyes changing, we mean an oblique diameter change. This oblique change, mediated by the rolling outwards of the two frontal bones is augmented, not only by the malar and zygoma, but by the ethmoid.

The ethmoid and occiput together, as a pair, and the sphenoid in the middle, roll the opposite way. The ethmoid follows the position of the occiput and pushes the vomer down. The vomer begins its descent because it is attached to the crest – the anterior medial crest of the ethmoid bone. It drops, and when the vomer drops it would normally encounter the superior border of the palatine surfaces centrally; while the external rotation of the malar bone and the accompanying changes of the ethmoid produce of necessity a rolling of the maxilla. It precedes the temporals, rolling outwards with the dental border, these drop, widening the nasals – so that the nasal structures flare out – producing the first peripheral physiological para-sympathetic endocrine impulse exchange.

Another point worth remembering is that the occiput and the upper cervical vertebrae may be considered as one unit functionally. These bones provide anchorage for many extradural muscles around this area. Here occipital influence is observed affecting the mobility and function of the dural tube, while the dura mater, is firmly adherent to the posterior parts of the second and third bodies. How important it is then to have a balanced occiput! It is not an exaggeration to suggest that it is invaluable to good health, and a balanced sphenoid comes into the same category.

The occiput affords many attachments for muscles and is particularly susceptible to their hypertonic states. The effects of hypertonicity do not stop at the occiput, which whenever affected by such a state is often rendered immobile, but has great influence over the dural membrane system. Both the tentorium cerebelli and the posterior part of the falx cerbri find anchorage at the occiput, and so do the posterior and inferior aspects of the falx cerebelli.

By these attachments occipital influence is mediated to the straight venous sinus, the posterior sagittal sinus, the occipital sinus, the transverse sinus, the confluence of sinuses. A mal-positioned occiput, therefore, can be very crucial. It can obstruct the fluid flow in the venous sinuses, and even the re-absorption of C.S.F.

And what else do you need to take into consideration when you put your hand on the patient's head, intending to correct whatever you see? There may be an enzyme or diatetic pattern elsewhere that you have not taken into account. If by force you create that desired release the treatment could be worse than the disease. Our supreme aim is to be part of the solution and not part of the problem. You may send that patient away confused. He may even be suicidal. Certainly he will have a headache, depression, be sleepy or drowsy. On the other hand he may experience a temporary state of euphoria. This latter is induced by the inter-action between endorphine and enkephalin. These all result from the liberation of chronic toxic residual states.

This is exactly the reason why you put your hands on that patient's head and wait. Wait until the head tells you what to do. The cranial rhythmic impulses will speak to you through your hands – despite what you are seeing – and all you have to do is co-operate with it. With your tactile capacity follow that gentle motion, stick with it. It will never disappoint you. It will never release itself at any greater speed than that with which it can cope.

For instance, suppose you are endeavouring to reverse a vomeric depression. How would you do about it? There is a grave danger of being heroic! So you proceed with the utmost caution remembering that you are, as it were, in a minefield.

Gently open the mouth and put your second fingers on the inferior border of the sphenobasilar symphysis and apply slight pressure. Do not push, the desired result will come as you exercise dexterity and patience. Failure to do this here could cause rupture of the veins of Galen (situated inferiorly to the Circle of Willis) and that would be fatal.

Only in children under seven years of age would you use direct action technique. Always use indirect action technique – called exaggeration. When you liberate those structures by this method there is a recoil motion. The minimal kink is increased and it is then that you let go, and it will spring back beyond the point of starting. It could be from ten degrees back to forty, the compressive state – hence that stress.

Whenever we think cranially it is imperative we must also think of the principles applicable to the fluid systems of the body – remembering in particular that these correlate to all the other systems, not least of which is the cranio-sacral.

ANDREW TAYLOR STILL

'Keep your searchlight forever on the brain, for from it we derive all power.'

'Fascia "the framework of life." It surrounds each muscle, artery, vein, and nerve, and all organs of the body. By its action we move, and by its failure we die.'

'Find it, fix it, let it alone!'

'Give me anything but a theory that you cannot demonstrate!'

CHAPTER THREE

Primary Respiratory Mechanism & Cerebrospinal Fluid

The concept of the Primary Respiratory Mechanism was the foundation stone on which Dr Sutherland based the motion that is peculiar to the cranio-sacral system. The fact that the inner layer of dura was repeated so many times was a sure pointer to the solution to his quest – that of discovering the source of movement of these structures.

Incidentally, the P.R.M. is not to be confused with the diaphragmatic excursion to which it is secondary. It is the mechanism by which long bones roll out on inspiration, and prostaglandin is released in the tissues. It is concerned with the interchange of nutrients and waste products in the tissues. It is also the trigger for endocrine activity.

Sutherland perceived that the functional efficiency of this mechanism had to possess a source of balance, an automatic shifting suspended fulcrum. His investigations revealed that this ubiquitous phenomenon is located in the falx cerebri and the tentorium cerebelli along the straight sinus (also called The Sutherland Fulcrum to commemorate his contribution to our understanding of this phenomenon). This sinus runs obliquely inferoposteriorly from the end of the inferior longitudinal sinus to join the superior sagittal sinus at its most inferior part immediately posterior to the tentorium cerebelli, and the basal vein. It is separated from the fourth ventricle by the cerebellum. It has been suggested that the small mass of pacchionian, bodies found at the anterior end of this sinus may act as a monitor (a ball-valve) to the flow and distribution of C.S.F.

As Sutherland saw it two basic motile phenomena are peculiar to the concept of cranial osteopathy. One of these is the motion perceived at the cranial sutures and the other a definite set of rhythmic impulses occuring within the cranium. These were unsuspected previously and, he felt, were largely responsible for maintaining homeostasis.

This postulation was added to by Magoun and others, and subsequent scientific measurements of the body impulses have borne out the truth of their discoveries. There are several detectable motions within the body, and more are still being found. But basically we are concerned with those which come under the heading of the Primary Respiratory Mechanism. These are all concerned with motility/mobility of

13 THE STRAIGHT SINUS AND ITS NEIGHBOURS

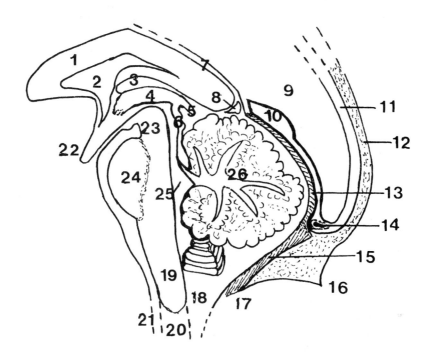

1   Corpus Callosum
2   Septum Pellucidum
3   Third Ventricle – Choroid plexus
4   Hypothalamus, Thalamus & third ventricle
5   Pineal body
6   Laminae quadrigeminae
7   Inferior Sagittal Sinus
8   Basal Vein
9   Falx Cerebri
10 Straight Sinus
11 Superior Sagittal Sinus
12 Occipital bone
13 Tentorium Cerebelli
14 Transverse Sinus at Confluence of Sinuses
15 Falx Cerebelli
16 Inion
17 Foramen Magnum – posterior border
18 Cisterna Magna
19 Medulla Oblongata
20 Spinal Medulla
21 Subarachnoid space (spinal)
22 Optic chiasma
23 Mesencephalon
24 Pons
25 Fourth Ventricle
26 Cerebellum

14 CRANIAL EMBRYOLOGICAL DEVELOPMENT

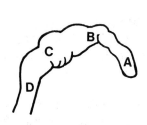

Approximately three weeks

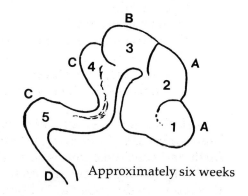

Approximately six weeks

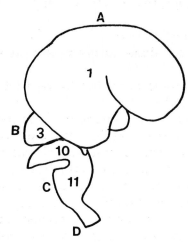

Approximately three months

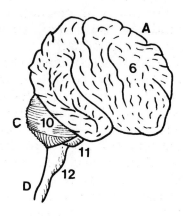

Pre-birth

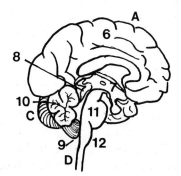

In the Adult

A, B, & C represent the earliest stages of the development of the brain. 1–5 the later stages. 6–12 the final structures achieved!

a) the cranial bones
b) the brain
c) the spinal chord
d) the intracranial and intraspinal membranes
e) the sacrum and ilia – involuntary motion (as distinct from the voluntary, or postural mobility of the ilia upon the sacrum).
f) the wave-like fluctuation of C.S.F.

Basically, oligodendroglial activity may be observed in the tissues of the brain and central nervous system. This activity is in existence from before birth and continues throughout life and even for some time after death. It is said that during neurosurgery a motion may be observed in the brain – and this has been described as 'vibrant' 'incessantly active.'

Magoun records that four types of observable pulsatile motion may be found in the fluid systems of the body:

one coinciding with the contractions of the heart,

a second which synchronizes with respiration – the changes in pressure at inspiration and expiration.

The third and fourth are cyclic pulsations unrelated to the first and second and not yet fully scientifically evaluated.

Magoun further contends that the embryonic development of the central nervous system with all its pulsatile activity, remains as this third motion.

Incidentally, embryologically the brain, ventricles, spinal cord and canal arise from the neural tube. The cephalic end becomes the parts of the brain and the ventricles. During the development of the neural tube, the cephalic end is sub-divided into three by membraneous tissues to form the prosencephalon (fore-brain); the mesocephalon (mid-brain); and rhombencephalon (hind-brain); and the cavities between these parts are modified to become the ventricles.

Imagine these three membraneous tissues as tennis balls, placed close together in a sock. Because of their shape not all of the surfaces will be in contact. The intervening spaces are called the ventricles. The rest of the neural tube becomes the spinal cord. The central canal being contained in its cavity.

So, on Magoun's premise it is conceivable that the brain possesses an inherent motility of its own, and it is through this motility that the cranial approach to treatment is directed.

In passing, these rhythms should not be confused with the much faster waves found in E.E.G. examinations – alpha, beta, gamma, etc.

It appears reasonable to suggest that cerebrospinal fluid may well be the second of these obscure fluid phenomena in the brain tissues. C.S.F. is the cranio-sacral system's hydraulic fluid. It is contained within a semi-closed environment where it fluctuates with a wave-like motion (unlike the

TABLE A CRANIAL EMBRYOLOGICAL DEVELOPMENT

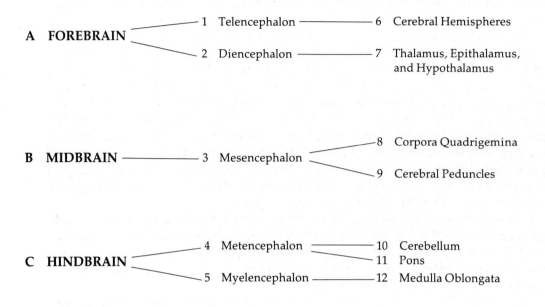

D SPINAL CORD

A, B, & C represent the earliest stages of the development of the brain. 1–5 the later stages. 6–12 the final structures achieved.

circulatory manner of blood) according the laws of the primary respiratory mechanism.

Its environs are vented only by the arachnoid villae which permit its return to the venous system. It may be found throughout the connective tissues of the entire body, and is identical with blood distribution.

The constituents of C.S.F. are dependent on the composition of the blood from which it is filtered. It comprises proteins, glucose, urea, trace elements, and various acids, etc as well as hormones (brain C.S.F. carrying neurohypophyseal secretions). About 100mls of C.S.F. are found cradling the brain and spinal cord. This 'cushion' reduces the gross weight of the brain – usually said to be about 140g – to a mere 50g net weight within the body, thus finely balancing and protecting the brain from injury from without, and undue pressures from within. It is clear and colourless, and among its many physiological activities it harmonises and co-ordinates the functions of the viscera. This is of the highest importance, as this 'Fluid commands vital influence over even the life-blood' (Denis Brookes).

It does not require much imagination to see the magnitude of the crises that can occur if C.S.F. fluctuation is restricted. And where would the restriction begin? In the cranium, of course. When all the osseous structures are in physiological balance the outflow or pumping of C.S.F. to the various destinations will be the normal result.

50% of this fluid is produced by the Choroid Plexus, the remainder mostly arises from the lateral ventricles and the cerebral vessels from whence it flows through the cerebral acqueduct into the subarachnoid space below the cerebellum through three pathways. Making its way into the very small central canal of the spinal cord, the C.S.F. fluctuates about both the brain and spinal cord within the subarachnoid space, invades the arachnoid villae, before returning to the venous blood system via the foramen of Magendie (apertura mediana ventriculi quarti) and the foramen of Luschka (apertura lateralis ventriculi quarti) and the superior sagittal sinus.

It is postulated that C.S.F. does not flow as does the blood or other fluids. Pascal's Law throws some light on this subject 'The pressure on a confined fluid is transmitted equally and undiminished in all directions' like the effect of dropping a stone in a pool of water; the waves spread from the centre of the force at the same speed in all directions.

Its behaviour in some ways is like electricity in that it has a phase relationship of positive and negative 8–12 cycles per minute, reciprocating with the C.N.S. motility, functionally. It has already been noted that the C.N.S. is inherently motile.

Opinions vary among researchers, but Bowsher postulates 'the entire C.S.F., its behaviour, circulation (distribution) sustenance and even the reason for its presence would be better understood if it were practicable to observe this system as it really is.' It defies definitive investigation. If its closed

15 VENTRICLES OF THE BRAIN & CEREBROSPINAL FLUID DISTRIBUTION

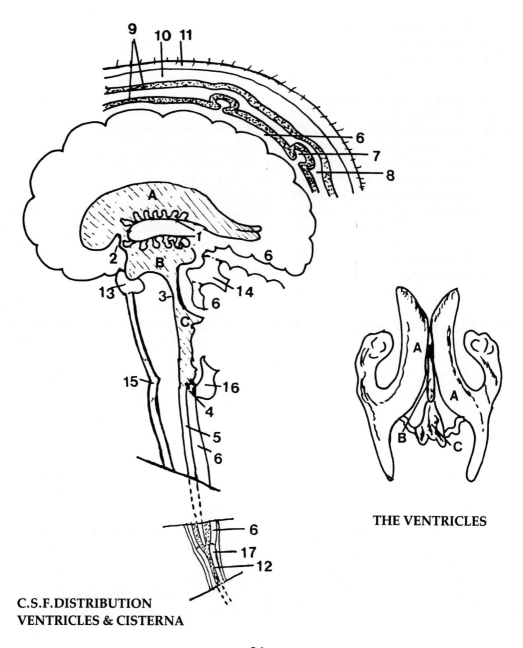

C.S.F. DISTRIBUTION VENTRICLES & CISTERNA

THE VENTRICLES

PRIMARY RESPIRATORY MECHANISM & CEREBROSPINAL FLUID

15 VENTRICLES OF THE BRAIN & CEREBROSPINAL FLUID DISTRIBUTION

A Lateral Ventricles (2)
B Third Ventricle
C Fourth Ventricle

1–8 Distribution of C.S.F. from blood stream through ventricles and back to blood stream.
1 Choroid Plexus
2 Foramen of Munro
   (intraventricular foramen)
3 Aqueduct of Sylvius
   (Cerebral Aqueduct)
4 Foramina of Magendie
   & Luschka
5 Chordal Canal
6 Subarachnoid Space
7 Arachnoid Villa
8 Venous sinus (Saggital)

9 Dura Mater
10 Parietal Bone
11 Scalp
12 Pia Mater

13–17 Cisterna – Location of main cisterns in sub-arachnoid space. These are formed where a 'ballooning' of the space allows C.S.F. to collect
13 Interpeduncular
14 Superior
15 Pontine
16 Magna
   (Cerebellomedullary)
17 Lumbar

hydrodynamic environment is broken into the resultant altered pressure changes that automatically ensue, obscures accurate observation; the integrity of the internal pressure being invaluable to its proper working. To quote Selye 'The structural organisation of life can often be studied by dissection after death, but vital processes can only be explored in living beings.' Might this not be the reason why many a neuro-pathological state remains veiled.

The normal activity of the brain itself is not yet fully understood.

Nevertheless, it is generally agreed that it maintains, as it were, a hive of activity within the skull, and does not have any muscular agency as assistance for promoting articular mobility as is manifested in other parts of the body. The brain involuntarily moves within its osseous chamber and exhibits a rhythm which involves dilation and contraction of the ventricles during respiration.

It is through this ventricular contraction and dilation that the fluctuation of the C.S.F. is effected. This gives rise to a chain reaction in that the arachnoid and dural membranes also move, and through the reciprocal tension membrane the basilar articulation also received impetus for mobility.

It is during inhalation that the ventricles dilate thus occasioning the expanding of the convolutions of the hemispheres. As this is taking place the third ventricle dilates into a 'V' shape, and the fourth ventricle into a diamond shape, together with the spinal cord drawn upwards.

There is relaxation of the convolutions with the ventricles contracting, the spinal cord dropping downwards with the C.S.F. again fluctuating. The upward and downward movement of the spinal cord does not involve the spinal canal as such. The movement is minimal, but nonetheless an inherently functional imperative that occurs like the inflating and deflating of a balloon.

In that the dural tissues are as structural supports for the main venous pathways to the jugular veins any restriction affecting the jugular veins will automatically result in a build up of C.S.F. pressure. This is attested to by the lumbar puncture spinal fluid test. Therefore quite often when cranial membraneous articular strains occur there may be undue restruction of the dural and arachnoid membranes and intracranial vessels. This is inhibiting to the C.S.F. fluctuation and the normal behaviour of the ventricles and convolutions.

Many disease processes are attributable to an inbalance in the constituents of the C.S.F. This is not difficult to visualize for, according to Gray, this fluid does not only structurally support the brain and spinal cord; it is the main nutrient to the brain, man's most valuable anatomical possession.

Attention is drawn to the evenness of pressure C.S.F. maintains upon the brain and spinal cord. Varying between 5–15 millimetres with pulse and respiration this pressure is of primary physiological importance. The dural envelope being fairly rigid and inexpansible, the variation of C.S.F. pressure is in direct correspondence with the nervous system, which converges on the internal jugular veins for 95% of its drainage. Proper nerve function too, is dependant on whether C.S.F. is of the correct chemical balance and where there is ample fluctuation of this fluid the medulla is never congested, and the C.N.S. centres are always stimulated.

To summarize:-

Integrated with all other fluid systems the C.S.F. under the direct influence of the P.R.M. remains dynamic and semi-closed; especially adapted for the selective passage of fluid from the vascular system into the ventricular system of the brain.

The C.S.F. is contained in the dural membrane and any outflow or intake of this fluid is monitored by the choroid plexus and arachnoid villae, which themselves are limited to sustained physiological patterns. As we shall see in a later chapter the behaviour of this C.S.F. can not only be felt but influenced by the cranial osteopath.

Involuntary motion of the sacrum between the ilia is a respiratory phenomenon occuring around the second sacral vertebra. The pelvic ligaments facilitate this motion in synchrony with the entire sacral mechanism, without any change in the basic tension peculiar to that area.

Cranial articular mobility is concerned with the tentorium cerebelli and the falx cerebri (which terminates anteriorly at the crista galli of the ethmoid). The position of these dural sheets is very significant and involves the straight sinus. The straight sinus (or sinus rectus) runs almost vertically between the junction of the tentorium cerebelli and the falx cerebri, joining the superior and inferior sagittal sinuses at their inferior end.

It is situated superiorly behind the Basal vein and is separated from the fourth ventricle by the cerebellum. Together these anatomical structures are a powerful membraneous band, which is continuous with the falx cerebelli and extends to the sacrum and the second sacral vertebra.

Recall that below the foramen magnum and C2 & C3, there is no firm dural attachment – apart from the dentate ligaments – until S2, where the sacrum moves in Sutherland's respiratory mechanism. Two phases are peculiar to the respiratory mechanism

1) Inhalation/flexion
2) Exhalation/extension

Let us look again at what happens in respiratory activity. Inhalation and shortening of the dural tube occur simultaneously. At the same time the cerebral hemispheres are also very active, opening up laterally, and moving upwards, resulting in the constituent parts of the brain being condensed. The form and functional activity of the ventricles especially the third and fourth, together with the choroid plexuses, are urged into action that facilitate the interchange of blood and C.S.F. flow. It should be noted, therefore, that Flexion is enhanced by inspiration, and is not dependent on it.

16 THE DURAL MENINGES
Cranial Respiratory Excursion Response

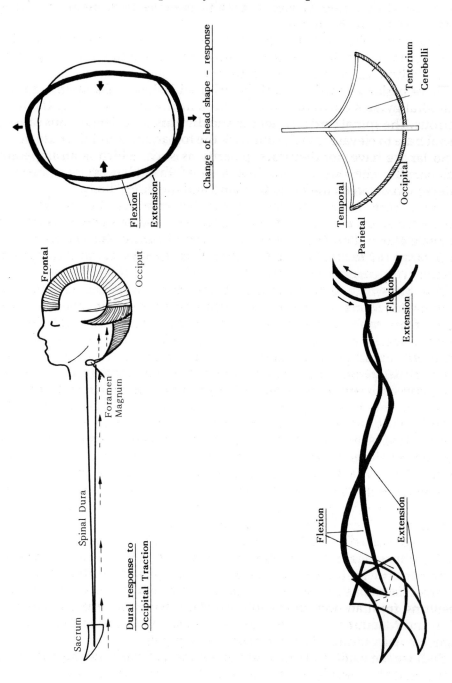

The result of this activity is that the sella turcica and hypophysis provide just the right stimulatory medium for the endocrine system. In synchrony with these activities there is also a cranial osseous movement involving the dimensions of the head itself.

From front to back (glabella to inion) its measurements diminish while there is expansion from side to side (bitemporally) with a corresponding lessening in depth from the vertex to basicranium.

There is also a broadening of the orbit with the nasal alae enlarging as the temporal gyrates outwards and upwards lifting and propelling the temporal petrous. The spinal cord now tenses and diminishes in length thus causing the sacral base to elevate into flexion with the top anterior and the base posterior.

So far we have not discussed polarity as such, which is an imperative to balance. To cite one or two instances of this phenomenon there is the interaction between the Pituitary gland and the Pineal body.

These create a 'slack tension' mechanism between themselves. This also occurs between the tubular long bones and the calvarium which interact between themselves both in form and function. Cranially there is a valid basis of polarity correlating the limb system with sphenobasilar mobility and the primary respiratory mechanism.

The practically inelastic state of the dura mater renders the sacrum vulnerable. We need to be well acquainted with the sacrum – particularly its involuntary mobility between the ilia. It is important to study the relevant muscles and ligaments. There are muscles and ligaments that in a hypertonic state will cause great difficulties in the cranial mechanism. For instance, consider the piriformis. In hypertonus it can cause side-bending torsion and even immobilisation of the sacrum. As a direct consequence the occiput will also succumb to sidebending and torsion and so will the sphenobasilar symphysis – perverted mobility being mediated through the dura to the cranial base. And what about the iliacus? A hypertonic iliacus will certainly flex the sacral base in a forward position. When this happens the cranio-sacral mechanism will automatically suffer imbalance. (See Chapter 14)

How does this apply practically? The dura mater and periosteum have a sensory nerve supply similar to the capsules and linings of any other articulation. Therefore when there is a strain of the dura resulting from a fixation or malosseous adjustment there may well be reflex symptoms.

The effects of increased pressure on articulating facets are well known. There is no reason why there cannot be a reflex pain resulting from say, a L5 and a lordosis; in a similar way there is no reason why there cannot be a reflex pain resulting from an occipitomastoid junction, when there is osseous fixation. They are the same type of joint having the same sensory nerve supply with the same physiological and anatomical rules applying.

Because the vault is founded in membrane and the base is cartilage, there is functional accommodation of the vault to the base during motion.

17 CRANIAL VENOUS SINUSES & ARTERIAL SUPPLY

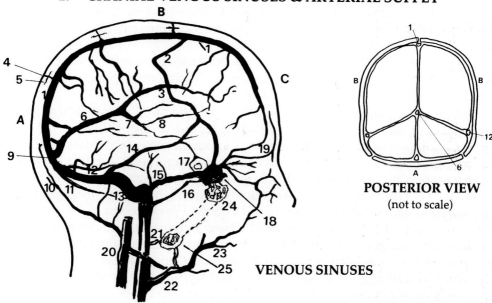

VENOUS SINUSES

POSTERIOR VIEW
(not to scale)

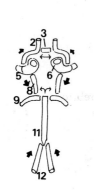

CIRCLE OF WILLIS

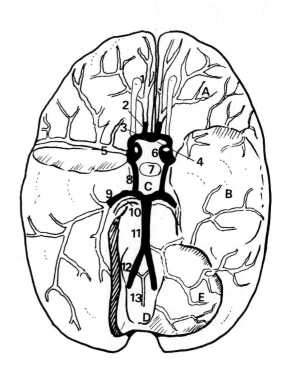

ARTERIAL SUPPLY

PRIMARY RESPIRATORY MECHANISM & CEREBROSPINAL FLUID

17 CRANIAL VENOUS SINUSES & ARTERIAL SUPPLY

VENOUS SINUSES

A Occipital bone
B Parietal bone
C Frontal bone

1 Superior Sagittal Sinus
2 Superior Saggital Veins
3 Inferior Sagittal Sinus
4 Emissary Veins
5 Diploic Veins

6 Straight Sinus
7 Great Cerebral Vein
8 Internal Cerebral Vein
   (both 7 & 8 are known as
   Great veins of Galen)
9 Confluence of Sinuses
10 Occipital Vein
11 Occipital Sinus
12 Transverse Sinus
13 Sigmoid Sinus

14 Superior Petrosal Sinus
15 Inferior Petrosal Sinus
16 Basilar Sinus
17 Circular Sinus (Ridley's sinus)
18 Cavernous Sinus
   (Part of Circular Sinus)

19 Supraorbital Vein
20 External Jugular Vein
21 Internal Jugular Vein

22 Common Facial Vein
23 Anterior Facial Vein
24 Pterygoid Plexus
25 Pharyngeal Plexus

ARTERIAL SUPPLY

A Frontal lobe – Cerebrum
B Temporal lobe – Cerebrum
C Pons
D Medulla Oblongata
E Cerebellum

1 Olfactory Bulb
2 Anterior Cerebral Artery
3 Anterior Communicating Artery
4 Optic Chiasma
5 Middle Cerebral Artery
6 Internal Carotid Artery
7 Hypophysis

8 Posterior Communicating Artery
9 Posterior Cerebral Artery
10 Cerebellar Artery
11 Basilar Artery
12 Vertebral Artery
13 Anterior Spinal Vein

PAUL E. KIMBERLY

'The mobility of the brain can only pass through its full cycle when the articulations are freely mobile.'

'... the fluctuation of C.S.F. which puts in the hands of the osteopathic physician using the cranial concept, a method more potent than any therapeutic agency yet established.'

'Most of the resistance to the cranial concept has been because of a preconceived idea that the skull is immobile rather than due to consideration of the media through which it operated.'

CHAPTER FOUR

Body Fluids

In Chapter One specific reference is made regarding the body's dependence on its fluid systems for its proper functioning. In various other places we have spoken of the role of the vascular system, cerebrospinal fluid, etc.

Body fluids can be divided basically into two types, those which operate in a 'closed' (or semi-closed) system and those that do not. We would associate blood, C.S.F., joint (synovial) fluids and acqueous humour with the former. The latter 'free' fluids include lymph, interstitial (which might be referred to as 'pre-lymph'), extracellular, glandular secretions, gastrointestinal contents, (chyle, bile,) etc. However, all fluids, whether they originate in the vascular system or not, must return to it.

Fluids therefore, change from one place to another by various means, filtration, absorption, osmosis, diffusion . . . across cell, capillary, and vessel walls, membranes, etc. The density/concentration/specific gravity is different in each case, depending on fluid/solid ratios. The chemical messengers present (such as cyclic A.M.P.) hormone and enzyme activity, etc. may alter the density of a particular fluid passing through a particular area.

The average person consists of almost two-thirds liquid (which can be sub-divided into one third plasma and interstitial fluids – extra-cellular – the remaining two thirds being intracellular). The other one third of body weight consisting of protein, fats, minerals, and so on.

E.C.F. (extracellular fluid)/I.C.F. (intracellular fluid) ratio is different in children from adults. It is this factor that allows children/infants to dehydrate more quickly proportionately. A little less than a tenth of body weight is blood – half of this is plasma – the pale, straw coloured liquid portion.

Lymph is one of the most important circulating liquids and no account of body fluids would be complete without some discussion of the lymphatic system. This system consists of vessels, ducts, glands, (nodes) which have a contractile rhythmic excursion of their own – the more lymph present the greater the contractibility. Having no pump it is dependant on muscular activity to maintain a steady flow. Lymph begins as a tissue fluid (interstitial fluid) that arises from blood plasma and is gathered up in the lymph capillaries. Like blood, lymph possesses coagulability and consists of liquid and solids, and like plasma it is usually straw-coloured though in the presence of pathology it can appear slightly pink from the presence of erythrocytes (red blood cells). It is slightly alkaline and conveys hormones, enzymes such as glycerol, esterase, and diamine oxyidase (histaminase) to the cells. Cancer cells are also metastasized by lymph transportation. It can therefore be seen that blood and lymph are very similar but that concentrations of calcium and phosphates, sugars, fats, urea, and other mineral elements, etc. increase lymph's specific gravity in some areas and varies the concentrations of the two fluids.

Lymph also helps maintain the concentration of urine being secreted by the kidneys. About seven and a half pints of lymph are circulated daily. From the smallest lymphatic vessels (lymphatics) which run beside the capillaries and like them pick up salts, sugars, and waste products, etc. holding and transporting infective material – lymph is channelled into larger vessels (which contain nodes) and ducts until it drains into the right and left sub-clavian veins (brachiocephalic junction). Lymph vessels are both deep and superficial. The former lie beside the large veins, the latter are distributed throughout superficial fascia. The lymphatic system then, is the means by which interstitial fluid levels are kept constant.

Lymph nodes are particularly concerned with the immune system. They are like railway stations along the lines of communication culminating in groups – termini or collecting points, at cervical, axillary, inguinal, and abdominal (cisterna chyli) stations. Within them are phagocytic (macrophage) cells whose specific function is to fight bacteria. These nodes are also glands. Their credibility as glands derives from the fact that they produce leucocytes (white blood corpuscles) and plasma proteins from lymphocytic breakdown. These glands also produce antibodies. These actions are monitored by A.C.T.H. produced by the adenohypophysis. Such small vessels are also found in the small intestines and are called lacteals, where they absorb fat particles into the vascular system. Adenoids, tonsils, and other similar groups of glands are all lymph nodes and their removal in diseased states is most undesirable. Instead of surgical intervention the cause of the pathologic state should be ascertained and an effort made to cleanse the system as a whole and the lymphatic system in particular. Of course, this is not the only part of the body to be concerned with defence/immunity action. As has been discussed elsewhere the endocrine glands, spleen, liver and intestines play their part.

The nodes are about the size of peas and are situated at the junctions of the larger lymph vessels. They are the first line of defence in body infection. Their action is obvious in infection at the extremities. An untreated cut, wound etc. say on a foot – will result in hard, shotty, glands in the groin, or behind the knee, indicating bacterial activity being 'held' at those railway stations. Without this protective mechanism the human organism could not survive for

BODY FLUIDS
18 LYMPHATIC SYSTEM

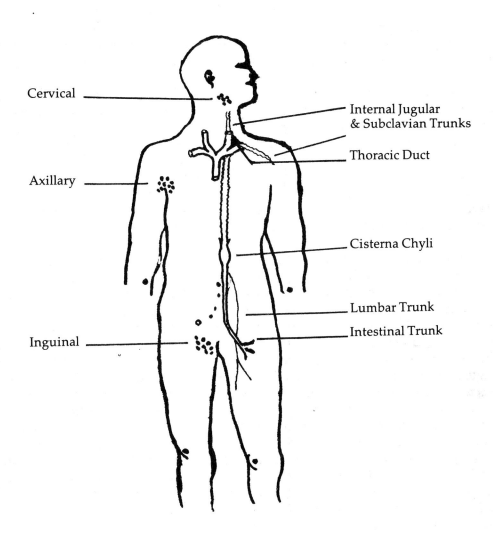

TABLE B

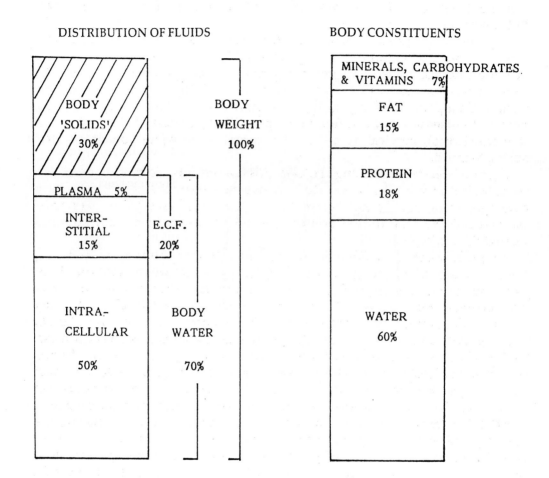

long. It would be most vulnerable and would ultimately be overtaken or succumb to disease processes. Infection would be able to directly attack vital organs giving the body's remaining healing mechanisms an impossible task.

It should be noted that no nodes are found in bone marrow, the spinal cord, or the brain.

The lymphatic system is prone to inflammation (coxsackie virus, etc.) new growth – melanomic multiple malignancies, Hodgkins disease (enlargement of lymph nodes, spleen and general lymph tissue), lymphocytic leukemia; tuberculosis; benign cysts; lymphadenomatosis (hypertrophy of lymph tissue). Enlargement of any group of lymph nodes, vessels, etc. is often a pointer to disease – mumps (epidemic parotitis), glandular fever (infectious mononucleosis), cervical adenitis, sore throat – are some conditions that spring to mind.

If lymph is in stasis, creating acidosis, this is a precursor to more generalized pathological states, arthritis, cancer, anaemia, for instance. At any lesion site, a sprained wrist say, lymph stasis is the first visible sign of structural 'pervertion' not only in and around the cells, but also in the surrounding related tissues/organs.

Lymph flow being conditioned by muscular reflex, any aberration involving their structure will hinder lymphatic drainage e.g. joint dysfunction, spasticity or contracture of muscles, trauma... Hence every effort should be made to clear obstruction as soon as possible, else healing will be slow to take place. Oedema is that visible accumulation of tissue fluid. Mostly occuring in the lower limbs, where gravity and faulty venous return enhance its occurrence, it is also found in the abdomen and upper thighs in cardiac and pulmonary conditions (ascites/peritoneal dropsy). This is occasioned by blockage of the thoracic duct causing back pressure (chyliform ascites). Oedema can also be seen below the eyes in cardiac and kidney disease, in the legs when pulmonary congestion is present. Pericarditis is excess lymph fluid in the serous pericardia. Inadequate drainage is always one of the precipitating factors to oedema. In excessive or chronic oedema as well as puffiness, pitting occurs. (A finger pressed into oedematous tissue leaves an impression when withdrawn. These pits may fill almost at once or remain for some hours). Such oedema can be toxic.

It is particularly important for articular areas in close proximity to the sub-clavian veins – where the lymph is drained into the circulation – to be functioning well. That is to say at the clavicular/sternal/costal junctions. Because of the variations in pressure between lungs, the heart, and its great vessels – this being caused by various factors, movement of the diaphragm, inflation of the lungs, the pumping action of blood from atria to ventricle, and ventricle to aorta, lymph is given impetus to return from the abdominal and lower limbic region, as well as from the head and upper limbs. Hence, treatment of the lymphatic system in stasis (as opposed to purely local drainage of an injured part of the body) is best facilitated by exaggerating these

ESSENTIALS OF CRANIO-SACRAL OSTEOPATHY

19 LYMPHATIC DRAINAGE

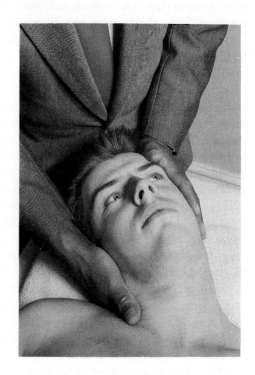

Thoracic Pump

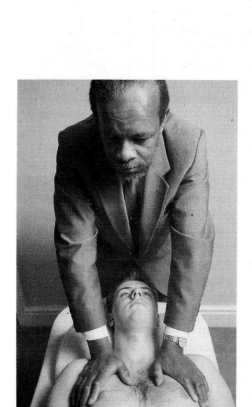

Thoracic Inlet

thoracic rhythmic pumping actions to facilitate free lymph flow. This action also stimulates heart and circulatory action, and other organic function, promoting a healthy even flow of fluids around the body. Most toxic, inflammatory, coryzaic, asthmatic, cattharal states respond well to this procedure – in fact so do most sluggish, chronic, pathological states. Clearing out the system in this way brings renewed activity and health to every cell in acute and sub-acute conditions also.

So, any congestion at these diaphragmatic/pectoral sites precipitated by a crowded diaphragm, retarded respiratory excursion, faulty posture etc. will hinder the lymph flow and noxious elements will be retained in the tissues – defective circulation in extremities can result in peripheral ischaemia in the lungs, emphysemic complications.

Primary lymphatic drainage is best accomplished with the patient supine and the operator at the head of the couch. With the palmar surface of the practitioner's hands in contact with the patient's anterior chest wall, below the clavicles, and thumbs aligned either side of the sternum. Keeping the arms straight give short sharp thrusts inferoanteriorly – caudally – at around thirty times a minute. Such pumping action should move the chest wall in order to be effective, but treatment should not exceed three minutes. Certain conditions contra-indicate lymph drainage:- lymphatic types of cancer, t.b., sarcoma, osteoporosis – including menopausal osteoporosis. Care should also be exercised when treating patients with barrel chests (seen in emphysema and kyphosis) and, of course, with elderly frail patients.

This may be preceded by stimulation of individual neuroendocrine gangliform contractions in head and thorax, and freeing sutural restrictions at nasion, lacrimals, maxilla, etc. Do not forget to check both sterno-cleido-mastoid muscles for undue tension. Like the Psoas they are harbingers of toxic matter. Incidentally, it is always a good rule to check these muscles prior to cranial vault and base treatment.

Soft-tissue manipulation to lesioned areas, or the whole body, is also valuable except that where there is haemorrhage (varicosity, open wounds, etc.) such treatment should be confined to proximal areas. Such attention to lymphatic stasis can precipitate an 'apparent' crisis, which may last from a few minutes to about thirty-six hours, after which there will be a significant amelioration.

As many diseases emanate from sub-diaphragmatic origins (i.e. stomach, gall bladder, liver, spleen, solar plexus, kidney), inadequate drainage here has been known to hasten fatality. As the diaphragm helps drain the abdominal, and to some extent the pelvic, cavity it is as well to know how to treat the area.

Sit the patient on a chair with both legs outstretched. If necessary use a stool to support the feet. Ask the patient to exhale and then pull in/contract the abdominal muscles and diaphragm; then to inhale whilst holding these muscles taut. The operator can place his hand on the patient's abdominal wall

TABLE C   BODY FLUIDS

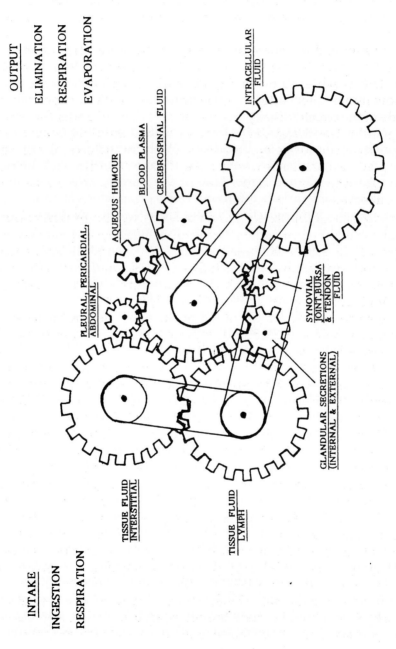

to assist. This exercise can be augmented by 'forced' inspiration with mouth closed and nose pinched.

Repeated 4–5 times (and two or three times a day at home) this will reduce oedema, relieving pelvic congestion, enteritis, constipation, threatened appendicitis, etc. and is not known to have any contra-indications. It creates alternating areas of positive and negative pressure, influencing venous, as well as lymph flow.

The liver, spleen, and appendix are related to the lymphatic system, as we have seen and specific drainage of liver and spleen should form part of our programme. This is achieved by having the patient supine as before – in fact this can follow immediately after thoracic drainage – with the operator at the left-hand side of the couch initially. He places his left hand under the patient's posterior right chest wall and the palmar surface of the right hand over the patient's right hypochondriac/epigastric area. Slowly and carefully compress the liver area and have the patient take a deep breath (which will also help the compression), hold to a count of six then release suddenly in a reflex move. Repeat this three times.

To drain the gall-bladder merely place the finger tips of the right hand just under the bottom of the right-hand portion of the rib-cage – about two inches from the ziphoid process. With the right hand lying flat and the left hand over the top in support 'stroke' posteroinferiorly – strokes about four to five inches in length – and repeat three to four times. A 'gurgling' sound indicating that the gall bladder is emptying its contents is usually heard.

To treat the spleen and pancreas stand at the other side of the couch and repeat the manoeuvre over the left hypochondriac/epigastric area two or three times, holding to a count of about ten each time.

The foregoing procedures will well reward any practitioner who cares to use them on patients with conditions already discussed but the most therapeutic cranial manoeuvre to drain the lymphatics is to open the thoracic inlet. One method of achieving this is to drain the cervical/thoracic area which creates a 'knock-on' effect to the brachiocephalic junction. With the patient and operator in the usual position for cranial treatments the practitioner should place one hand low down on one side of the patient's neck, enveloping the entire lateral cervical area, with the thumb anterior pointing forward across the sternocleido junction. The other hand is placed in a similar manner on the other side of the neck, a little higher, embracing the occipital/mandibular area – the thumb being positioned almost along the line of the jaw. This assymetrical hold allows the practitioner to laterally flex, or rather side-bend the neck to the farthest possible point with perfect control, allowing the chin to point towards the patient's opposite shoulder.

The lower hand is the fulcrum, the upper one supports. Ask the patient to take a deep breath and then increase the curve; let him exhale, and repeat the side-bend until maximum lateralization is achieved – whereupon the operator gives a short travel, medium velocity, final thrust, increasing the concavity. There will often be an audible 'clunk' denoting a satisfactory resolution. Repeat the procedure for the other side of the neck.

Although full lymphatic drainage is contra-indicated in some conditions, as we have seen, such will respond well to soft-tissue manipulation and long 'stroking'/brushing movements across areas of skin – in the direction of lymph flow to detoxify the body. Fingers (or a soft natural bristle brush) may be used to stimulate the flow and remove dead cells from the skin, allowing the skin to 'breathe' more freely. The lower limbs are taken first, from the toes upward, then the abdomen, stroking up towards the heart. Then the upper areas are dealt with, head and arms again working toward the mediastinum.

Pressure is minimal, around 5 lbs being used – just enough to cause 'stretching' of the skin. The extent and duration of such treatment will, of course, be bounded by the patient's tolerance, age, etc. Other detoxification methods such as controlled fasting, homoeopathic remedies, colonic irrigation, will also aid lymphatic drainage. There are also many other soft-tissue, neuromuscular, osteopathic and 'Chapman's reflex' techniques, which are not covered in detail here, that are designed to assist lymphatic drainage. Most of these are valuable and all have the right idea behind them namely, restore fluid integrity and harmonic rhythms, and you will have gone a long way toward achieving homeostasis.

We are not, primarily, flesh and bone; by that we mean hard, solid substance. We are essentially a collection of interacting rhythmic, pumping fluid arrangements which, when functioning perfectly, maintain the human body in health.

JOHN HUNTER

'There is a circumstance attending accidental injury which does not belong to disease – namely, that the injury has in all cases a tendency to produce the disposition and means to a cure.'

There is no such thing as a hereditary disease, but there is a hereditary disposition for a disease.
I believe the cure consists in the removal of the cause.'

'The various effects of the mind upon the body are almost without end. . . There is not a natural action in the body, whether voluntary or involuntary that may not be influenced by the peculiar state of the mind at the time.'

CHAPTER FIVE

Cranio-Sacral Balance & Fluid Mechanics

Balance is probably the most important phenomenon in osteopathic thought and practice. In cranial osteopathy this is particularly apparent. The over-riding pre-requisite to homeostasis therefore must be that the cranium and sacrum are in balance.

Two supportive quotations may be cited here from men of some eminence among osteopathic educators. The first is from Perrin T. Wilson, past President of the American Osteopathic Association. 'When all parts of the body are perfectly adjusted in position and action it can best meet its environmental changes of temperature, food, mental strains and difficulties to which it is subjected.' Note that the emphasis here is really on adjustment. We shall certainly be looking at this in greater depth as we proceed.

The second quotation is from the late H.H. Fryette, that venerated osteopathic legend whom we cannot afford to ignore. In his 'Theory of Movements' he postulated 'when all parts of the body are properly aligned and balanced in relation to each other, a state of equilibrium exists in which the body works most efficiently.'

You have noticed, haven't you, how these postulations agree on the fundamental necessity of proper adjustment. This applies as much to the cranium as to all other parts of the body – involving motion – cranio-sacral motion, together with postural articular changes. There must be anatomical and postural harmony between sacrum and cranium. This is vital, especially when we are concerned with lesion patterns – internal or external rotation, flexion, or extension.

These usually involve the whole mechanism, and your potential as a creditworthy cranial practitioner can be stretched to its limit when faced with such cases. You will have to be aware that within this mechanism there are certain areas which, under some conditions, are subject to restriction. These restrictions can immobilize the reciprocating balance of the whole structure. You will also have to know what specific techniques you must use to unlock that particular structure or articulation in order to restore mobility to the area, that balance may be established and proper function restored.

20 DURAL MENINGES

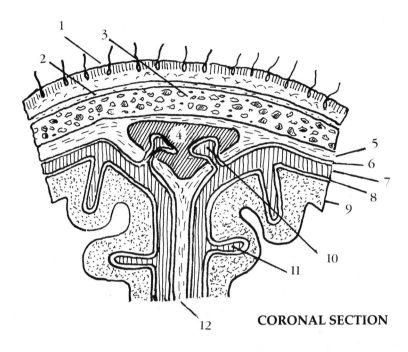

CORONAL SECTION

1. Scalp
2. Periosteum
3. Parietal Bone
4. Superior Sagittal Sinus
5. Dura Mater
6. Arachnoid Mater
7. Subarachnoid Space
8. Pia Mater
9. Cerebral Cortex
10. Arachnoid Villae
11. Arachnoidal Trabecula
12. Falx Cerebri

For example, there is currently a high incidence of hypertension in our society. Sooner or later you will have to handle one or more of these cases. How will you treat them? Or, if you are already handling this type of patient, how successful have you been? If you are not doing as well as you might why not check the basicranium. Check the occipito-atlantal joint. Disturbances here, suggestive of imbalance around the upper cervicals and the petrous portion of the temporal bone, will most likely yield the solution, and with your cranial technique you can bring relief to the suffering.

It is in the floor of the fourth ventricle that you will discover the resources for raising and lowering blood pressure. It is also within this area of the intracranial mechanism that we find we can control all the physiological centres of the body. Remember that the expansion and contraction of capillary walls takes place through the action of the autonomic system.

It is not possible to arrive at cranio-sacral balance without fascial

21 SPHENOBASILAR SYMPHYSIS

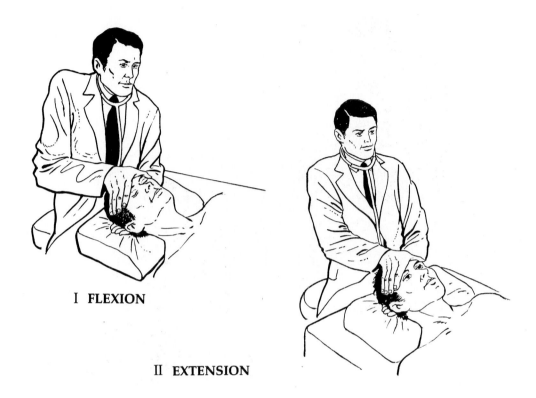

I FLEXION

II EXTENSION

involvement. Fascial malfunction together with that of other tissues sub-occipitally is always involved in the cause of lowering the tension in this area and there is a good chance of blood pressure normalizing.

This might sound like throwing a spanner into the works but the story of the cranio-sacral balance is really the story of the entire anatomical structure together with its multifarious systems – and basically the function of the anatomical structure is dependant on fluid flow.

Fluid flow is as important physiologically as oil is to a motor car. If the oil lines are blocked the engine will not function efficiently. So with the body – nutrition, waste removal, energy conservation, conduction, or storage – all depend on an efficient though intricately balanced fluid flow, for the whole mechanism to be sustained in homeostatic integrity. You may ask where in all this the blood circulation is concerned? What has it to do with balance? The performance of the ventricles balances exactly the friction loss of energy, as the blood courses through the vascular system. A perfect balance exists between the volume of blood through any part and the whole of the circulation.

22 SPHENOBASILAR SYMPHYSIS

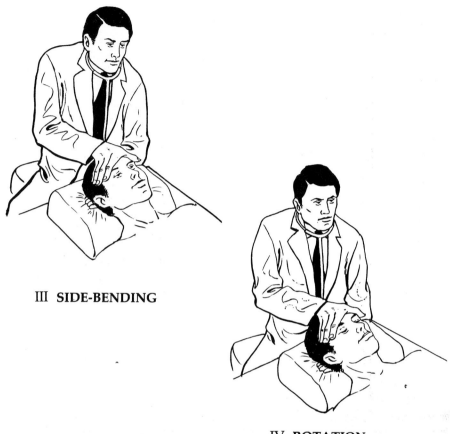

III **SIDE-BENDING**

IV **ROTATION**

There is an equivalence of blood flow through all the arteries to the flow through all the veins. In the event of there being any interference with this fine balance you can imagine the consequences – disequilibrium of the entire mechanism.

You may have a patient come to you complaining of digestive problems. You may examine him. You may question what he had for breakfast, lunch, or whatever. You interest yourself in his dietary habits and do your usual palpation here and there perhaps for lesions, but all in vain. Don't stop there. Mobilize your thinking. Let it expand and deepen, taking in the possibility of fluid entrapment and the inter-relationship of the different systems within the body; then you almost certainly will find there is an obstruction to normal fluid flow.

You ask where you might check for this. What about the occiput? Check it for

23 CRANIAL PALPATION

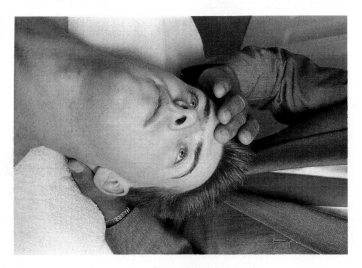

Checking for
forehead restrictions

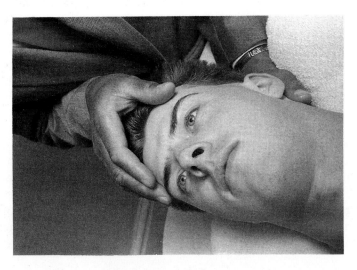

Checking for motion

balance with the sacrum. Mobilize that occiput and the problem should be over. Equilibrium in fluid pressure will be re-established in the various proximal and distal parts.

Incidentally, when you are examining your patient with digestive trouble, he might also complain of back-ache. Palpate his spine and no doubt you will find several tender places without there being any specific lesion. What is the first thing you begin to imagine? It's plainly and simply due to a build-up of undue pressures in the presence of fluid bombardment. I am convinced this is the very reason why so many ailments fail to respond to what is usually regarded as normal procedures or treatment. Many practitioners concentrate on the obvious local symptoms, and not on the underlying fluid status.

Remember, fluid balance (according to the laws of physiology) is the state of the body in relation to the ingestion, metabolization, and excretion of fluids – water, electrolytes... Therefore that indigestion, backache, etc. is often the result of metabolic imbalance. An American friend of mine puts it like this 'when your intake exceeds your output, your upkeep becomes a blow-out.'

How true this is! In osteopathic language though, we can be content to emphasise that obstruction to normal fluid flow may not only cause aggravation at the place where the obstruction is, but will adversely affect other systems and organs that depend upon it.

What is one of the most prevalent ailments affecting the public today – what prevents thousands from enjoying a full life? Isn't it backache? How often we see the folk coming into our clinics twisted in all shapes. Some of us might lay much store by the detection of the so-called 'slipped disc' in some of these cases. Cranial osteopathy doesn't acknowledge this. Craniosacral balance attests to the fact that we are concerned with a system which is subject to the laws of fluid mechanics.

Of course, there are mechanical problems. There are those conditions that will yield to the violence of the crack, the pull or the push with amazing results. But it is always useful to understand what is happening. We cannot divorce physiological function from fluid flow in some form or other. The presenting symptoms will indicate the destabilizing area of fluid entrapment and enable us to treat our patients cognisantly.

When a patient comes to us listing to one side, for example, we dare not think of him in mechanical terms of fixed bolts and screws. In the light of our knowledge of pressure changes within the cranio-sacral system we can lay that patient on his back, and with tactile dexterity contact the cranium, and reverse the result of perverted physiology. We must treat cognisantly or else the results can be disastrous where they might easily have been otherwise.

Perhaps it is time to consider some lesion states or patterns in the cranio-sacral mechanism. A piriformis contracture or hypertonus affecting the sacrum may result in a side-bending or torsion of the cranial base. This anomaly will persist or be recurrent as long as the sacrum is allowed to remain uncorrected. Conversely, lesions of the cranium can produce somatic and visceral disturbances, and cranial base dysfunctions often result in sacral anomalies. These can be ascending or descending lesions, the difference between which can only be determined by careful analysis with due regard to menigeal distribution.

The golden rule is that we must resist the temptation of accepting the obvious as diagnostically conclusive. A check for disturbances elsewhere often discloses the primary anomaly. This is especially so in the case of flexion, extension, sidebending and torsion lesions affecting the cranial base.

The sacrum usually conforms to the occipital pattern of distortion. For example, if the sacrum is tipped so that one side is posterior and inferior the cranium will go into torsion with the occiput low on the same side.

One of the most profound aspects of the cranial concept is that we are dealing with minute analysis, and every patient presents a separate and distinct challenge. At best the osteopath's aim is not to correct C2/3, D5/6, the wrist joint, or whatever, but to re-establish balance in the whole individual. This is the hall-mark of all his procedures, and he realizes that any departure from homeostasis will have a bearing on the cranium.

Detection of the causal factor is usually dependent on the degree and extent of the disturbance. Some cranial lesions are not at all obscure. Many can be discerned even without palpation or sutural tests. When you understand what the norm should be the anomalous will be obvious.

Is there any room then, for wondering why, in our practices so many conditions fail to respond to conventional treatments? The osteopath with the requisite knowledge of his subject is never satisfied merely treating the area where discomfort or pain presents. He checks through the system back to the causal factor which – as we have been discussing – is fluid obstruction.

As touched on before it is well to remember that the body's fluids are contained in specialized vessels according to the particular system or systems for which each type of fluid is designated. If at any time there should be an extraordinary demand for fluid of one kind or another, or for depletion; production may be either sped up or lessened, by virtue of the inherent fluctuant capacity of the hydraulic system as a whole.

An even simpler explanation for this self-adjusting or 'rhythmstat' mechanism becomes clearer when we recall that the body operates as a unit whether in health or disease.

HARRISON H FRYETTE

'Dare to be different! So many would rather be orthodox than right.'

'One's success in Treatment is governed very largely by one's diagnosis.'

'When a doctor says, "Yes, I had a case exactly like that one yesterday," he has made his first mistake.'

'It is the hours of study and the minutes of treatment that get the best results.'

CHAPTER SIX

The Significance of the Sphenoid in the Cranial Concept

The Sphenoid is of primary significance in the rhythmic accommodative motion of the cranium. It is also very important to the mobility of the basilar area; as well as to the vault and facial areas. Any malposition of the Sphenoid will change the shape of the face, and orbital cavities.

If for no other reason than its direct physiological relationship with so many other bones of the cranium, the Sphenoid is unique. Its location, borders, surfaces, margins – in fact, its whole anatomy – and muscular attachments, are responsible for this distinct prominence over the rest of the cranial bones. It is the only bone in the human body that articulates with twelve others. (Frontal (1) – treat as two, Parietals (2), Occiput (1), Temporals (2), Zygoma (2), Ethmoid (1), Palatines (2), Vomer (1); including the spheno-basilar articulation which Sutherland discounted originally as having a disc between. This number can, of course, be considered as 'thirteen' in those people who have a patent metopic suture). Therefore the Sphenoid's significance as a mechanical 'corner-stone' is clear.

The Sphenoid as located at the base of the skull, assists in forming the anterior, middle, and posterior cranial fossae. Its base is formed in cartilage, and the rest in membrane. In shape it is like a bat with outstretched wings comprising a central portion, or body. This is hollow, and therefore compressable, containing the sphenoidal sinuses, olfactory grooves, sella turcica, and dorsum sellae. There are also attachments for the Greater and Lesser Wings.

The Lesser Wings project laterally from the body with the optic foramen between. The great wings project laterally to the Pterion – the junction of the Parietal, Frontal, and Temporal with the Sphenoid.

The pterygoid processes with their medial and lateral plates extend inferiorly from the sphenoidal body and articulate with the palatines; through referral their relationship with the temporomandibular joint is often overlooked in cranial considerations as being 'outside' the main cranial osseous areas; but it is often necessary to deal with a lesion here before reparation may be established at the cranial base.

It is crucial that the muscular attachments of the Sphenoid be given special consideration by any student of the craniao-sacral mechanism. They can, and often do, cause malfunction if abnormal tonus is present. This is usually of great clinical significance mainly because of the number of articulations that are involved.

The relationship of the Sphenoid to the sacrum is also crucial. The sphenoid is to the skull, as the sacrum is to the ilia.

Is it any wonder then that Sutherland chose the Sphenoid for his model of the centre of the cranio-sacral concept? From a mechanical point of view it was quite acceptable – at least one thing was clear. The effects of any motion affecting the sphenoid would automatically be found throughout the cranium.

Furthermore, by dura-osseous connection, and C.N.S. relationship all parts of the body would be influenced by such a motion – under the auspices of the primary respiratory mechanism and fluctuation of the cerebro-spinal fluid.

Subsequently opinions as to the validity of Sutherland's model have varied; especially in relation to the spheno-basilar joint. But when the facts are carefully examined, the pioneer of the cranio-sacral concept is not worthy of even the least castigation. What he has done has paid tremendous dividends, adding nothing but depth, colour, and vigour to the situation.

The accusation that instead on naming the joint a synchondrosis, he chose to classify it a symphysis, does not imply that he did not know what he was doing. If he had categorically named it a synchondrosis he would not have been able to intelligibly illustrate the undoubted pliability in this area. His main concern was with function, not mere anatomy! If ever it can be said that the end justifies the means, it is here; for it is generally agreed that throughout life there is a measure of pliability at the sphenobasilar joint.

Bravo, Sutherland! He used the subtlety of an anatomic incongruity to demonstrate the phenomenon of sphenobasilar motion; side-bending rotation, flexion, or extension.

It is worth noting, that, according to Magoun, 'in the inhalation phase of the primary respiratory mechanism, the mid-line bones of the skull (occiput, sphenoid, ethmoid, and vomer) are moved physiologically into flexion, about a transverse axis of rotation through the body just in front of and on the same plain as the sella turcica.

The frontal (which sits superiorly on the sphenoid) – the zygoma and maxilla – in fact all the facial bones with the exception of the mandible – follow the swinging motion of the sphenoid by rotating externally.

The zygoma's action being at a 45 degree angle, this pulls the inferior border of the orbit posteromedially, therefore increasing the orbital oblique diameter. At the same time the other paired bones of the vault are rotated externally. Extension and internal rotation follow, in the extension phase. This certainly vindicates Sutherland's pioneering work in establishing such an intriguing yet vastly complex concept.

The Sphenoid's Great Wings manifest tremendous influence over the bones

24 SPHENOIDAL MUSCLES

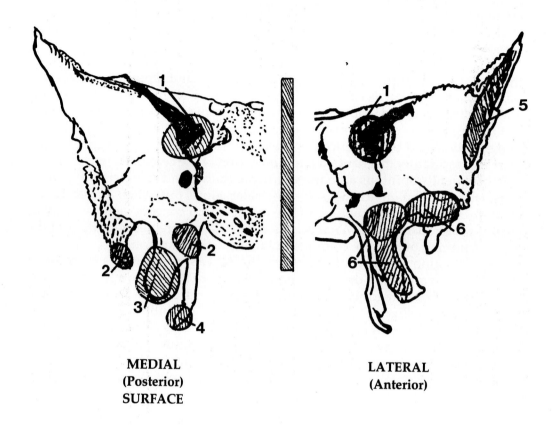

MEDIAL
(Posterior)
SURFACE

LATERAL
(Anterior)

1 Orbital Rectus, Superior Oblique
   Levator Palpebrae Superior
2 Tensor Palatine
3 Medial Pterygoid
4 Superior Constrictor
5 Temporalis
6 Lateral Pterygoid

THE SIGNIFICANCE OF THE SPHENOID IN THE CRANIAL CONCEPT

TABLE D   SPHENOIDAL MUSCLES LIGAMENTS AND FORAMINA

NAME	ORIGIN	INSERTION	INNERVATION	FUNCTION
MEDIAL PTERYGOID (Pterygoideus Internus)	Lateral pterygoid plate - posterior surface & maxillary tuberosity	by tendon into angle of mandible and medial surface of ramus	Branch of 5th Cranial (mandibular)	closes jaw and grates teeth
LATERAL PTERYGOID (Pterygoideus Externus)	by two heads – superior: infratemporal crest & zygomatic fossa of great wing; inferior: lateral pterygoid plate, lateral surface	mandibular condyle T.M.J. capsule	Branch of 5th Cranial (Mandibular)	moves mandible forward, downward & side to side
SUPERIOR CONSTRICTOR (Constrictor Pharyngeus)	Medial pterygoid plate - posterior surface, inferiorly Hamulus, pterygo mandibular raphe	mandible – mylohyoid ridge; muscous membrane of lateral base of tongue	Branch of 10th Cranial Pharnygeal plexus	constricts pharynx – aids swallowing
TENSOR PALATINE (Tensor Veli Palatini)	Medial pterygoid plate scaphoidal fossa Auditory tube – cartilagenous lateral wall Spinous process (with internal lateral ligament)	(passes through – between – medial pterygoid muscle & plate) by tendon via hamulus to palatine – horizontal plate and aponeurosis. occiput – pharyngeal spine via median raphe	Branch of 5th (mandibular)	tightens palate opens auditory tube NB: lesions here can greatly affect hearing & function of ear
TEMPORALIS	Great wing – temporal fossa & fascia	mandible – anterior coronoid process (& to Frontal & Parietal)	Branch of 5th	closes jaw NB: sphenobasilar side-bending affected by lesion to this muscle
ORBITAL RECTUS (Superior, inferior, medial, lateral)	from tubercle of lesser wing at optic foramen	Sclera of eye	3rd Cranial (except for Lateral rectus – 6th Cranial)	eye movements
SUPERIOR OBLIQUE	Lesser wing – superior border of optic foramen	Sclera	4th Cranial	eye movements
LEVATOR PALPEBRAE SUPERIOR	Lesser wing – optic foramen	top eyelid	3rd Cranial	raises eyelid

67

TABLE D (continued)

LIGAMENTS		
SPHENOMANDIBULAR (Internal Lateral)	angle of spinous process of Great Wing	Lingula of mandible medial to T.M.J.	a thin flat band of aponeurosis – covering part of Meckel's cartilage
PTERYGOMAXILLARY	internal pterygoid plate at apex	internal oblique line of mandible – posterior end	separates Buccinator and superior pharyngeal constrictor
PTERYGOSPINAL	lateral pterygoid plate (superior border)	sphenoidal spine	—

FORAMINA	LOCATION		VESSELS CARRIED
OPTIC	between two roots of lesser wing and sphenoidal body		Optic nerve & opthalmic artery
SUPERIOR ORBITAL FISSURE	between greater and lesser wings and sphenoidal body		branches of middle meningeal and lacrimal arteries superior opthalmic vein oculomotor, nasociliary, and trochlea nerves and fibres of internal carotid plexus
ROTUNDUM (Superior maxillary)	Great wing (anteromedial part)		maxillary branch of 5th cranial nerve
VESALII (Sphenoidal emissary)	Great wing (medial to ovale)		present in less than 50% of skulls. Transmits vein from cavernous sinus to pterygoid plexus
OVALE	Great wing (posterolateral to rotundum)		accessory (meningeal) artery emissary veins (from cavernous sinus to pterygoid plexus) mandibular branch of 5th cranial nerve. Occasionally the lesser petrosal nerve
SPINOSUM	Great wing (at posterior angle)		a short canal carrying middle meningeal vessels branch of mandibular nerve
PETROSAL (Innominate)	Great wing (medial to spinosum)		if present carries lesser petrosal nerve – instead of the ovale

There are several small foramina to be found in the sella turcica for passage of nutrients to the inner table. External orbital foramina occur in the great wing for the passage of deep temporal arterial branches.

The list of Sphenoidal foramina can be augmented if the various canals or fissures which occur between the parts of the sphenoid and other bones such as the palatine, vomer, maxilla, temporal and occipital are included. These are the lacerum (sphenoidal fissure), the pterygomaxillary fissure; and the palatovaginal, vomerovaginal and pterygoid canals.

THE SIGNIFICANCE OF THE SPHENOID IN THE CRANIAL CONCEPT

of the Vault; this is to say frontal, temporals, parietals, and occiput. Functionally, the Sphenoid is associated with the basiocciput, ethmoid, vomer and petrous portion of the temporals in the cranial base. These in turn articulating with the other bones of the cranium leave us in no doubt of the sphenoid as the centre of cranio-sacral balance.

Some authorities regard certain bones of the cranium as three modified vertebrae manifesting characteristics resembling those of the spinal column. The first of these three is the dorsum sellae, the second the sphenoid, and the third the occiput. Therefore functionally these can be considered as part of the

25 SPHENOBASILAR TORSION

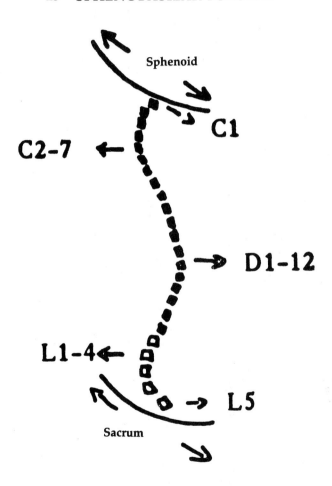

Effect on Spinal Column
With displacements to high and low sides

26 SPHENOBASILAR SYMPHYSIS

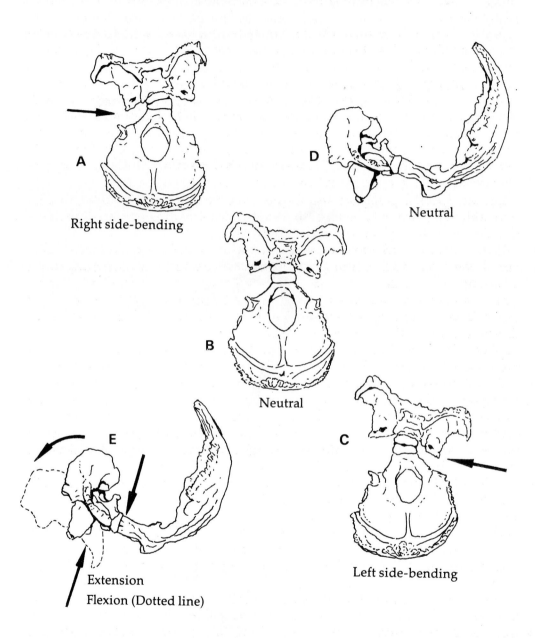

A Right side-bending
B Neutral
C Left side-bending
D Neutral
E Extension
   Flexion (Dotted line)

SUPERIOR (A, B, C) & LATERAL (D, E) ASPECTS

spinal column. These are related to the internal secretions of the hypophysis cerebri. The anterior lobe supplying detoxication, and the posterior lobe pharmacology.

Remembering the pituitary's position in the sphenoid's hypophyseal fossa (sella turcica) it is not difficult to visualize the chaos that is likely to follow should the sphenoid be in malfunction.

Physiologically it is imperative that the sphenoid must be balanced in relation to all the structures with which it is in contact. Normal health demands this. Whenever you contact the sphenoid with your fingers you are in effect touching all parts of the cranium – and influencing the entire human organism.

It must be borne in mind that there is always a natural measure of flexibility permitting the sphenoid, in common with other cranial osseous structures, to change its shape in conformity with its immediate environment.

Certain specific palpatory techniques may be employed to determine its normal range of articular extension, flexion, side-bending and rotation at the junction with the basilar process of the occiput.

With the patient supine we can begin to test for these various movements. For flexion, have one hand cradling the occiput and the palpating hand spanning the frontal – thumb and middle finger on the Great Wings. Inclination towards the patient's feet is achieved by moving your body weight over this hand and forward – rather than by movement of the hand itself. It is a directional inclination – not a forceful one.

What the sphenoid is doing will soon begin to register in your hand as a pumping felt underneath the palm of your hand within the patient's skull.

To test for extension the hold is the same but now the movement is reversed. Ease your body backwards so that the inclination of your hand is directed superiorly. Side-bending movement is tested by a similarly achieved contralateral inclination – from superior external orbital rim to parietal prominence, on both sides. Rotation requires a lateral movement – inclining from one side to the other, as if lifting the lid off a kettle.

In health all movements should be equal and the pumping felt underneath your hand should also be equal – a lack of movement, or a reduced pulsation in any one position indicates a sphenobasilar lesion.

The lesions may be the result of trauma; – birth, accident, referred. The greater or lesser wings may be jammed. One side of one wing may be elevated or depressed, side-bent, or rotated. The other wing may be in the same plane or torsive.

The second cranial nerve is susceptible to malfunction through osseous interference with its normal behaviour. Consider the number of people wearing glasses. Many of these are not the victims of second nerve conditions alone. The sphenoid can sometimes be blamed. The optic nerve in passing through the cranial cavity occupies a groove on the sphenoid. When the bone moves into flexion or extension, the mechanical action on the nerve may well

27 SPHENOBASILAR SYMPHYSIS

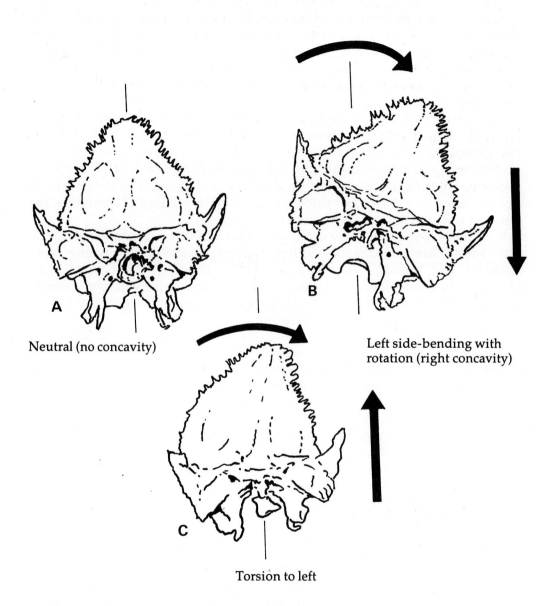

A. Neutral (no concavity)
B. Left side-bending with rotation (right concavity)
C. Torsion to left

ANTERIOR ASPECT

disturb its function. Eye problems such as cataract, myopia, etc. respond well to an oblique widening of the orbit via the sphenoid.

As touched on earlier, as well as its articulation with so many cranial osseous structures the sphenoid also influences the dural meninges by receiving the anterior inferior poles of the falx cerebri at the clinoid process. (The anterior superior poles attach to the crista galli of the ethmoid – which owes much of its own movement to its close proximity to the sphenoid; the posterior poles attach to the occiput and the lateral poles to the petrous portion of the temporal).

The maintenance of correct tension in this 'tent' which covers the brain maintains basal articular movement and acts as a balance-spring to the whole of the body.

But the greatest contribution the sphenoid makes to homeostasis is observed at the spheno-basilar junction.

KENNETH E LITTLE

'I like to compare the cranial articular mechanism to the works of a fine watch each part of which is meshed with one or more other parts. One bearing . . . jarred loose or one wheel out of adjustment affects the functioning of the whole mechanism and impairs its efficiency.'

'We may consider the sphenoid as two wheels joined by an axle, and the occiput similarly as an axle with two wheels.'

'In Cranial diagnosis and therapy, a sense of contacting the bony surfaces through the skin and superficial tissues must be attained.'

CHAPTER SEVEN

The Endocrine Umbrella

Whatever else we may speak of in the body as a whole, whether Cranial, Osseous, Ligamentous, Muscular, Neuromuscular or Circulatory; and whatever importance we may attach to these in our particular sphere of work, we have always to remember the Endocrine Umbrella.

The subject of Endogenous Endocrinology is so vast, however, and has been covered so extensively in books wholly devoted to the subject, that we can only hope to touch on it here. We will merely look at aspects that particularly concern the cranial osteopath, keeping in mind – as Denis Brookes used to say – 'You will never be a successful cranial osteopath without a good knowledge of the Endocrine system.' How true that is! Dr Sutherland, of whom he was an inveterate protege, regarded the functional efficiency of this system as dependant on the physiology of the brain.

Given therefore that a purely mechanistic approach to diagnosis and treatment cannot possibly supply the answers to the questions that cranial evaluation demands, we must also take account of Still's words as quoted by Sutherland. 'The brain of a man is God's drug store, and has in it all liquids, drugs, lubricating oils, opiates, acids, and every quality of drug that the wisdom of God thought necessary for happiness and health . . . The brain is an electric motor'.

Significant to our understanding of the endocrine system as a whole is the Pituitary gland (Hypophysis Cerebri). Best and Taylor record that 100,000 fibres link this gland to the Hypothalamus, which itself is a control centre in the autonomic nervous system for the regulation of metabolic processes.

These communicating fibres are nothing less than a complexity of nerves and blood vessels. These are influential in maintaining a healthful reciprocal balance affecting every cell of the body.

28 THE ENDOCRINE SYSTEM

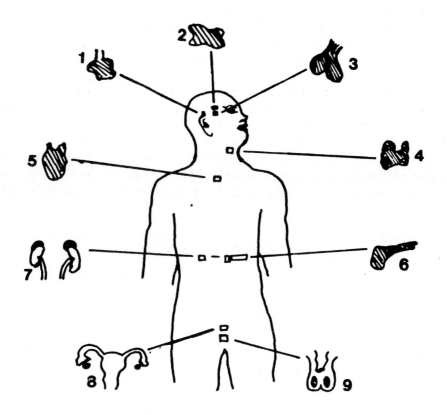

APPROXIMATE LOCATIONS

1 Pineal Body
2 Hypothalamus
3 Pituitary (Hypophysis)
4 Thyroid & Parathyroids
5 Thymus
6 Pancreas
7 Adrenals (Suprarenal)
8 Ovaries (Gonads)
9 Testes

The whole pituitary gland, which some of us, Cushing, for example, used to consider the conductor of the endocrine orchestra, would now appear to be in the position of leader, or first violin, with the Pineal body wielding the baton.

Our concern is with this inter-relationship, the interchange of activity – the distribution and interchange of fluids between the hypothalamus and the

THE ENDOCRINE UMBRELLA

Pituitary, and the Pineal; and the rest of the orchestra – thymus, thyroids, adrenals, gonads, etc, and their ultimate effects upon the rest of the body. We cannot divorce these effects from the cranio-sacral concept. They are the reason for its existence, indeed the divine reason. Any impairment of the endocrine system will automatically result in some chemical or mechanical malfunction – the pineal-pituitary inter-relationship acting as a braking system against purely physical development at the expense of the spiritual.

This book is not, as we have said, devoted to an 'in-depth' discussion of hormone secretion, enzymes, amines, and the like – suffice it to say, homeostatically the body's internal economy cannot function correctly without the efficiency of its fluid systems.

The blood is the main fluid, conveyed as we know by arteries and veins through the pumping of the heart. There is also the lymph system, in glands, channels, and ducts; and the cerebrospinal fluid, probably the most important factor in our cranio-sacral consideration – is conveyed by collagen fibrils.

29 LEMNISCATE ACTION

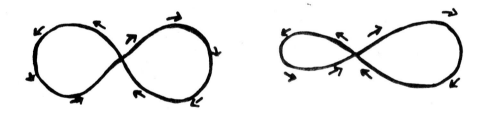

FIGURE OF 8 POLARITY

Note: Either side of the octate is not necessarily equal

We must also think of polarity – the ebb and flow of movement around a central still point – a lemniscate – a fulcrum – that describes a figure of eight. Perhaps we can best illustrate it this way. Imagine two bodies each of which has its own magnetic field of attraction. There is between these an area where the magnetic pull is equal and opposite in both directions . . . herein lies the still point. This phenomenon obtains in the cranium as well as in all other parts of the human organism – a still point amidst the incalculable complexity of motion, not a fixed point, but one that is in a state of constant shifting and adapting in relation to its fluctuating fulcrum. This does not mean that both sides of the octate have to be the same size. The size is dependant on the pharmacological or biochemical insistence.

It is difficult, if not impossible, to speak constructively about these functions without referring again to the hypothalamus, although it is not strictly speaking an endocrine gland. Its activities relative to the different hormones can often provide valuable information regarding appetite, emotions, blood pressure, temperature, and the like. Any undue stress through side-bending, rotation, or torsional patterns at the sphenobasilar symphysis will doubtless mediate undesirable effects as far as hypothalamic/pituitary relationship is concerned.

Cranio-sacrally speaking, this is of particular significance, as we continue to consider the endocrines, the physiology of body fluids, and how they affect the musculo-skeletal system, etc. Under constant threat from cranial lesions, and controlled by hormones from the adrenal cortex are those activities relating to the cardia; rate, output, blood pressure, and the integrity of the myocardia. Also that most potent vasopressor, epinephrine which is secreted by the adrenal medulla and governs carbohydrate metabolism together with A.D.H. (Anti Diuretic Hormone) from the hypophysis cerebri's posterior lobe, influences water metabolism.

For instance, just think of the chaos that ensues once there is a breakdown in pineal function – the results can be hydrocephalus, gait disturbances, diabetes insipidus, hypopituitarism, precocious puberty, impotence, lack of sexual drive, adiposity . . . remember, the pineal gland is at the very hub of cranial activity. It is the starting point for the endocrine structure, and is the still point for the mobility of the cranial mechanism; ligamentous, osseous, membraneous. All these have one central point around which they work, and it is the straight sinus to the fourth ventricle, directly in line with the pineal gland.

Now let us move on to the rest of the endocrine orchestra and remind ourselves of a few facts on each part of the system.

PINEAL BODY

The pineal body (L. Pinealis – small pine cone) or Epiphysis Cerebri, was for a long time shrouded in mystery and is still not clearly understood. It is one of those structures that is constantly included in, or left out, of endocrine lists (as is the hypothalamus and the pancreas). Though obscure it is of tremendous importance in craniosacral considerations. It is the key to many pathological states and can be said not only to coincide with the ageing process but to monitor it.

It is a cone-shaped structure deep within the brain: part of the epithalamus in the diencephalon, in close proximity to the corpora quadrigemina and the acqueduct of Sylvius, beneath the corpus callosum. It arises from the roof of the third ventricle embriologically and attaches to the posterior and habenular commissure.

The pineal is innervated by sympathetic and parasympathetic fibres. It is composed of glial and parenchymal cells, the cells of secretion being called pinealocytes. They have a bulbous finish on the blood vessels from which they appear to empty their contents into the blood stream – though it is postulated that the pineal secretes directly into the C.S.F. (cerebrospinal fluid) through the foramen of Munro via the third ventricle – the concentration in C.S.F. being greater than in blood plasma.

Descartes, the French philospher and mathematician of the 17th century, considered the pineal to be the seat of the soul, the 'third eye,' and tradition teaches that it is not only the centre of wisdom but the connection between our real selves and our physical bodies. Be that as it may, it is known that the pineal is an imperative to human physiology.

The pineal's function is to act as an antagonist to the pituitary gland through lemniscate action. It is highly vascular and has many different functions. It is the only source of melatonin (5-methoxy-N-acetyl tryptamine) as derived from seratonin and H.I.O.M.T. (hydroxyindole-O-methyltransferase) and it also contains histamine which has a marked effect on acid secretion and may be under the control of cyclic A.M.P. It is also believed to contain gonadotropin inhibiting peptides. Pineal secretion also enhances the production of prolactin (milk secreting hormone). The pineal absorbs iodine almost as much as does the thyroid gland.

The fact that H.I.O.M.T. is also found in nerves surely means that hormones or neurohormones operate from the pineal body throughout the entire human organism. H.I.O.M.T. therefore, is imperative to homeostasis, and is the catalyst for the neuro-mechanism. The pineal is outside the 'blood-brain' barrier and is often visible on X-Ray due to the presence of 'pineal sand' (calcium phosphate and carbonate). This gland is generally larger in infants than in adults. Like the thymus it used to be thought to calcify at puberty. The pineal is subject to tumours, and can be displaced by malignancies occurring in other brain tissue.

We have just touched on melatonin. Note that this is found both in C.S.F. and plasma and is metabolized in the liver. Light inhibits melatonin synthesis as soon as the eyes register daylight, allowing seratonin release which converts to melatonin by the action of H.I.O.M.T. but light has an opposite effect on melatonin in plasma.

ESSENTIALS OF CRANIO-SACRAL OSTEOPATHY

30 BI-TEMPORAL ROLLING

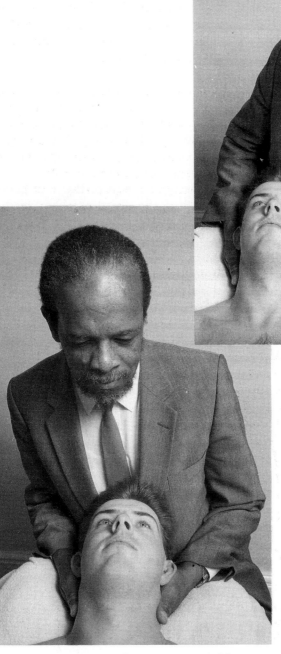

This is to say, melatonin release occurs in the absence of daylight, under the stimulation of noradrenaline. (It is also stimulated by immobilization, stress, and hyperglycaemia). It is a sexual inhibitor/excitor as well.

In the animal kingdom it is noticeable that many do not mate during the autumn and winter as the day (light) time is shortest then. Male animals store testosterone when light is lacking and the female oestrogen. Mating time is usually in the spring. Even though some animals do not possess a pineal body they do have what is called a 'third eye' which stands in place of the pineal in function.

In the human being pineal time, or light, is not all-affecting. There is what is called S.A.D. (seasonal affective disorder). Too much melatonin has a devitalizing effect. It has been found in some psychologically disturbed patients that their 'depression' is very marked, even suicidal, during the autumn and winter and yet almost disappears during spring and summer. This had always been put down to psychological or climatic factors.

When these patients' days were artificially lengthened by their sitting for a few minutes per day in front of very strong light panels – the depression lifted and there was a marked improvement in their mental state. They almost immediately became very optimistic, active, and extremely happy individuals. The 'day-light' had to be of high intensity to achieve this.

Later research showed that body rhythms are often diurnally set at 25 hours – not quite a circadian rhythm. Getting up too early (before the sun catches the eyes) can leave a person 'half-awake.'

Therefore when it is dark noradrenalin is released from the sympathetics, close to the pinealocytes. The retina being aware of the light changes, transmits this to the C.N.S. and onward to the cervical ganglion and adrenal medulla. Pineal activity correlates to that of the adrenals in the promotion of skin pigmentation. The main function of the pineal though, seems to be development of the sex glands and their activity, and body growth. That is to say, the pineal stimulates growth if light is allowed in to act on the P.W.F. (pineal weight factor) – thus inhibiting melatonin.

Incidentally in children the pineal retards sexual activity (along with the influence of the hypothalamus). It defers this function enabling the individual to grow and develop first. When a pinealoma is present, therefore, there can be sexual retardation or precocious puberty. Many everyday complaints with which we, as practitioners, are concerned, stem from pineal dysfunction.

For instance, coronary occlusion: Chapman says 'an innominate lesion produces an endocrine problem.' If you reduce the sacral lesion, (which you will undoubtedly find present in most cardiac conditions) you will inhibit the production of L-dopa under the influence of the pineal. This will allow the level of lipoprotein to be increased, which is necessary for organ cell function. Generally speaking, patients with cardiac problems, new growths, pancreatitis . . . have reduced lipoprotein levels. These lipoproteins control vitamin E in

31 THE ENDOCRINE GLANDS

THE PINEAL
1. Acervuli (Calcific nodules)
2. Pineal Stalk
3. Retinohypothalamic tract (Leading to optic tracts)

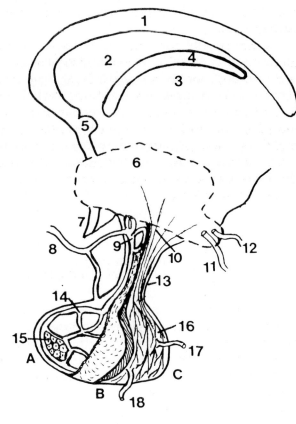

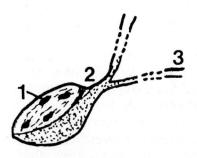

THE PINEAL

THE THALAMUS, HYPOTHALAMUS & PITUITARY

THE PITUITARY
A Anterior Lobe
B Intermediate Lobe
C Posterior Lobe

1. Corpus Callosum
2. Septum Pellucidum
3. Thalamus
4. Fornix
5. Anterior Commissure
6. Hypothalamic Area
7. Lamina terminalis
8. Superior Hypophyseal Artery
9. Portal System
10. Infundibulum
11. Hypothalamic Artery
12. Hypothalamic Vein
13. Pituitary Stalk
14. Sinusoids
15. Cells
16. Nerve Fibres
17. Inferior Hypophyseal Artery
18. Inferior Hypophyseal Vein

the body in the sense that vitamin E cannot function when the lipoprotein level is depressed. Giving vitamin E artificially does not stimulate the body's defence in the same way. All it does is pervade the tissues.

Again, in hypertension (high blood pressure) it is possible to use bi-temporal rolling to affect pineal function. This is accomplished with the patient supine and the practitioner at the head with both hands encompassing the patient's temporal squama at the mastoid process. The thumbs are the only part of the hands that are engaged. Neither the patient's head nor the practitioner's hands should move during this procedure. It is the practitioner's body that moves from side to side. (His chest should just about the top of the patient's head).

Incline laterally and hold to a count of 10, then incline to the other side and hold to a count of nine. Repeat this manoeuvre slightly reducing the angle of inclination on each occasion whilst also reducing the count to 8, 7, 6, 5, 4, 3, 2, 1. Hence, on 1, the practitioner's body should be almost in the mid line. Gently disengage as this procedure is now complete. The blood pressure should be recorded both before and after bi-temporal rolling – it will usually be found that the systolic has reduced by 20mmHg, and the diastolic by 10–20mmHg.

Incidentally, peripheral oedema is often seen to reduce dramatically with these measures, as oedema is, of course, quite frequently a concomitant of cardiac malfunction.

PITUITARY GLAND

The Pituitary gland or Hypophysis Cerebri is situated in the sella turcica (Turk's saddle) of the sphenoid bone. It is shaped somewhat as the head of a golf club, is small – about 1.4cm in diameter at its widest point, and weighs about 1.5 gm. It is attached to the base of the brain by the pituitary stalk, posterior to the optic chiasma. The internal carotid artery supplies the pituitary and it is innervated by the superior cervical ganglion.

The posterior lobe is connected to the tuber cinereum by a small process called the infundibulum. This tuber cinereum consists of gray matter. It lies between the optic tracts and comprises part of the floor of the third ventricle. The main part of it secretes substances which enter the blood vessels of the pituitary to control the anterior lobe's hormones.

This tuber cinereum and the infundibulum form part of the hypothalamus. The hypothalamus comprises the lateral wall and the floor of the third ventricle. Although it is described as a particular structure it is, in fact, part of the brain, and includes the optic chiasma and the hypophysis. The main function of the hypothalamus is seen to be the control of homeostasis by governing temperature, appetite, sexual behaviour, water balance, sleep, and hormonal function.

The hypothalamus controls the pituitary in as much as it sends regulatory impulses to that gland, both for the production and release of hypophysiotropic hormones. These are such as originate in the anterior lobe and have their effect on the thyroid, adrenals, sex glands, etc.

To the unsuspecting the pituitary gland might appear to be a single unit, but it is, in fact, in three parts, two of which are the main lobes having special and distinctive characteristics. One of these lobes is the adenohypophysis or anterior pituitary gland, which embryologically derives from the Buccal epithelium (Rathke's pouch – from the name of the man who in the 1830's published such a clear account of the development of the pituitary).

This lobe consists principally of the pars distalis (the rest is the pars tuberalis). Hormones secreted by the two main types of cells (acidophils and basophils) of the anterior lobe are:-

1) Growth hormone (G.H.) – Somatotrophin (S.T.H.) – aids fat breakdown in tissue (adipose) and acts on muscle and bone to promote growth. G.H. is inhibited by somatomedins from the liver and other tissues which in turn are activated by G.H.
2) Prolactin (Lactogen) is secreted by acidophils. Acts on mammary gland which is exocrine.

The remainder of the secretion from this lobe is from basophils. There are five of these:-

1) Thyrotropin (T.S.H.) regulates thyroid activity
2) Adrenocorticotropin (A.C.T.H.) regulates adrenal cortex
3) Follicle stimulating hormone (F.S.H.) regulates gonads
4) Luteinizing hormone (L.H.) regulates gonads
5) Melanocyte stimulating hormone (M.S.H.)

All these hormones are transmitted to target organs and stimulate these to release other similar hormones.

Before leaving the subject of the type of cells found in the anterior pituitary, there is a third type present – chromophobes – which comprise approximately half the glandular tissue. the activity of these non-staining cells does not appear to be fully understood, but they are said to produce A.C.T.H. and that hypersecretion of hormones from the pituitary gland may be related to chromophobic tumours.

The other main lobe is the neurohypophysis or posterior pituitary, an outpouching which arises embryologically from the diencephalon. It is not really a gland and has no nerve cells but receives nerve fibres from the hypothalamus, and is joined to the hypothalamus (in the third ventricle) by the infundibular portion of the pituitary stalk. The neurohypophysis used to be thought of as the origin of hormones containing anti-diuretic action, but it is now realized that it is only their store, as they have no secretary organs of their own. It is the neuron secretion from the paraventicular and supraoptic nuclei branches of which pass from the hypothalamus down through the neurohypophysis from which they are released as and when necessary into the blood stream and E.C.F. (extracellular fluid).

A.D.H. (vasopressin) monitors the water content of the body and the blood particularly. In dehydration, hyperglycaemia, haemorrhage, etc. A.D.H. is made available by osmosis immediately the water balance is depleted to an unacceptable level. It also has a vaso-constrictive action by contracting the lumen of vessels to increase blood pressure during blood loss, and facilitates increased peristalsis.

Like A.D.H. oxytoxin is a polypeptide of nine amino acids. It is not present in the male, but in the female it acts on the uterus to promote contractions of the gravid uterus to expel the foetus. It also stimulates lactation.

The third part of the pituitary is the pars intermedia, an intermediate, or not clearly defined region that lies between the two lobes, and is often classified with one of them.

However, the fact that all three parts of the pituitary gland derive from different organs is significant. They are diverse in their morphology and hormonal secretion. And it is not without meaning that the names of the two main lobes are 'adeno' and 'neuro' hypophysis. The former signifies glandular tissue and the latter nervous. The anterior lobe's sinusoids taking up hormones via the portal veins from the hypothalamus and the posterior lobe via secretory neurons.

The importance of the entire pituitary gland in human physiology is concerned with hormone secretion. In our patients, emotional stress will manifest itself in different forms, not least of which might be worry, fear, anxiety, anger; and in this regard something more must be said about hypothalamic-pituitary function. It is largely a negative feed-back system producing or synthesizing chemicals from the glands it has supplied from the blood.

Each chemical so synthesized is peculiar to one particular gland or pituitary hormone. These chemicals are passed into a portal system from the axions of the nerves in the hypothalamus. This is known as the pituitary portal system which takes them down into the pituitary gland from whence they are secreted. Hence another name for the anterior lobe of the gland is the neuro-endocrine transducer.

Or put another way, it converts neurological impulses into chemical secretions. These are such as arise from the cerebral cortex, emotion, fright, . . . the hypothalamus being activated by these, build up proteins from the available chemicals.

Through this portal system these neurosecretions have the effect of speeding up the production of releasing factors. These are important to defence – latent forces and mechanisms; antibodies, agglutinins. . . They are soon brought into action, as and when required. Nevertheless, their presence and efficiency are all dependent on the cranio-sacral system being in balance and functioning well.

We have already briefly outlined some of the functional disorders that result from pineal-pituitary or hypothalamic insufficiency, but they are only part of a long chain.

THYROID GLAND

The Thyroid gland comprises two lobes held together in a fibrous capsule whose posterior region envelops the four parathyroids. Its scitiform tissue is basically a mass of alveoli called acini or follicles, and is located in the neck embracing the 2–4th cricoid rings in front and the region of C6 behind.

The cavities of the acini are laden with a sticky substance, colloid, which is basically of the same composition as the acini (homologous). This colloid originating from the lining cells is the purveyor of the thyroid hormone. This hormone may be considered as two active principles, thyroxine, which increases the rate of cell metabolism and contains 4 iodine atoms; and tri-iodothyronine which has 3 atoms and is much more active than the former. It is in the colloid that both tri-iodothyronine and thyroxine (thyroxinum) are synthesized and held in thyroglobulin suspension until secretion. This gland also secretes thyrocalcetonin in small amounts in adults. This polypeptide hormone is in larger amounts in children where it aids bony growth; and in pregnancy and lactating mothers where it maintains bony integrity. It is the antagonist of parathormone – inhibiting bone re-absorption, lowering the level of calcium and phosphates in plasma (in hypercalcemia) and is probably controlled by cyclic A.M.P.

It is through the function of this thyroid secretion (along with other factors already discussed in the pituitary/hypothalamic complex) that most of the very important systems and developments such as metabolic rate, growth, maturation, oxydation in the cells and tissues, are regulated and controlled. The thyroid is highly vascular because its supply comes directly from the external carotid artery, and it is richly supplied with four vessels (two superior and two inferior). This gland is concerned at many levels with nervous activity, and its overall regulatory function is imperative to homeostasis. It also aids carbohydrate metabolism.

In children thyroid insufficiency – hypothyroidism (infantile or congenital myxoedema is of real clinical significance. Their mental and sexual development is characteristically retarded, being often deaf, misshapen, limp and fat, having diminished intelligence, and sometimes a freakish expression. Unless correct therapeutic replacement measures are applied as soon as the condition is detected these children do not attain normal height and are termed 'dwarfs' or 'cretins'. These unfortunate people are the consequence of insufficient thyroid secretion in infancy.

Myxoedema is another condition which is peculiar to hypothyroidism, this time in adults. Cosmetically this can be very menacing as its characteristic features are so undesirable; thickness, dryness and puffiness of the skin, pale conjunctiva, accompanied by sparseness and brittleness of the hair, and mental dullness. There is also a tendency to a hoarse deep voice. These patients move slowly, as their pulse and temperature are sub-normal and they are always cold. They are usually of full stature, in that the disease does not strike until after normal growth and development have taken place.

Mostly occurring in women hyperthyroidism in adults is a well-known pathological state of two kinds basically, toxic adenoma and exopthalmic goitre (thyromegaly) caused by the pituitary secreting too much thyrotrophic hormone (T.S.H.). This puts the thyroid gland into 'over-drive'. It is possible that the reason the pituitary oversecretes is stress – emotional and mental stress, hence it is often seen following bereavement, divorce, menopause, etc. Hyperthyrotoxic people are marked by one or all of the following symptoms: tachycardia, fine tremors, loss of weight, irritability, nervousness, hyperthermia, exopthalmosis (wide-open eyes), proptosis (protruding eyes), increased metabolic rate, extreme sweating (hyperhidrosis) enlarged pulsating thyroid gland, goitre. The opthalmic complications are caused by the pituitary oversecreting a hormone which governs orbital fat. In thyrotoxicosis (which is also known as Graves or Stokes Disease) the systems of the body appear to have 'gone wild' – working at an excess rate.

As has been indicated thyroid function is under the control of the Thyroid Stimulating Hormone (T.S.H. – thyrotrophin) of the anterior pituitary. This trophic hormone is also regulated partially from a sophisticated feedback system of thyroid hormone, and partly through the hypothalamus by way of nerves.

The thyroid gland needs iodine as much as a fire needs fuel to adequately perform its functions. When iodine is ingested it is taken to the thyroid where it is soon changed into iodide, which, after a complex series of change and suspense, is eventually released as thyroxine, triiodothyronine, diiodotyrosine, and monoidotyrosine into the cytoplasm.

When iodine is in short supply this gland increases in size and loses its characteristic buoyancy. Its tissue becomes retrograde and the quality of the secretion contained in the acini impoverished.

ESSENTIALS OF CRANIO-SACRAL OSTEOPATHY

32   CRANIAL PROCEDURES

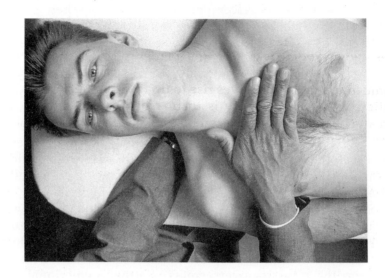

Treating the Thyroid

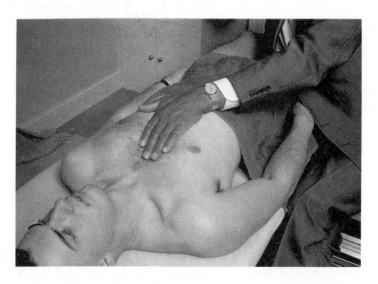

Sacral flexion with Ziphoid process accompaniment

Parenchymatous goitre in itself might not be critical, but cosmetically it can be very disturbing. There are two main types of goitre, the one already described and simple goitre; which is not identifiable with general thyroid dysfunction. In any event both types may appear in either malfunction state of the thyroid – hyper or hypo thyroidism.

Best and Taylor record that goitre is usually the result of lack of iodine in food and drinking water. Hence in different parts of the world – or parts of some countries – where iodine is lacking, the incidence of goitre is not rare and often has a local name such as 'Derbyshire neck.'

It is time to consider what gives rise to thyroid malfunction and how it may be rectified. In a word toxicity is to blame, incurred through the gland's function as a detoxifier. It is affected by the residue from metabolic and other processes – noxious efferents that must be cleared.

How may we achieve this? We must mobilize the relevant articular structures – sternoclavicular junction, including the sternum and first and second ribs; and restore fluid flow balance by certain cranial measures.

Of course, if the thyroid has not received T.S.H. from the anterior pituitary that is again a cause of malfunction and is often termed 'pituitary hypothyroidism.' Malfunctions may also present as Thyroiditis – as inflammation of the gland is termed – and this can be of several kinds. Probably the one with which we as practitioners are most familiar is de Quervain's Thyroiditis; a granulomatous (large single nucleur cells in an enlarged mass of colloid and fibrous tissue) which is accompanied by sore throat, hyperpyrexia and lassitude.

Another form sometimes seen is known as Hashimoto's thyroiditis and is actually a struma lymphomatosa – a progressive goitrogenic degeneration of the epithelial tissue which becomes replaced by fibrous and lymphoid tissue.

The thyroid gland is said by some authorities (probably on the principal that replacement therapy is available) not to be an imperative to life; but its absence would certainly make life very inconvenient.

The practitioner should note that both thyroid and parathyroid tissue can be found in varying amounts in other places than described in this text. Such tissue has been found in the floor of the mouth, the tongue, the tissues of the throat, around the mediastinum and upper ribs, and at the ovaries. Its functional capacity is questionable but should be taken into consideration when assessing a patient's toxic state.

One way of treating the thyroid locally is to be seated at the patient's head as he is supine on the couch. Place the palmar surface of your left hand underneath his upper dorsum – in contact with the spines of the thoracic vertebrae. At the same time your right hand should be resting on the manubrium. You are now in a position to evaluate, then wait and procure the requisite point of balance.

This treatment concerns the sternocleidomastoid muscle at its origin at the

33 THE ENDOCRINE GLANDS

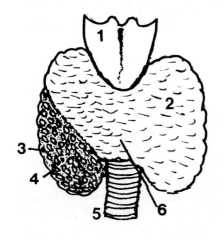

THYROID GLAND

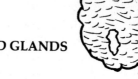

PARATHYROID GLANDS

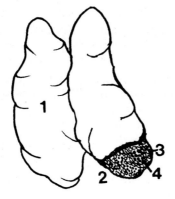

THYMUS GLAND

THYROID GLAND

1 Cartilage
2 Lobes
3 C. Cells
4 Colloid follicles
5 Trachea
6 Isthmus

PARATHYROID GLANDS

1 Cartilage
2 Trachea
3 Oesophagus
4 Parathyroids
5 Thyroid

THYMUS GLAND

1 Cortex
2 Medulla
3 Hassel's corpuscles
4 Granular cells

manubrium, the sternum, first and second ribs, and the rest of the musculature involved with the thyroid – sterno/thyro/hyoidal; stylo/palato/pharyngeus, etc.

PARATHYROID GLANDS

There are usually four parathyroid glands (epithelial bodies) held by connective tissue in close proximity to the posterior surface of the thyroid gland. However, both their number and their actual location are extremely variable. Despite the similarity in name, they are vastly different both in structure and function from the thyroid itself, but are essential to life.

Oval or rounded in shape, they usually present as flattened discs weighing about 50mg each and red/brown in colour. They develop from pharyngeal entoderm as part of the foetal branchial (gill-like) complex. These parathyroids are composed of columnar cells with extensive capillary vascularity. Both their blood and nerve supply are also variable, usually from the inferior thyroid arteries and cervical plexus respectively.

They possess two types of epithelial cells. The 'active' or chief cells have a clear cytoplasm and are numerous. These are the main source for the secretion of parathyroid hormone (parathormone, P.T.H.). The larger 'inactive' cells are less numerous and have oxyphil in their cytoplasm and possess an abundance of mitochondria.

Parathormone exerts a vital influence on the regulation of ionized calcium and phosphorus metabolism. Phosphorus (phosphate) is absorbed from the intestinal tract and is most active in an antacid environment.

The importance of this secretion cannot be overstressed, especially when it is recalled that both calcium and phosphorus are integral parts of all tissues and fluids. This hormone also stimulates the use of Vitamin D in the intestine and aids its conversion to 25–hydroxycholecalciferol the liver, and 1,25–dihydroxycholecalciferol the kidney.

Calcium is not only crucial to the formation of bone and teeth and their maintenance (in fact 99% of calcium is found there) but also plays an major role in neuromuscular behaviour. It acts as a stabilizing factor in membranes, enzymes, and blood.

Phosphorus (phosphate) also is crucial to bone and teeth formation and, again like calcium, the normal human body requires 800–1200mgs per day. The amount of phosphate absorbed from the intestine is dependent on vitamin D and calcium being present. Carbohyrates, fats, and proteins all rely on phosphorus to produce cell growth, repair and division, and for neural activity. It is found in all protein foods (meat, fish, eggs, seeds, nuts, etc.).

Calcium and phosphates together are excreted in urine, but phosphate monitors renal reabsorption of calcium for it is taken back to the parathyroids to stimulate the secretion of parathormone all over again. If this lemniscate balance is not maintained certain pathological conditions will ensue. For instance, if too much calcium is allowed to pass the renal threshold – without the requisite phosphate catalyst action being present, it may calcify, forming renal stones (usually of calcium phosphate, oxylate, or urate formation), and the parathyroids will draw calcium from the bony deposits causing demineralization (resulting in 'softening' and deformation).

Another possible condition of imbalance is osteitis fibrosa cystica caused by over-activity of parathyroid glands, the symptoms of which are excessive levels of parathormone in blood, multiple bone cysts and sometimes a tumour or tumours of the glands themselves. A general hyperparathyroidism may also be blamed for calcium kidney stones, loss of muscle integrity, demineralization of bone and hypocalcemia. Heart muscle activity and coagulability are subject to the level of parathormone in normal plasma as well. When there is a lack, there can be hypercalcemic tetany occasioning cramps, spasms – and convulsions in severe cases – as the lack of calcium causes irritability in the muscles. This condition has been known to occur following thyroid surgery, due to accidental removal of the parathyroid glands. How crucial then is parathyroid hormone influence on homeostasis, and even to life itself.

THYMUS GLAND

Located in the anterior superior mediastinum, a little above and in front of the heart, and behind the sternohyoid and sternothyroid muscles the thymus is closely associated with the pericardium, venae cavae, and pulmonary veins, though separated from them by a layer of fascia.

It is grey/pink in colour and has two unequal longtitudinal lobes joined across a median – not unlike the thyroid. It is considered by some to be lymphoid rather than endocrine, and is indeed part of the lymphatic system. These two lobes have a cortex and medulla. The cortex is of lymphoid tissue, while the medulla is of lymphocyte cells called Hassel's (or Leber's) corpuscles. These are the residue of earlier times, being tiny circular bodies which were epithelial tissue during development.

In the child the thymus is larger than in the adult and in a baby can extend from the lower border of the Thyroid to the level of the fourth rib. It may weigh around half an ounce.

It was long thought that the thymus had no further function after adolescence, but many physiologists now agree that this is not so. There is evidence that thymic activity – though grossly depleted – continues throughout life, and eventually the form of the gland changes to being more or less fibrous tissue.

It appears that this gland has the power to act as a braking system to life itself. As we have already seen, during the early years it flourishes. Then suddenly the brake is applied, in the sense that the gland's deterioration commences. Is it not significant that this coincides conveniently with the ageing process of the entire human organism? I believe it monitors that ageing.

To what could we best liken this phenomenon than to an electric battery in a motor car? Its life span is finite, and so is the usefulness of the car. The moment that battery fails the vehicle is useless; likewise the body, the moment the thymus fails, the host dies. To coin a phrase 'the thymus gland is the harbinger of death.'

Through the medulla the thymus produces lymphocytes known as 'T' (cellular) lymphocytes (as distinct from 'B' (humoral) lymphocytes produced by the liver and spleen which do not enter the thymic tissue at all).

For general purposes T & B lymphocytes are indistinguishable. Both are concerned with the immunological system and tend eventually to gather in bone marrow and lymph nodes – the thymus distributing immature (potential) T types to lymph organs, nodes, tissue, etc. where they secrete a substance that attacks certain foreign cells, tumors and microbes. T lymphocytes appear to develop through the action of thymosin, which along with other peptides is also produced by the thymus. Cellular haemoglobin is also found there. It would appear that T cells are the more powerful, as they can inhibit the action of the B cells, but they have an affinity to each other in the blood stream.

Prior to puberty thymic secretion is crucial to the immunological response but scientific teaching has been that when this hormone is not present, or if the supply is manifestly depressed there will be susceptibility to infection or even death. In fact, chronic illness denotes weak thymic activity, for the thymus dominates the lymphatic system, and is itself sensitive to physical and emotional stress factors which may hasten atrophy of the gland. The greatest functional capacity of the thymus (and therefore its greatest propensity to malfunction) is its role in immunological response. Under-secretion impairs immunity to infection, toxicity, etc. We see this particularly in diseases such as A.I.D.S. (Acquired immunity deficiency syndrome). If the body has no method of fighting the disease – death quickly ensues.

And what causes Aids? Many theories have been advanced, but the most probable cause is a virus labelled HTLV 111(LAV). This damages the special T lymphocytes which normally 'fight off' intruders. It is particularly interesting to note that not all infected persons succumb to the virility of the infection; or the disease can be present in the body for a long time before the destructive effects are manifested. The symptoms can range from lymphopoiesis, tiredness, and fever; to skin tumours, pneumonia, and death.

Other pathological conditions occurring in thymic dysfunction can be Myasthenia Gravis (pseudoparalytica) which presents as a lack of control of muscular activity, muscle fatigue accompanied by a paralysis that does not incur atrophy nor does it usually produce pain. It can affect anywhere in the body, but is usually confined to the facial muscles (lips, tongue, throat, etc) and more particularly the eyelids, causing a characteristic 'droop' – an inability to keep the eye open. This condition is often associated with over-growth of thymic tissue (hyperplasia). 'Sudden death syndrome' mostly seen in infants, is also associated with an enlarged thymus (and other lymphatic tissue) and because enlargement constricts surrounding structures it can often produce respiratory distress.

A word about immunity in general. This can be natural or acquired. Natural immunity is built up in utero, by being breast fed, or by genetic mutative constitutional factors. Acquired immunity can be from exposure to certain diseases/conditions, prophylatic immunization, etc.

Artificial suppressants to immunity include irradiation, anti-lymphocytic agents, and specific antibodies – chemotherapy – often designed to stop the body rejecting artificial implants, transplants, etc. Hence patients treated this way will be immediately susceptible to gross infection.

THE PANCREAS

Although the Pancreas is now counted with the Endocrine (ductless) glands it is also an Exocrine gland.

Located transversely behind the stomach, between spleen and duodenum the lower medial portion (or head) of the pancreas is very large compared with its upward projection (the tail or uncinate process) that ends in close proximity to the left kidney.

The exocrine (acinar) aspect of the pancreas is for the secretion of several enzymes in the hormone Secretin (pancreatic juice) said to be the first hormone ever found, over a litre of which reaches the duodenum daily via the pancreatic duct. The enzymes include Trypsin, Elastase, P. Lipase, and P. a-amylase, and are concerned with cholesterol, amino acids, fatty acids, etc.

It is argued that Secretin itself aids in the production of insulin and helps reduce duodenal acidity. Two other hormones are secreted in the mucosa having influence over Insulin release, one is labelled C.C.K.-P.Z. (cholecystokinin-pancreozymin) also found in the cerebrum; and the other is Gastrin. It appears to be linked to seratonin and norepinephrine and apparently only plays a part in insulin secretion if the stomach is ingesting a large amount of protein material (not starch or sugar). It is also dependent on vagal activity.

More importantly, from our point of view in this chapter, is the Pancreatic endocrine activity.

THE ENDOCRINE UMBRELLA

34 THE ENDOCRINE GLANDS

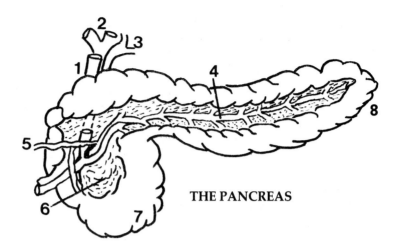

THE PANCREAS

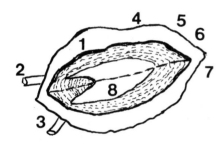

THE ADRENALS

THE PANCREAS

1 Common Bile Duct
2 Portal Vein
3 Hepatic Artery
4 Pancreatic Duct
5 Accessory Duct
6 Head
7 Uncinate Process
8 Tail

THE ADRENALS

1 Capsule
2 Adrenal Vein
3 Adrenal Artery
4 Cortex
5 Glomerular zone
6 Fascicular zone
7 Reticular zone

Glucagon is made in the Alpha cells and Insulin in the Beta cells. These come together in groups and are then known as Islets (or corpuscles) of Langerhans – named after their discoverer a German pathologist of the nineteenth century. Although found in the pancreas in large numbers these islets only make up a fraction of the weight of the organ.

Other cells present in these groups are Delta cells producing a hormonal peptide Somatostatin (or G.I.H.) which is also secreted in the medial portion of the pituitary and in duodenal mucosa. This controls secretion of gastrin, secretin, glucose assimilation, etc. Two un-named groups of cells are also involved, one of which produces P.Polypeptide.

Glucagon is associated with fat and protein breakdown, and is dependent on several inhibitory and stimulatory factors to function effectively. Inhibitors include insulin, glucose, somatostatin, and ketone bodies. Stimulatory influences range from C.C.K., cortisol and certain amino acids to factors such as stress, infection, and possibly a variety of drugs. It also has an affinity with cyclic A.M.P. on heart muscle. Its relationship to ingestion of food should be studied further to understand the gastric function as a whole. For instance, fasting (or starvation) causes a great increase in output of glucagon.

The two-chain polypeptide insulin is perhaps best known since the work of Banting and Best in the 1920's, to isolate the substance from dogs to use as replacement therapy in cases of Diabetes Mellitus (Willis disease) where a deficiency in carbohydrate oxidation renders the islets of Langerhan inefficient in regulating glucose metabolism.

Most practitioners will be familiar with the symptoms – thirst, polyuria, fatigue, glycosuria, ketonia – hypo or hyper reactions. If untreated, extremes can result in coma and/or death. (Medical treatment usually consists of daily/weekly injections of one kind or another or/and strict dietary regime). The smell of acetone in urine or on the breath of a suspected diabetic patient is often the first clue to ketosis being present.

Insulin secretion is in response not only to the rise in the levels of blood (and stomach and duodenum) mucosal glucose, but also to vagal excitability – both parasympathetic and sympathetic nervous activity are involved. Tissues need insulin in order to make use of glucose – adipose, cardiac and skeletal muscle particularly – also the pituitary and aorta, etc. The liver depends on it for efficient storage of glycogen; too small an amount and glucose is disgorged into the circulation creating hyperglycemia. The only tissues, perhaps, that are not glucose dependent are erythrocytes, cerebral, and the tubercles of the kidney.

Other pathological states are found in the pancreas which we will not discuss here, only to say that it seems to be a major site for malignancy.

THE ENDOCRINE UMBRELLA
ADRENAL GLANDS

The adrenals are well known as the fight, fright, or flight mechanism. There is one of these glands on top of each kidney consisting of two parts, one enclosing the other, and each part appears to be functionally different. Pyramidal, each gland is from one to two inches long, and very rich in blood supply. The adrenals are regulated, not only by trophic hormones from the pituitary, but by the sympathetic branch of the autonomic nervous system.

Within the endocrine system, apart from the pituitary gland, the adrenals secrete the largest number of hormones. Unlike the pituitary, which is under the direct control of the nervous system, the adrenal is controlled by the autonomics. Nevertheless, both these glands coincide in their reaction to every type of stress, glucocorticoid secretions being influenced by the pituitary function. The inter-relationship of these two glands illustrates the interdependance of the entire endocrine system.

The inner part of the adrenals is called the medulla, and around this is tissue called the cortex. The cells of the adrenals are chromaffin and are closely related to the sympathetic ganglia. The medulla comprises nerve cells and cells which secrete adrenaline (epinephrine). They also produce nor-adrenaline (nor-epinephrine).

This secretion is the direct result of stimulation of the splanchnic nerve, and should there be over-stimulation, depletion of stored adrenaline results. This can be crucial, especially when it is recalled that coagulation of blood, acceleration or deceleration of the heart activity, and adjustment of blood pressure are all parts of the general physiological defence mechanism/reaction, under adrenal administration.

Adrenal secretion is also subject to the behaviour of the medulla oblongata, and it is undeniable that adrenalin function engenders states of excitement. It is an imperative to the performance of function that demands special effort whether defensive or offensive.

The cortex secretes cortisones – corticosteroids (aldeosterone, glucocorticoids, cortisol, etc. and sex hormones, mostly androgens) which assist in controlling renal function and influence the metabolism of water and salts. They also facilitate the metabolism of carbohydrates, assist in sexual development, store vitamin C, oppose thyroxine, and promote lactation. Hypofunction of the cortex – often associated with atrophy of this gland, or T.B. (tubercular) lesions elsewhere in the body, may result in Addison's Disease (hypocorticalism). This disease is characterized by one or all of the following symptoms:- pigmentation, muscular weakness, loss of weight, tiredness, abdominal pain, diarrhoea, digestive disturbance, low blood sugar and blood pressure. Also, because of the relationship between the adrenals and the gonads (re. secondary sexual characteristics) men may suffer impotency and women amenorrhoea. Both may loose body hair and become dehydrated due to salt imbalance.

Secretion of the hormones of the cortex are under the control of A.C.T.H. (Adrenocortico-trophic-hormone) of the pituitary gland. Hyperfunction of the cortex is neither uncommon or difficult to recognise, as evidenced in Cushing's Syndrome. Although this is usually due to over-action of the supranenal cortex it can also arise from a tumour of the adenohypophysis (anterior pituitary).

Occurring mostly in females it is characterized by re-distribution of body fat (to the face and torso), muscle wastage, inability for wounds to heal, and disturbances to metabolism which produce bruising and purplish skin (striae), tiredness, insomnia, hypertension, hyperglycaemia, osteoporosis, increased hairiness in the female, and decreased masculinity in the male. We must also not forget the classic 'moon' face. In fact, it is the opposite to Addison's disease. (See also notes on Pineal – P.79).

Phaeochromocytoma (Pheochromocytoma) is a benign tumour of the adrenal medulla (chromaffin tissue) distinguished by an extreme rise in the blood pressure from increased secretion of epinephrine and nor-epinephrine. It is also marked by gastro-intestinal disturbance, retinal haemorrhage, headaches, anxiety, fear, vomiting, nausea, florid or wan complexion, abdominal or thoracic pain, and tingling of the extremities. Treatment of such diseases can be via the pituitary, creating a 'knock-on' effect to the adrenals.

THE GONADS

The gonads are common to both sexes. They are the collective name for the organs of reproduction. In the male there are two of these called testes; and in the female there are also two called ovaries.

In early foetal life these are found on the posterior abdominal wall next to the kidneys (and are indistinguishable from each other).

From this embryological siting they must later 'descend' to their respective anchorings for the remainder of life; the testes to the scrotum, and the ovaries into the pelvic bowl at the fimbria of the fallopian tubes.

The gonads are (relatively) inactive until adolescence when, under the influence of gonadatrophins from the anterior pituitary they begin to function. In the female adult the ovaries are two almond shaped glands lying on either side of the uterus in the ovarian fossa on the lateral wall of the pelvis. Each is about 3cm long, 1.5cm broad, 10cm thick and is attached to the posterior surface of the broad ligament.

The surface of the ovary is made up of a single layer of germinal epithelial cells, but its inside is made up of a multitude of tiny structures and graffian follicles. These are the maturing follicles which contain the ovum set in two main layers of cells, the inner granulose and the outer theca interna. These are present in the sexually mature female and are under the influence of F.S.H. from the hypophysis.

There are various stages of development in ovarian activity but for our purposes in this book we shall concern ourselves mainly with its hormone secretion and the menstrual cycle.

At puberty the internal secretions of the ovary promote certain definite changes called the secondary sexual characteristics, menstruation, broadening of the pelvis, development of the breasts, and changes in the emotions. These are peculiar to adolescence, and are, of course, in preparation for the role of motherhood.

Two ovarian functions begin to take place, ovulation and hormone secretion. The ova develops in the ovaries and is discharged into the pelvic cavity between the folds of the broad ligament.

At menstruation, on the first day, numerous graffian follicles commence growing and developing. As this increase persists the secretion of oestrogens and progesterone also commences and usually only one follicle reaches maturity and makes its way to the surface of the ovary. The follicle surface soon loses its integrity conveniently for the mature ovum to be released into the pelvic cavity. This is called ovulation. It normally takes place prior to the beginning of the next menstruation.

The menstrual cycle lasts about five days, but there are exceptions, some of which are due to maldevelopment. This ovarian activity continues unabated until the menopause at about age forty-five years. Something more should be said about F.S.H. This hormone works in conjunction with L.H. which is also a secretion of the pituitary gland. Commencing at puberty these two secretions (known as gonadotrophic hormone) affect the testes in the male and the ovaries in the female, equally.

F.H. is produced locally in the graffian follicle, and lutein hormone in the corpus luteum. In the male testosterone is produced in the testes (under the influence of L.H.). It is also found in small amounts in the female.

The testes hang from the pubis and perineum and corresponds to the ovaries of the female. They are small ovoid glands that lie in the scrotum (a skin covered pouch). They are held outside the body in order to keep them at a lower temperature (95°F) for the development of sperm is best at this temperature.

Incidentally, this throws an interesting light on some male 'infertility.' Since the advent of artificial fibres and skin-tight clothes it has often been found that the scrotum is too hot for sperm to mature properly.

One should question the suspected infertile patient regarding this, and advise loose fitting cotton underwear. This has been found to be a desirable solution on many an occasion, and has obviated the use of extensive tests. A similar state pertains (and there is degeneration of tissue) if the testes remain 'undescended,' or in tight restraint anatomically.

Internally, the testes comprise a multitude of irregularly placed tubules (the convoluted seminiferous tubules). Interstitial cells (Leydig's cells) secrete into the testes. There are a complexity of lobules, tubes, lobes, ducts; and a plexus – the rete cords – and on the posterior side of the testis is the epididymis. The upper part of this is much larger than the lower part or tail, from which arises the vas deferens, occupying the posterior aspect of the testes entering the abdomen and linking with the ducts of the seminiferous tubules – those on the outside being of two types, cuboidal and columnar, the latter are the cells of Sertoli. These cells are in cytoplasmic folds. They hold glycogen which feeds the spermatids and allows them to mature, whence they are released into the tubular lumen. The cells themselves owe their maturity to F.S.H. stimulation, which in turn is activated by a negative feed-back principle, by Inhibin, a hormone produced by the Sertoli cells. These cells are also said to secrete oestrogen.

Two specific functions are performed by the testes, spermatogenesis and the secretion of hormones. Fructoze – produced by the seminal vesicles also helps with the production of sperm. Testosterone is the most significant as it is responsible for the sex attributes, secondary organs and characteristics. Small amounts of the female influence – oestrogen is also secreted.

Testosterone is not only related to maleness or sexual behaviour. It is partially responsible for the regulation of metabolism and is crucial to protein anabolism and musculoskeletal growth, development, and strength. It also aids in the closing of the epiphyses, and these have a bearing on height. When there is an abnormal increase in the height of a young person this is partially attributable to late epiphyseal closure, and the reverse is true for the short person.

Another function of testosterone is concerned with fluid and electrolyte metabolism. It has an effect on the kidneys' ability to cope with the reabsorption of sodium and water, and elimination of potassium. Testosterone is also inhibitory to the secretion of gonadotrophic F.S.H. & I.C.S.H. (interstitial cell stimulating hormone) in the female L.H. (Luteinizing hormone).

As we have already seen 4VC is an hormonal stimulant and therefore has very good effect on gonadal anomalies. Freedom of the physiological motion of the pituitary and the rest of the endocrine orchestra is of the utmost importance in cranial effectiveness. It is a potent antidote to uterine inertia, hence, do not use 4VC on a pregnant woman; though it can, of course, be beneficial during labour.

THE ENDOCRINE UMBRELLA
35 THE ENDOCRINE GLANDS

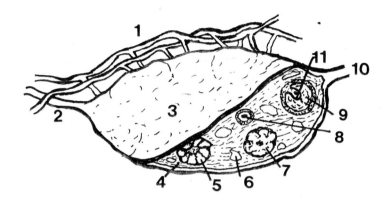

OVARY

1 Ovarian Arteries & Veins
2 Ovarian Ligament
3 Epithelium
4 Connective Tissue
5 Early stage Corpus Luteum
6 Capillaries
7 Mature Corpus Luteum
8 Primary Graafian Follicle
9 Mature Follicle
10 Suspensary Ligament
11 Ovum

ESSENTIALS OF CRANIO-SACRAL OSTEOPATHY

36   THE ENDOCRINE GLANDS

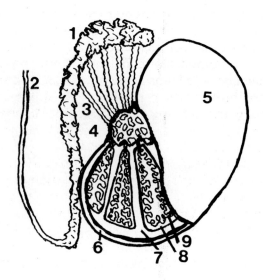

TESTIS

1 Epididymis
2 Vas Deferens (Seminal duct)
3 Efferent ductules
4 Rete Testis (in Mediastinum)
5 Tunica Albuginea

6 Tunica Vaginalis
7 Septum
8 Lobules
9 Seminiferous Tubules

THE ENDOCRINE UMBRELLA

The forgoing, a brief survey of glandular inter-relationship, is but a glimpse into the vast array, indeed the complexity of endocrine interplay. It cannot be overemphasized that the orderly functioning of all the body's physiological systems are dependent on hormone activity from the glands of internal secretion, the pituitary acting as a collector of news regarding the effects of the secretion of all the other glands and reacting accordingly. In this way the entire metabolic process, growth, reproduction, etc. are not only regulated but co-ordinated. In this chapter we have endeavoured to cover the specific role of each of these endocrine glands and how they relate to one another in order to effect homeostasis throughout the body. In our clinics we do not see people in homoeostatic balance, only those with 'disturbed homeostasis ever need us' – as Hans Seyle puts it. He also says in *The Stress of Life*: 'It is the responsibility of the central nervous system, augmented by the action of the pituitary and other endocrine glands, to combat stress with a complex machinery of checks and balances for adaptation to environmental changes.' This balance embraces all body functions, musculo-skeletal (and other 'mechanical' activities) as well as electrical and chemical.

Cranial treatment, the subject of this book, normalizes pituitary secretion, and on the basis of the peculiarity of the influence of this gland in the system, there is improved endocrine function throughout the entire organism.

We have seen that in the cranium there are numerous rhythms, impulses and cycles, many of which are hidden from normal observation; mainly because they are not anticipated, and do not accord with physiological preconceptions.

Nevertheless, they are the purveyors of life itself. Conversely, if they are perverted, they can be the heralds of disease and death. These impulses are influenced by various factors including loss of sleep (and here we may again think of the possibility of pineal insufficiency) fear, loss of oxygen, increase of carbon dioxide, fevers; and of great significance is the possibility of restriction of motion at the sutural level of the occiput, temporomastoid, sphenobasilar symphysis; and frontosphenoid articulations.

Consider the clinical implications of occipital motion restriction – schizophrenia can possibly be one of the results; while in severe spheno-basilar symphysis locking, there can be – and often is – a manic depression, and involutional mania where the frontosphenoidal restriction is severe. Basically these conditions are a result of breakdown in the integration or synchrony of motion and balance in the body systems.

All the anatomical structures, and indeed the whole human organism then, is subject to endocrine regulatory activity; the cells are harmonized and maintained in physiological and functional balance through a cross-fertilization of hormone influence.

When this balance is upset it might not be obvious for a long time until pathology is manifest either in certain organs, glands, or evidenced by disturbances in the nervous system.

Lesions of the cranio-sacral system are often responsible for disturbances in the functional state of the hypothalamic-pituitary complex. The extent of the effects of these lesions can best be measured in the light of altered supply of cerebrospinal fluid throughout the body. If this fluid does not arrive on time and in the correct amplitude, at all the centres and structures to which it is vital, health is bound to be impaired. Dr Still left us in no doubt of this 'withering fields must be irrigated with the waters of the brain.'

When the cerebrospinal fluid is equably and efficiently distributed to all the cells, the nervous system is enabled to produce the requisite impulses, thus affording improved glandular function, and energy, together with digestive and circulatory amelioration.

Another helpful statement of Dr Still was that 'each part is as great and useful in its place as any other.' Sutherland, too maintained this concept, as illustrated by his refusal to demonstrate cranial technique to those of his students who did not have a sound knowledge of the cranium. When he was confident that they were familiar with the articular surfaces of all the cranial bones, only then was he free to instruct on limitation of movements occasioned by lesioning, and what was involved in their correction.

What he appeared to have in mind was that it wasn't just a matter of correcting this or that lesion, when faced with the sick and suffering, but of being aware of the endocrine physiological effects that are likely to ensue. He would doubtless point to the hypothalamic-pituitary activity within the internal environment of the body.

So, it bears repeating that when pathology is well established, whether in an organ or the nervous system, cranio-sacral structural lesions may well be responsible. Patience will often prove a useful adjunct, as the response to therapy is often slow. It is encouraging, however, that cranio-sacral therapy is often beneficial in stopping the progress of most pervasive pathology.

OLIVE M STRETCH

'... the Pituitary is not the Master gland, but is part of a chain and is affected by the other links of that chain.'

'The dura, diaphragmatic sellae, falx, and tentorium (in motion) all tend to bring the pituitary into proximity to the sphenobasilar symphysis.'

'We cannot isolate our treatment, we cannot treat regionally, at any stage of human life, from birth to the declining years of the aged, our thinking and treatment *must* involve the whole man.'

CHAPTER EIGHT

Fourth Ventricle Compression

Fourth ventricle compression (4V.C.) is a most valuable part of our cranial armamentarium. Its application is simple and the results are usually very rewarding. Seldom is it contra-indicated, only where there is respiratory distress (asthma, hay-fever, etc.), haemorrhage (profuse bleeding), or in the presence of recent trauma or shock involving the cranium (head injuries, fractured skulls), aneurysms, cancer, or on the pregnant woman (as it can induce uterine contractions).

Normally, no one can be too ill to receive 4V.C. and as Magoun writes 'if you do not know what else to do, compress the fourth ventricle' – and, in my experience that is exactly so. 4V.C. is the most effective, most comprehensive, therapeutic procedure known to the profession. It is second to none; it co-ordinates and regulates the viscera. It has tremendous influence over the autonomic and neuro-endocrine systems in restoring balance and efficiency.

Some of the conditions which may benefit from this procedure are fluid stasis – oedema of the limbs, ascites, high blood pressure, uterine inertia, sore throats, circulatory problems, joint inflammation; peripheral ascaemia and paraesthesia; headaches, migraine; arthritis, psychological disturbances; hyper-activity, depression. . .

When you compress the 4th ventricle you are reaching the whole C.S.F. system via the 3rd ventricle and then the 1st and 2nd (lateral) ventricles and it is through the mediation of the C.S.F. that the results of this wonderful technique are achieved. The fluctuation effects balanced interchange of body fluids. Hence 4V.C. may be beneficially applied in the presence of the most complicated lesion. It is dependable in cases where tissue tone is in question and may be of great assistance in preparation for certain articular adjustments.

The patient should be supine, as for many other cranial procedures, and should be made to feel warm, comfortable and secure with a thinnish pillow underneath the head and halfway beneath the scapula.

Elevating the shoulders will prevent any likelihood of fluid constriction occurring in the neck during the treatment.

FOURTH VENTRICLE COMPRESSION

The best results will be achieved if the patient is relieved of all possibility of suspicion should he be unused to the gentleness of cranial therapy.

Interlace your fingers fairly loosely, and without startling your patient slide your cupped hands underneath the occiput. Lightness of touch and accuracy are essential. The thenar eminences of your thumbs will now be in contact with his supraocciput. Have your elbows spread about six inches away from your body and the thenar eminences approximating, with the patient's head almost slipping out of your hands. You are now in the right position to start the compression.

I have for a good reason taken care in describing the hand placement. If you are applying pressure to the wrong area you will not get the right results. Caution must always be exercised to avoid the masto-occipital junction. If you happen to compress this region, to your embarrassment, the patient might suffer projectile vomiting.

So be careful.

37 HAND POSITION FOR 4V.C.

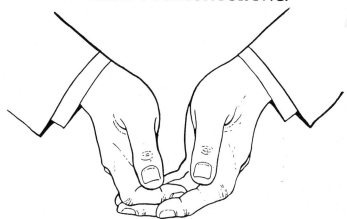

Now begin to apply even pressure of a few pounds by pressing your thenar eminences against the patient's supraocciput. Maintain this for a minute or two and he will most likely begin to feel some sensation in his hands and feet. They may be warm and tingling, and his breathing may change from normal to slow and even.

The lessening of subcutaneous fluids allow for more distinct skin creases and a change to a peach-like complexion. The evenness of the respiratory activity occasioned by this compression (or 'idling' of the fluctuation) will minimise until it is hardly noticeable.

38 FOURTH VENTRICLE COMPRESSION

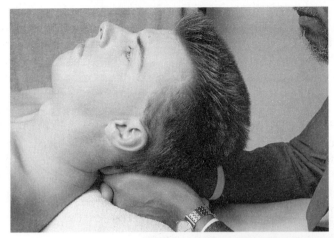

Usual method

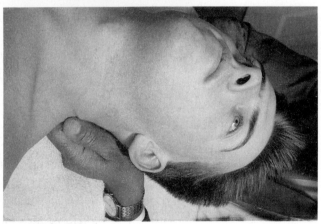

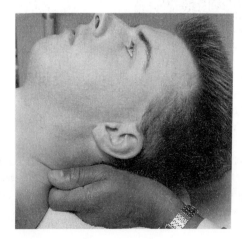

Second method

FOURTH VENTRICLE COMPRESSION

Watch the patient's forehead for slight moistening. As soon as you see this sign it is time to slowly release your pressure. You have achieved what you intended.

Another pertinent sign indicating urgency for cessation of the compression is if the patient sighs. This sometimes precedes the moistening of the forehead and must not be ignored, but obeyed.

It is important not to overdo 4V.C. The whole operation should take no more than four minutes. If you overtreat, the patient will feel nauseous, disorientated, or at least have a head-ache. Therefore, as with other therapeutic measures, the very procedure that possesses such potential for good, if misapplied, can be disastrous or at the very least off-putting for the patient.

39 SACRO-OCCIPITAL BALANCING

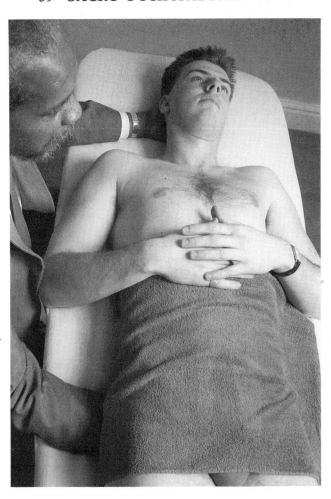

ESSENTIALS OF CRANIO-SACRAL OSTEOPATHY

40 CRANIAL TECHNIQUES WITH TWO OPERATORS

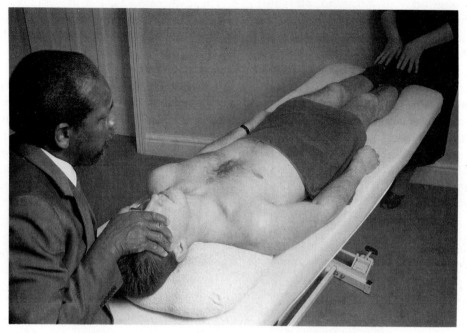

'Taking into' Flexion

II

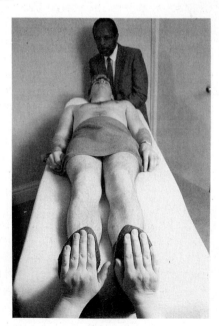

'Taking into' Extension

FOURTH VENTRICLE COMPRESSION

In the event of there being an adverse reaction to the treatment whether through ignorance of the specific procedure or some peculiarity that you do not readily understand, all is not lost. You can reverse the undesirable effects by working from the sacrum. You simply hold it in respiratory extension. Sit beside the couch at a level just below the patient's loins and slip your hand between his thighs and under his sacrum. Just cradle it in your hand which should be spread so that the tip of the middle finger approximates to L5.

Allowing your forearm to rest on the couch for steadiness, gently caress the sacrum. Do not try to treat or adjust anything. As the sacrum is held anteriorly you may enlist the patient's respiratory co-operation. Holding his breath in exhalation will facilitate a speedy resolution.

In resistant and complicated articular lesions 4V.C. can be of real advantage. Here, however, you have to exercise patience, as it may be necessary to apply this technique several times before a resolution is achieved. And as for membraneous and ligamentous tone, its value cannot be too highly stressed.

Space does not allow for a more definitive account of 4th Ventricle compression. Suffice it to say this technique can best be understood when considered in conjunction with the Primary Respiratory Mechanism and the fluctuation of the C.S.F. The full picture is only apparent when we relate this to the balanced interchange of fluids that is constantly occurring, realising that 4V.C. has great influence over the entire fluid system.

There is a second method of inducing compression of the fourth ventricle. This is sometimes useful when there appears to be no fluid motion after an appreciable time of compressing the bulb as in the first method. It can also be used on its own, but is a more 'mechanistic' approach.

Contact the mastoid junction of the occiput with the thenar eminences – making sure that the thumbs are aligned with the transverse tip of the atlas (under the lobe of the ear), and gently 'pump' in time with inhalation. When motion is established revert to bulb compression to complete the procedure.

Thirdly, as we have touched on before, ventricle compression can be effected from the sacrum.

Apart from acting as a moderator, this procedure is of great value – and is often the 'end' of choice, for treating infants and children up to six years old. This is especially so in hyperactive, educationally sub-normal and recalcitrant states. The most fractious child will settle down happily in your hand after a minute or two of this treatment.

In the adult, acute lumbar and sacral lesions can often be treated this way without any further osteopathic manoeuvre being necessary.

All these can be carried out by one operator. There are occasions, however, where, as in some other cranial treatments, 2 people working together can bring a 'fine tuning' to this procedure. If the two are synchronized in methodology there are heightened therapeutic results. It enables the practitioner to secure maximum effectiveness of C.S.F. distribution.

ESSENTIALS OF CRANIO-SACRAL OSTEOPATHY

41 CRANIAL TECHNIQUES WITH TWO OPERATORS

III

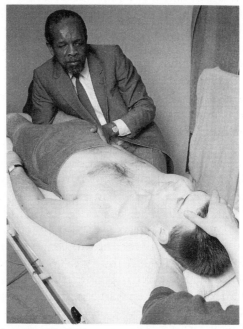

Sphenobasilar correction with sacral assistance

IV

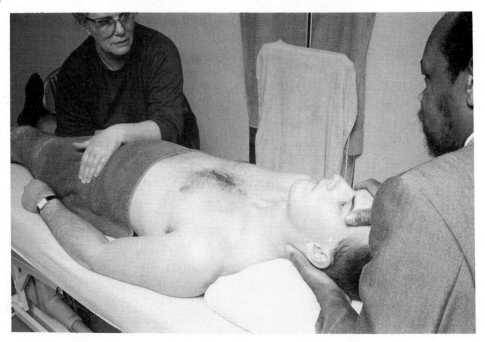

Spinal conditions, muscular rigidity, involuntary tremor syndromes, and so on, can all benefit. You can also nullify all those states that are additional to the primary arthritic presentation. This procedure is also beneficial in quadrant analysis.

Harold Ives Magoun made great use of one, two, and even three assistants working together on a patient; sometimes having one at the feet, one at the sacrum, and one assisting him at the head. We can also use pedic assistance. Either with another practitioner, or by the patient's co-operation. It is, of course, better to have a second person who understands precisely what you are trying to achieve – but, failing this the patient can be asked to dorsiflex or plantiflex the feet as desirable. This latter enhances the pumping action of the C.S.F. through the auspices of the P.R.M.

Yet another method of balancing C.S.F. distribution is available to the single operator. It is called 'sacro-occipital balancing.' By sitting at the side of the couch and cradling the occiput in one hand and the sacrum in the other (laterally) – you will be aware of weight in either hand, and this has to be in balance. In order to carry out this procedure have the couch covered with a foam 'mattress' – 3 to 4 inches thick is ideal. This will allow you to 'dip' one hand or the other; 'stretch' caudally or cephaladly; lateralize the occiput or sacrum, to achieve this balanced state. It is almost like using a spirit-level. As the C.S.F. distribution becomes equal one can mentally see, and feel, the 'still-point' of fluid motion achieved.

V

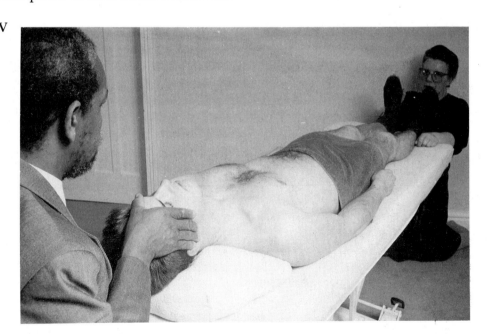

'Taking into' Contralateral Flexion

TABLE E

SUMMARY
FOURTH VENTRICLE COMPRESSION

Method

Contact
    at bulb
    at Occiput
    at Sacrum
Establish rhythm
Maximum duration – 4 minutes

Improves

C.S.F. Distribution
Metabolic State
Reduces oedema
Tissue Replenishment
Defence Mechanism
Immunity Response
Endocrine behaviour
Liver, spleen, & pancreatic states
Absorption of deposits – e.g. calcium
Differential diagnosis heightened

Indications of Efficacy of Treatment

Patient takes involuntary deep breath/sigh
Respiration & heart-rate slow/steady
Facial/forehead skin colour changes to 'peach'
    bloom & becomes moist
Patient often expresses feeling of well-being
    or peacefulness
An apparent relaxation of patient state

DENIS BROOKES

'We' (the practitioner) 'are like structural engineers . . . if the chassis is right, the car has a good chance – though the petrol may be wrong – but if we can put the chassis right . . . it will run well!'

'One of the key symptoms in the low back problem is 'confusion.' If ever you get a patient who is confused, you have got a chronic psoas problem.'

'The lymph system is the key system. Fascial bands direct lymph flow.'

'Release of dural membraneous tension will always facilitate the tendency toward fluid balance.'

'In the adult the three sickles of the dura occupy so commanding a position in the cranial hypothesis that they have been named the Reciprocal Tension Membrane.'

CHAPTER NINE

Cranial Diagnosis and Evaluation

Cranial diagnosis makes full use of the principles which are common to the osteopathic profession. In all our work observation must be primary and tactile capacity must be an imperative.

Despite the great advance in technology and science with the attendant benefits of diagnostic and therapeutic aids, which are so easily available to the profession, nothing can replace the well trained palpatory sense and skills of the human hand. It can best differentiate between one condition and another; and determine not only the condition but the course of action necessary to remedy it.

Every time that one touches a patient it should be a conscious experience such as will provide valuable information that cannot be gained by other methods of diagnosis. For this purpose the state of the patient is not the all-important thing. What really matters is that in touching him the practitioner is learning and developing his skill/art/science . . . to the benefit, not only of that particular patient, but all who follow after him. This is to say that the cranial osteopath will always be tending to become more and more efficient according to the greatness of the number and the variety of individuals he has palpated.

X-Rays are valuable, especially where there are gross pathological changes to be evaluated. In the laboratory it may be relatively easy to elicit blood sugar levels and alteration in body chemistry. Helpful information may be gathered at the flick of a switch or the touch of a button.

In our Clinics we may attach our clever machines to patients by electrodes, or whatever, and relieve their backache. But none of these devices have the ability to reveal minute differences in tissue tone, tension, temperature, elasticity, resilience, mobility, flexibility, extensibility, or reaction to stimuli . . . They cannot supply the host of vital essentials to adequate diagnosis that one touch of the sensitive hand conveys to the practitioner.

Cranial diagnosis demands that we be aware of the reason why each part exists. Until you can put your hand on a person's head and begin to distinguish pulsation, motion, and rhythm, cranial osteopathy is but a theory

42 DIAGNOSIS & EVALUATION – OBSERVATION

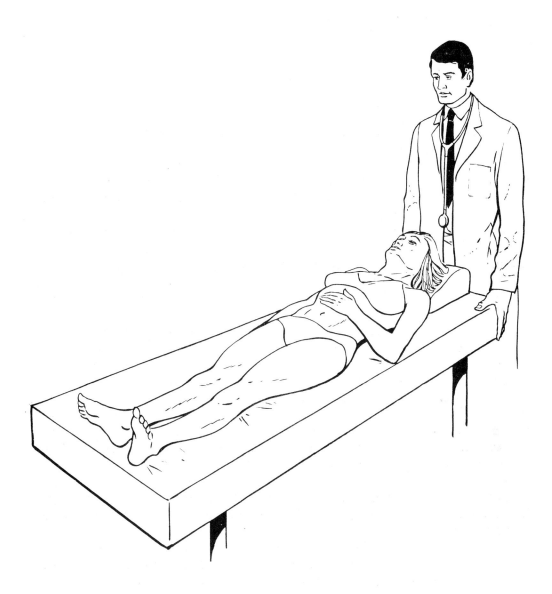

43 PEDIC ANGLES

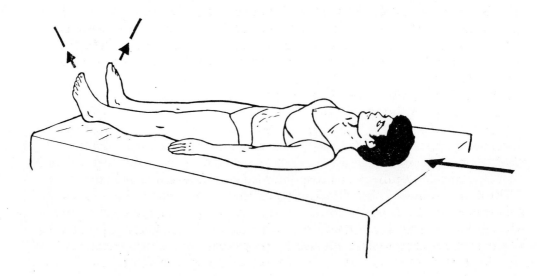

With patient supine and relaxed, note the attitude the feet assume. Record as illustrated below, from the head end – looking caudally.

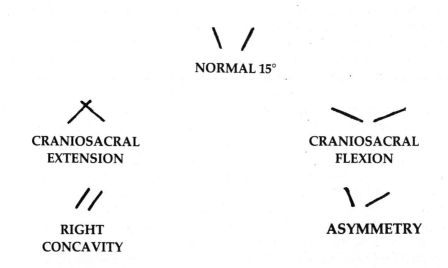

This quick method allows a record to be made before and after treatment, at each visit, etc.

or a dream. Whether you are testing for motion, or treating, lightness of touch is the golden rule. Success depends on your ability to exercise this particular finesse. You do not wish to override or 'blot out' what the tissues can tell you.

Ordinarily you should be able to feel rhythmic impulses in the human skull – occurring at around 10–14 cycles per minute in normal adults. Only gentle proprioceptive palpation will enable you to perceive this rhythm, which is not to be mistaken for circulatory or respiratory motion. For our purposes it is the 'Cranial Rhythmic Impulse' – C.R.I.

When palpating the head do not expect movement such as you find in joints in other parts of the body. All you may expect is pliability, resiliance, or a slight yielding suppleness where the sutural articulations occur. Unlike a coconut or dried out specimen skull, the head of our particular patient is not only live, but pliable, and the inherent motion does not result from bone moving on bone. There is a subtle yielding in correspondence with interarticular tissue.

These are some of the disadvantages that occur when there is lack of delicateness in handling the head. An immediate spontaneous self-protective barrier ensues. This is reflex action which is likely to offset accurate palpation. The tissues tense in order to resist the intrusive force. This tension, though only temporary mediates abnormal impulses to the central nervous system. The result of this is that the impulses which are being sought by palpation are being perverted, and your analysis will automatically be inaccurate.

During palpation any action that is likely to excite, or arouse emotion must be avoided. You, the practitioner, also need to be as relaxed as possible, not only during the examination of the patient, but also while treating him. Failure to adhere to this principle will transmit undesirable impulses to the patient and thus obscure precise appraisal and correct diagnosis.

Imagine you are about to start your first cranial investigation. The patient should be supine – warm, comfortable, and free from all undue anxiety. If this is a woman she ought really to remove all clips, pins, combs, etc. from her hair – and don't forget that earrings can be inhibitory to normal fluid flow.

Firstly, walk round the couch. Take a good look at the patient generally. Start at the head of the couch and observe caudally; then go to the feet and re-evaluate what you have seen. Are the feet lateralizing, inverted, everted, parallel; or is one grossly inclined to the one side? Cast your eyes from the feet to the face again. Is one nostril wider than the other? Are the orbits equal? Are the ear lobes at the same level; is one ear closer to the head than the other? Are the nasolabial and supra-nasal vertical folds parallel? Has the body assumed a concavity that is mirrored in the facial structure? If so, to which side? This is important in analysis of spheno-basilar correlation.

These brief observations will not help you to be more proficient in palpation, but ultimately, when it comes to making a diagnosis, they may be indispensable. We shall discuss more detailed observation in a later chapter.

44 FACIAL FORAMINA

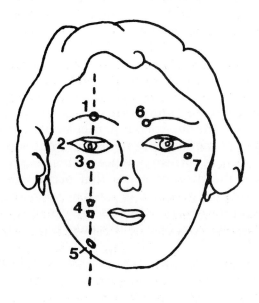

1	Supra-orbital Foramen	1 inch from mid-line
2	Pupil	
3	Infra-orbital Foramen	¼ inch below inferior orbital rim
4	2nd Pre-molar	
5	Mental Foramen	½ inch above mandibular inferior border

1–5 are usually in a direct vertical plane. However, it should be remembered that the angle of the mandible changes from obtuse in infancy to almost a right angle in the adult and back to an obtuse angle in old age. The mental foramen is found on the superior anterior surface in the aged.

6	Frontal Notch	½ inch from mid-line
7	Zygomaticofacial Foramen	¼ inch laterally from inferolateral angle of orbit

Be sure you are sitting comfortably at the head of the couch. It is recommended that both your feet be flat on the floor and you should be free from all undue strain. Your hands must be warm and dry before attempting to handle the patient's head.

Start with cradling the occiput in your left hand, leaving the other free to palpate. For the sake of steadiness your forearm must rest on the couch. Gently span the forehead allowing your hand to settle delicately upon the superficial tissues. Your thumb and second finger should now be resting on the great wings of the sphenoid. From this position you can, and certainly should begin to gather information. What about the skin? Is it hot, cold, dry, moist, rough, or smooth? Are the tissues under your palpating hand tonic or atonic? Is there evidence of fluid retention, toxicity, or tenderness? Any divergence from normal health in these superficial tissues will be evident, and relevant to the total picture.

It is already noted that in healthy persons the C.R.I. ranges between 10 to 14 cycles per minute. Cranial palation is largely concerned with this phenomenon. It is reliable for diagnosis. A firm but gentle hand placed over, and in contact with both asterion will elicit this inherent motion within the cranial mechanism.

In the event of the patient being psychologically disturbed it will be found that the C.R.I. rate is decreased but this is the opposite in the presence of fevers; the rate is increased.

The psychiatric case may also present with an almost rigid forehead, whereas the tissues in this area are usually elastic. Of course, as in fever, the severity of the clinical condition is proportionate to the increase or decrease in the rate of C.R.I.

Your observation and palpation must now move on to test for sutural motion. Still cradling the occiput with the left hand, begin to test for sphenobasilar abnormalities. At the sphenobasilar junction you can have many. By way of observation you will doubtless already have noted certain irregularities. There might be torsion to the right or left with sidebending right or left. There might be a vertical strain with a lateral strain. All or any of these conditions might be present. They may even present in a compounded form in flexion or extension. These can be really complex.

Keep in mind that, when it comes to treatment, we are not aiming at symmetry, but normalization of sutural mobility and consequently adequate fluid flow. Gently rest your third finger on the patient's forehead medially about an inch above the nose. Here you are about to test for restriction, so lightly move your finger superiorly and inferiorly to judge the tissue. Move it to the fullest extent without releasing contact. Have you more movement one way than the other? Are you aware of roughness and 'jarring' one way, and easy smoothness the other? The direction that is not as resilient as it might be denotes restriction. Then test the oblique angles – from glabella to frontal ossification points, in the same way. You may suspect the cranium to be in extension if the restriction is superior. The head may be elongated and locked in that position. The reverse of this obviously, would be flexion.

Earlier we mentioned the use of X-Rays. These are not diagnostically valuable in cranial osteopathy. At best they can only be supportive – for instance, for examination of the great wings, or the level of the fossae... As the patient walks through the door your diagnosis should start. You would not, of course, say he has this or that condition. However, you will begin to formulate certain ideas.

As a matter of fact, people coming into my clinic are often surprised at how few questions they are asked regarding their condition, and what I do for them is often as deceptively simple.

You should be able to do the same – even if your patient is on a couch in the dark, you should still be able to diagnose, evaluate, and treat him by that very 'touch' that tells you everything. The invisible is more articulate than the visible.

Certain visible influences can always be exluded because they are pretentious. They are what the patient projects, their hair style, perfume, clothing, speech . . . You do not have to know what is wrong with the patient. As already noted you begin by handling the head. You feel for animation, warmth (not heat or temperature). In fact you can put your fingers on anybody's arm and start to interpret what you feel.

Suppose you put your hand on a table you are bound to feel something. It might be wet, sticky, hard. Remember there are different degrees of hardness. With the tips of your fingers you can tell the degree.

Now for the head – if you happen to feel something you cannot define, try again. Ultimately you will differentiate between skin and bone. You will feel muscle outline and fatty tissue. Let them tell you what they will.

You will feel the same pattern of C.S.F. in the limb system as you feel in the head. With your fingers correctly placed, by now you should be feeling the impulses with the base of your fingers. You feel impulses with the epicritic sensation. So, as you envelop the head, place the second finger over the great wing, the third finger on the S.S. pivot. This is to say on the squama of the temporal bone and the styloid process, and the fourth finger on the S.M. pivot, at the termination of the temporal bone at the mastoid process. Place the fifth finger just behind the OM. suture. So you have one on the great wing, one on the anterior pivot, one on the posterior pivot, and one on the occiput. (The thumbs should not be in contact with the skull). These are the four finger positions around which you will feel sphenobasilar mobility. Regard this particular combined operation as concerned with bone and fluid. You will feel the great wings moving laterally, superiorly and inferiorly; you will recognise them just pushing very gently against your fingers.

When there is a specific lesion the bony movement will be restricted, but the fluid movement will be augmented. So a pushing, pounding sensation against your fingers in this position from within – over a suture – indicates not mobility, but a lesion.

In that there is a contradistinction in your palpable epicritic analysis between bone and fluid your interpretation will enable you to decide on the course of action that might be necessary. If you so desire you can now take the occiput into flexion. Ease your four fingers down taking the occiput with your little fingers anteroinferiorly in one composite movement.

Now, to test for orbital obliquity you may put one finger on the oblique external inferior attitude of the orbital rim. Put another finger – of the other hand – on the medial aspect of the frontal orbital rim, and feel whether the rim is presenting an abnormal ridge. You will also be able to discern the state of the vomer. Is it depressed?

Ask the patient to take a deep breath. Observe whether, while he is breathing in, the impulses that appear under your hands are lateral or not; or on one side only; or forward and not backward – anterior or posterior.

Do not be disappointed if you are at first unable to feel all the phenomena presented in this text. You may have to practice what you have learnt for some time before it begins to make sense. As soon as you are able to differentiate between the impulses peculiar to bony mobility, you will pass over a significant line of demarcation – from hoping to experiencing, and cranial osteopathy will have gained another convert!

For the sake of clarity even at the expense of being repetitious, the C.S.F. mobility is felt as a soft rubber ball pushing against your fingers – pulse-like. Bony movement is not like that. When there are two phenomena present then you may sense ligamentous or membraneous mobility. You are then feeling on the periphery that which takes place in the middle of the head.

As these membranes shift, and they are shifting all the time – they provide a fulcrum. Each head has a changing fulcrum. The object of this fulcrum is for adjustment, accommodation to the production of C.S.F. This is really an adjustment to fluid capacity and the distribution of it.

The membranes dividing the brain accommodate the distribution of fluid. This accommodation is particularly important to the maintenance of the functional capacity of the straight sinus. The fluid consistency maintains it, operating in that balanced midline, perpendicular plane. This is why the head is inexorably trying to maintain a level upright position. Even as you talk, you alter the roof of your mouth; you alter the fascia; from the laryngeal structures to the styloid process of the temporal bone in the occipital base. Hence, there is membraneous adjustment to accommodate your speech through the floor of the sphenobasilar symphysis. There are bony, fluid, membraneous, and articular patterns – all of which are palpable at the spheno-basilar symphysis.

Holding the head intelligently will reveal to you what is happening inside. The head will tell you what its lesions are. For example, suppose there is a left occipitomastoid lesion with all the attendant consequences down the distribution of the 9th, 10th and 11th cranial nerves; deglutitional problems and the like, if you hold that head you would find a pounding on that side. Now continue holding the head a while in that position already described, and you will find that the whole head moves, but not the part that indicates the lesion – that will be rigid in your hand.

So you will have two conditions to consider, a pounding coming to the

45 CONCAVITIES

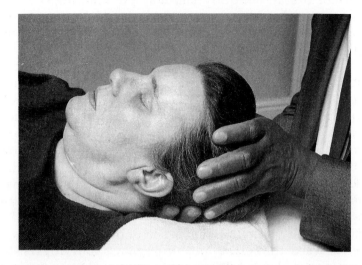

Top of concavity

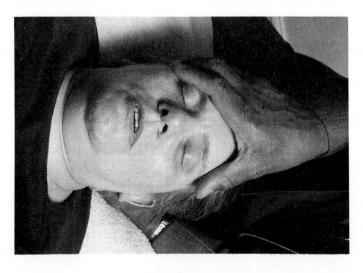

Middle of Concavity

surface, which is fluid; and also a rigidity and some degree of mobility peripherally. When you understand palpating these fluids, you will know whether the lesion is in inspiration or expiration. The best way to know this is to get the patient to hold his breath. Then there is no diaphragmatic excursion, so now you can decide on the potency of that rhythm (pounding); as well as all the other palpating factors. Also discern whether it is in excursion or not. This might not appear to be simple, but it is really.

Think of it this way. If you cross your thumbs over the top of the two parietals, they will expand towards the lambda. If you feel the lambda moving away in that direction you would know that the parietals are going into flexion quite well. Even without any previous knowledge of the patient, you would know that he is potentially asthmatic, migrainous, eczematous...

Let me suggest a little experiment you might perform on yourself, to illustrate this very brief excursion into cranial diagnosis. This will allow you to experience the cyclic changes in cranial capacity that occur during the description just given.

In a supine position on the couch clasp your hands over the sagittal suture. Apply firm pressure over the postero-inferior angles of the parietals, and the lambdoidal suture. Whilst holding steadily, breathe out all you can – to the very last degree, and then breathe in to the fullest extent possible. Repeat this breathing in and out, and slowly release the compression. You will doubtless realise the outward movement of the postero-inferior position of the parietals as well as the expansion of the brain.

What you have experienced is more or less central to the cranial concept. The inhalation phase of the P.R.M. involves an uncoiling and thickening of the C.N.S. Simultaneously the osseous chamber shortens and widens, while the vault lowers. All the cranial structure is involved in this operation.

Inferiorly the bodies of the parietals and the squama of the temporals move laterally, while the saggital suture lowers and the tentorium cerebelli flattens, with the mid-line of the frontal drawn posteriorly by the falx cerebri. The lateral angles of the frontal and greater wings of the sphenoid circumduct antero-inferiorly, while the spheno-basilar symphysis elevates to shorten the antero-posterior diameter of the skull.

ESSENTIALS OF CRANIO-SACRAL OSTEOPATHY

46   SAGITTAL SPREAD

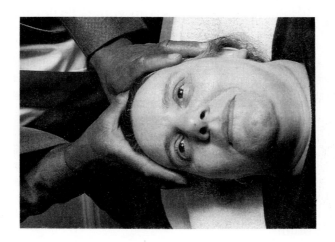

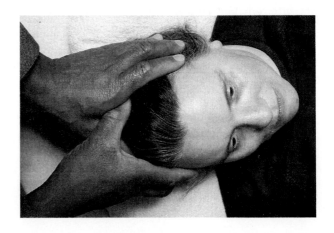

LEON E PAGE

'Diagnosis is the clinical interpretation of Pathology.'

'The object of treatment is to aid the natural body defences as far as possible, and to remove all deleterious influences from the body and its environment.'

'The question of naming the disease is of secondary importance.'

CHAPTER TEN

Lesions – Vault & Base

Usually lesions are, in the cranial sense, neither primary nor secondary, but multiple almost from the moment they occur. That is to say that immediately a lesion occurs accommodative factors come into play – whether or not treatment is undertaken – as the body attempts to regain homeostasis.

Consider the symptoms of an extension lesion, for example. They range from small eyes, high palate, buck teeth, crowding of the jaw; to inward rotation of the maxillae and nasal recession. The latter is typical, and is due to vomeric compression as a rule, occasioning narrowing of the posterior nasal orifices.

What about a fractured skull? In the event of a vault fracture will treatment correct it? There is something very particular about cerebral tissue that must always be borne in mind. The adaptation capacity of the human brain is like that of the liver. Whatever the injury, that osseous tissue will repair provided about 70% of the brain tissue remains functional.

However, it is not advisable to hasten to attempt correction of a lesion in this area. There may be a secondary distorted mechanism with a fracture involved. There may also be a compensatory accommodative sphenobasilar lesion, and you may think you are obliged to do something about it. The problem is that you can make the most beautiful face out of something mediocre, and then wish you had not, for you might have a lunatic on your hands.

Therefore it is good to know what you are doing. Where accommodation has occurred it is wise to proceed with caution. In the event of there being a chronic cranial birth problem, treatment of the vault is best avoided.

The vault is formed in membrane and is therefore plastic; while the base is formed in cartilage (with certain exceptions) and therefore corrections are direct. Of course, as we already know, many cranial lesions are the result of the birth pattern. Injuries sustained then often do not only remain as a potential health hazard, but actively participate in shaping the future well-being or otherwise of the individual. In this sense 'the child is father to the man!' We must now look into this in greater depth.

In that the bony plates of the head are mobile, as we have been seeing, they are therefore also capable of being moved in a perverted manner either from

LESIONS – VAULT & BASE

47 THE FOETAL SKULL & BIRTH

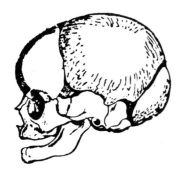

NORMAL FOETAL SKULL

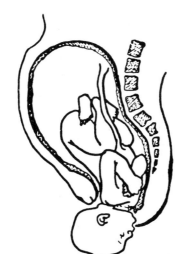

POSITION OF NATURAL DELIVERY

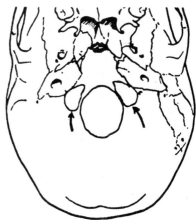

OCCIPITAL CONDYLES
Arrows show direction of displacement (anteromedial) as discussed in text

48 BODY ATTITUDES

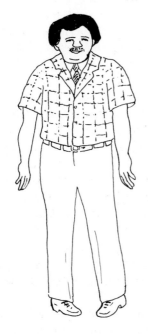
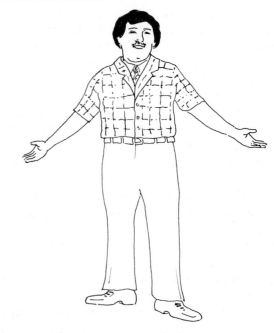

CRANIOSACRAL EXTENSION　　　**CRANIOSACRAL FLEXION**

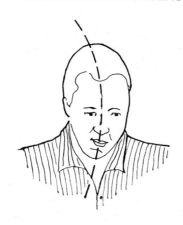

SPHENOBASILAR SIDE-BENDING
Right Concavity
('Banana' Head)

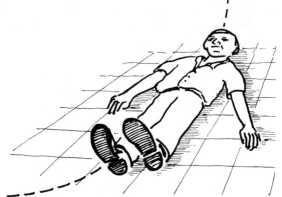

SPHENOBASILAR SIDE-BENDING
Right Concavity (N.B. Pedic Angle)

trauma or from pathological forces. It is necessary for the cranial osteopath to understand the mechanics of birth and the difference it makes to a child's development, and subsequently the adult's of whatever age, whether the birth was a 'natural' one or not.

When a baby is born, as you know, it is the moulding that takes place during delivery that gives the shape and bony relationship to the head. For various reasons – injudicious handling, forceps badly applied, the need for a caeserian section ... this moulding does not take place as it should. With some presentations the maternal contractions may not actually achieve this moulding and the skull may be compressed, elongated, flattened, etc. This is not always easy to assess at the time unless the doctor has knowledge of the cranial concept, or there is obvious brain damage. The anaesthetic the mother receives may also contribute to a 'lazy' birth. When the baby is delivered, it is its first cries that should complete the expansion and regulation of the entire infant structure, and there should be no restrictive areas that are 'jammed.' The P.R.M. begins at this point and undue haste in clamping/severing the umbilical cord will restrict or even prevent the expansion/regulation of the delicate bony plates. In many instances this accounts for the elongated head, together with mental dullness, as a direct consequence. A lack of moulding (and constantly placing the baby on one side only in a cot) can cause restriction of the sutures, which, in turn, causes pressure on the contents inside giving a potentiality to almost any malformation of the body, and a predilection to almost any disease state.

This is why many practitioners wholly deplore forceps delivery. The reasoning behind their thinking is that all things should be as natural as possible. But we must be reasonable, and be careful not to 'throw out the baby with the bath-water.' Forceps in the right hands can be of some benefit in bringing that infant into the world, especially if labour is prolonged, or movement (rotation) of the temporal and occipital bones is to be avoided. Any traction here can cause alteration of internal structures, e.g. the sella turcica containing the pituitary and hypophyseal stalk may be mal-positioned – occasioning endocrine malfunction in later life – even if no evidence is manifested in the baby's early years.

We must remember that forceps were not designed to extract, but assist delivery and therefore traction by forceps or by hand is always a less than perfect contingency.

So, when we are talking of lesion possibilities, we are not necessarily talking of recent injury. The patient who arrives at your clinic may manifest certain signs and symptoms. He may give you a history of the condition as he understands it; but time and time again you will find evidence of a long standing sutural restriction, so that he almost could not help developing the condition he now has!

Hence, one of the first questions one asks the mother of a child patient is 'What kind of birth was it' long, short, induced, forceps, difficult, or easy, etc. Embryologically the vault is formed in membrane to protect the contents of 'The Cranial Bowl' with layers of bone and dura which are intimately related throughout. It is that moulding and squeezing the neonate head (and to a

TABLE F   CRANIO-SACRAL LESIONS & BODY ATTITUDES

CRANIO-SACRAL DESCRIPTION	HEAD SHAPE	BODILY ATTITUDE	RESPIRATION	PEDIC ANGLE
EXTENSION	Dolicephalic 'Banana'	FLEXION Internally Rotated	Exhalation	Inverted
NEUTRAL	Mesocephalic 'Orange'	'Resting'	'Resting'	15° from mid-line
FLEXION	Brachycephalic	EXTENSION Externally Rotated	Inhalation	Everted

lesser extent the rib cage) down through the birth canal to a new world that determines not only shape and size, but also behavioural and functional ability in later life. The bony plates over-ride, expand, and come together again during birth to assume their 'permanent' positions.

Birth injuries are common and range from the frequent slight bruising of skin, to the still-born baby. Being born is still a dangerous business, despite our sophistication, and so much technological advancement!

The foetus may be too big for the birth canal. This may be an anatomical anomaly between a particular woman's body and the growing foetus, but sociologists and anthropologists agree that the whole morphology of Man appears to be changing with every generation. It is a truism that in the Western world in particular, it is getting difficult to tell the young adult female figure from the male! The female pelvis is tending to lose the rounded contours so familiar to all anatomy students.

Induced births and forceps delivery then, are perhaps, the main causes of undue distortion of membrane and cartilage in the infant skull. Incidentally, delivery trauma is also the cause of much maternal misery in the form of post-natal depression, backache, gynaecological disorders, pelvic disturbances, etc. Beware of the woman who says at her first visit to you 'I've never been well since the birth of my last baby' – of whatever she complains – this is a clue to the underlying pathology.

Injury to the infant at birth is often dismissed as merely something that will 'heal in its own good time' or the baby 'will grow out of it.' What a travesty of the facts as they really are! Much of the adult presentation then is adaptive, yet accepted as permanent. It is not necessarily permanent, it is most often pathogenic!

So the influences on later life can be enormous. Some antisocial, and even infamous, behaviour can be attributed to cranial lesions at birth. It is possible that many of those who fill our prisons today might not be there had they either had a 'natural' birth experience, or been assessed cranially immediately after being born, as happens in some places. The same might be said of the population of our mental institutions. Many were disabled at birth!

Another word about children in particular. We see so many who are educationally sub-normal, physically weak – stunted in growth either mentally or physically. There is a correlation between the size of the skull and the growth of the brain.

Think of the frontal bone, which overlies the behavioural centres of the cerebrum. If this is forcibly held in hand or forceps during birth, the subsequent distortion puts undue pressure on the intracranial mechanism.

Early neglect of such factors can be very costly both cosmetically and homeostatically. The cranio-sacral mechanism will be disturbed throughout infancy and into adult life. When we speak of the cranio-sacral system we necessarily include the nervous system, the impairment of which is also of grave consequence. Any injury to vascular/nervous vessels will often not adequately repair.

Let's recap. The sphenobasilar symphysis – that area at the base of the skull where the base of the occiput and the body of the sphenoid meet called a synchondrosis, or ossified joint – has the rudiments of a cartilaginous disc between and remains flexible; so that flexion and extension, side-bending and torsion are all possible here. Because the sphenoid articulates with eleven other cranial bones (all the vault and base, and most of the face) any change that takes place in the sphenoid is transmitted to the whole head and therefore to the whole body system. That is why the sphenobasilar symphysis is so important.

A supplementary reason for its importance is that just behind this area, at the condyles of the occiput (that articulate with the atlas) ossification first takes place. Now you can see how important it is that a baby is – let's say – 'born well!' If the symphysis is misaligned, or the condyles are driven anteromedially (condylo-atlantal compression) as often happens during the birth process, although no apparent injury has been sustained – that growing hardening skull has to accommodate to this rapidly ossifying malformation – and accommodation is always adaptation, and never as it was meant to be.

Therefore the problems that arise here contribute to, or are caused by, its unphysiological function.

Cranial osteopathy is quite often the best solution to the maladies described here – and the earlier it is applied the better. Of course, when treating babies and infants, even more gentleness and lightness of touch is necessary than when treating adults. But a little moulding of the baby's head is often all that is required to correct some of these anomalies; and this is achieved by the practitioner merely placing the palm of the hand on say, the right frontal, and allowing the head to do the work of restoring sutural harmony.

But perhaps the technique that is most frequently necessary in children (and often in adults, too) is CRANIAL BASE DECOMPRESSION with a view to disengaging the atlas from the occiput – posterolaterally.

But, before attempting any cranial work (especially on infants) please remember that, as with any skill, 'a little learning is a dangerous thing!' Any procedure that is powerful enough to do good also has the propensity for mis-use. So that, despite any one else's words to the contrary, I must caution you to thoroughly study the subject before using it on patients – or even friends!

The method of approach to correct this compressive anomaly is to sit with arms akimbo (almost parallel to the patient's shoulders) resting on the couch. Locate the condylo-atlantal articulation with the pads of your middle fingers. There should be just enough separation for your fingers to slip between the two structures. (That is, between the condyles themselves and the superior facets of the atlas). The rest of the fingers are not in contact with the skull.

Encourage the patient's co-operation in inclining the head forward, chin on chest, which will assist in separating the joints. Gently hold, merely inclining posterolaterally, and somewhat posteriorly (very carefully, you are not manipulating). You will most likely discern a greater pulsatile movement on one side than the other. Let this continue until you feel an evenness of motion and a still point, until the desired release is registered under your fingers. Then maintain this position for a minute or two at the end of which the patient should be asked to inhale deeply and then breathe out slowly to a count of three. A spontaneous relaxation of the tissue around the base of the neck will be perceived, whereupon you will realize that this aspect of the treatment is complete.

This is not a procedure to be undertaken light-heartedly, or without a clear diagnostic pattern being established. If this anomaly is present it has almost certainly been there since birth (the only exception would be from direct trauma to the back of the neck, at the base of the skull) and will therefore very likely not be the only lesioned state present. It is necessary then, to look for the accommodative factors that have taken place since birth in the body's attempt to compensate for this early injury.

It is therefore imperative to have more than a little knowledge of the subject to be sure of the order in which the various lesions should be dealt with. It ought also to be noted that, as with many other cranial procedures, it may be necessary to repeat the treatment more than once or twice to establish and stabilize the altered state.

You may now procede to evaluate and correct any corresponding occipito-mastoid lesion that may be present. Using the fourth finger to balance the squamosal part of the occiput, contact the mastoid tips of the temporals laterally with the index fingers. Lift these tips gently from the occiput simultaneously turning the squama with the other fingers. The correct placement of the fingers allows for the head to be balanced securely on your fourth fingers with the middle and little fingers ready to turn the squama and incline the temporals away. This entire procedure requires finesse and dexterity. Each digit although working separately, must be in unison with its fellow.

Now check the temporals for mobility. This is achieved by placing the palmer surfaces of your hands beneath the occiput (fingers interlaced as for 4VC) allowing your thumbs freedom of movement to contact the mastoid process. Your thumbs may be used to initiate turning of the temporals internally or externally as the case may require.

Returning to considerations of the spheno-basilar symphysis, we will now look at CRANIAL BASE DECONGESTION. The aim here is to mobilize the basiocciput, sphenoid, and petrous portion of the temporal and, incidentally, open up the foramen magnum – decompressing the condyles of the occiput and promoting drainage and fluid interchange.

ESSENTIALS OF CRANIO-SACRAL OSTEOPATHY

49   CRANIAL BASE TECHNIQUES

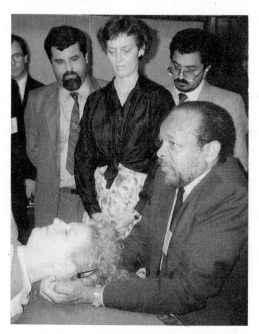

Decongestion

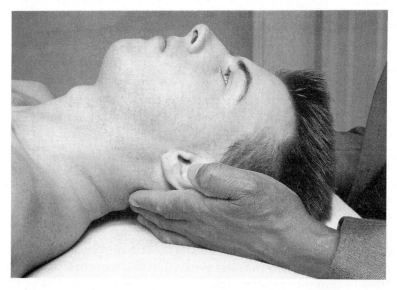

Decompression

LESIONS – VAULT & BASE

Recall our discussion of fascia and its importance to homeostasis. You will doubtless be aware of the sub-occipito-fascial interrelationship and blood pressure. Tension around the base of the skull, the condylar aspects especially being synonymous with high blood pressure, must be relieved.

The subtlety of cerebrofascial tensions must not be under-estimated. They have their influences over hypothalamic activity in respect of control and regulation of physiological behavioural patterns e.g. the autonomic system, water balance, the sleep-wake phenomenon. Therefore our consideration of the sub-occipital area is not circumscribed. Investigation should involve the sacral base, the upper thorax, balance abnormalities, and do not forget posture.

Lesions that affect these areas and behavioural patterns must first be attended to as these are usually primary. The laws of neurophysiology demand that our treatment be conducted this way round in order to arrive at homeostasis.

Cranially speaking, you cannot achieve relief by vigorous intervention. In fact, any attempt at such could result in tragedy, or at the very least, disappointment.

The technique to be employed in decongestion is to sit with both forearms on the couch, cradling the occiput with the fingers flexed (a half fist, so to speak) and pointing cephaladly – just below the nuchal line. Or, if this is a little confusing, another way of describing it is to say, place your open hands parallel, little fingers touching one another and all the fingers directed a little toward the palms – making sure that your fingers are in contact with the transverse processes of the atlas. Your thenar/hypothenar eminences will then be supporting the supraocciput – the right shape for accommodating the roundness of the back of the head. The whole area may be very sore and unpleasantly tender.

Incline posteriorly and slightly upwards (anteriorly). Your inclination should be firm, but not forced, else the patient's condition may be considerably worsened incurring nausea, persistent headaches, tremors, etc. owing to shock through injudicious handling of the delicate nuchal tissues. So, instead of acting as a release to these tissues – and the underlying dura whose attachment within this area is significant to the whole dura/fascial relationship – you will have induced constriction.

Therefore do not be tempted to force a release if the desired mobilization is not soon effected. When you first make finger contact you may feel that one or both sides of the occiput are tight and restricted; or one side may be soft and resilient. Simply hold and wait, the inherent capacity of the c-s system will bring the requisite release. As this begins to happen the head will fall back further onto your hands and you will discern that your fingers have protruded even deeper into the tissues. Go with this until the movement ceases and a spontaneous release is perceived. You will probably find the patient is now

50 VAULT LIFTS

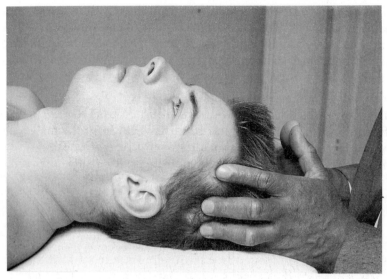

Parietal Lift

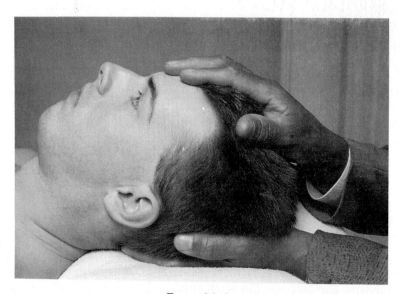

Frontal Lift

thoroughly relaxed and that there is an evenness of motion throughout the cranio-sacral system.

It is not unusual during this procedure for the head to lateralize, or laterally rotate considerably. There is nothing wrong with this. Allow it to happen, while you maintain your contact. When the treatment is finished the head will resume its proper stance.

Gently disengage your fingers allowing the patient's head to rest in your hands for a few moments. The treatment is now complete. Let us now consider some vault techniques and their application. In FRONTAL LIFT the idea is to lift the frontal anteriorly, thus mobilizing the frontofacial articulations: frontosphenoid, frontozygomatic, frontonasal, frontoethmoidal, frontomaxillary, frontolacrimal; and incidentally to affect the frontoparietal (coronal) suture.

With one hand cradling the occiput, lay the spread fingers of the other hand on the frontal in the sagittal plane. (The thumb is not engaged).

The very placement of your fingers creates sufficient adhesion to allow you to lift the frontal. The efficacy of the lift will be perceived as a pulsation under the fingers which should still be in contact with the skin.

An evenness of motion will soon become apparent – a 'stilling' of the pulsation. Hold this for about 8 cycles of the rhythm before disengaging your working hand. Then gently slide the other hand away from the occiput. This technique is very beneficial in congested facial fields.

An alternative method of freeing the frontal is to again cradle the occiput, and place the index finger and thumb of the other hand on the outer side of the frontal ossification points (emminences) and as stated previously incline anteriorly, holding steadily until the requisite pulsation has steadied, as before described.

To lift the frontal cephaladly, place the hands as described in the first method. This time very gently incline superiorly – you are only 'taking up the slack' on the skin, remember. The patient should hardly perceive any weight or movement of your hand in any of these procedures.

You will know when the treatment is finished when the 'stilling,' yielding movement underneath your fingers occurs, at which point you very delicately remove your hands.

This particular lift is most beneficial for some resistant forms of headache, migraine, nausea, frontal 'heaviness' (that feeling of extra weight in the head). The patient usually feels better immediately, and if he remarks on this whilst you are still treating him, gently stop, or you will lose the maximum benefit.

This lift also facilitates freedom of the falx cerebri, and therefore the whole dura, and enhances distribution of C.S.F.

SPREADING THE FRONTAL is achieved by placing the palmar surface of the fingers of each hand on the patient's temples just above the parietal squama, making sure that the index fingers are up against – but behind – the external orbital process. The thumbs should be resting one upon the other (crossed) on the metopic suture. (An alternative placement for the thumbs can be one either side of the metopic suture).

You are now in a position of readiness to spread and mobilize the frontal bone during the expansion phase of the cranial mechanism, by exerting pressure upon the glabella posterosuperiorly, while simultaneously inclining the external orbital process anteriorly. As with all other techniques timing and finesse are essential.

As to the parietals it is important to note that the frontal bone fits in between the two parietals at their inferior angles.

The frontal can be viewed as hanging by a hinge at its medial junction, and having the facility of swinging forward at its base.

This feature is of importance, especially where blows to the forehead are concerned as the frontal then tends to be wedged into the parietals, causing articular fixation at the great wings of the sphenoid, and that limits basilar mobility.

In PARIETAL LIFT therefore the object is to lift the parietals superiorly, freeing the squamosal suture, and the sphenoidal great wings in particular, as well as having a general effect on the coronal and lambdoidal sutures.

We know from our anatomy studies that the middle of the lateral borders of the parietals are bevelled externally (the squamosal border of the temporals being bevelled internally). Hence the parietals drop down behind the temporal squama.

Place the palmar surfaces of the fingers either side of the head – on the parietals, being careful not to encompass any of the sutures. The index fingers should be at the anteroinferior angles (at the pterion). The thumbs must be free of the scalp, but can be crossed above the head to facilitate steadiness.

Incline superiorly – gently, of course, and hold. A pulsatile motion will soon be evident. When this is felt on both sides equally, wait for about eight rhythmic impulses to elapse before gently disengaging your hands.

A direct action technique – PARIETAL SPREAD – is concerned with mobilizing the C.S.F. around the cerebral hemispheres, and facilitating sinus drainage via the superior sagittal sinus. By spreading the parietals, the sagittal suture is encouraged to open – as it does in the healthy subject during inhalation.

The finger hold is similar to parietal lift, but lower down – the little fingers on the temporomastoid, the middle and fourth fingers overlapping the squamosal suture. This time the thumbs are doing the work and are crossed in contact with the opposite parietal just anterior to the lambda.

Apply gentle pressure with the pads of the thumbs inclining infero-anteriorly (the fingers are only for maintaining stability). Because of the bevels of the lambdoidal suture and the wider serrations of the sagittal towards the lambda, this hold will allow disengagement.

LESIONS – VAULT & BASE

Respiratory cooperation can be enlisted – inhalation being the most effective, of course. As with other holds described in this chapter the ensuing pulsatile motion will equalize and reach a 'still-point' thus signifying completion of the treatment. Disengage gently, allowing the parietals to resume their normal state.

There may be times during any cranial technique when you are patently not achieving the desired result. It cannot be forced. If the result is not forthcoming you have either ignored the basic rules and have your hands in the wrong place; or you have more than likely put the cart in front of the horse.

Examine again. It may be that you have not evaluated the whole patient as well as you might. Did you begin your treatment with 4VC? This is often an entry into the system you are trying to influence, and should precede most treatments. Check the four quadrants. Check the spheno-basilar symphysis. How do you do that? Mentally divide the head (as seen from the top of the skull) into four sections. Our concern here is to see the effect of sphenobasilar lesions as evidenced by the position of the great wings at the pterion; and the position of the occiput. The latter is best observed at the mastoid process of the temporal (as the movement of the lateral squama of the occiput is followed by the temporomastoid process) and by the inflaring/outflaring of the pinna of the ear.

You may also prove which side of the occiput is internally or externally rotated (superior or inferior) by palpation. Simply allow the head of the patient (who is lying supine) to rest in your hands; with your fingers caressing the superior nuchal line and check for mal-position.

It is usual in flexion, extension or torsion lesions for the anterior and posterior quadrants (Plate 51, p. 142) on the same side to agree. That is to say in total flexion both sides (all four quadrants) are externally rotated; and in extension all are internally rotated. In torsion behaviour on one side is opposite to the other: left torsion has an externally rotated great wing and occiput on the left; and the opposite on the right (internally rotated).

Considering a side-bending rotation with concavity; or vertical strain lesions, the position is somewhat different.

Let's take vertical strain lesions first. The great wing will be in external rotation on both sides and the occiput in internal rotation on both sides – if this is a superior sphenoidal vertical strain. In inferior sphenoidal vertical strain the positions are reversed (the great wings internally rotated in extension, and the occiput externally rotated in flexion).

Side-bending rotations have a high and low side but the quadrants on the same side are in opposite rotation i.e. a side-bending rotation with a concavity on the left has a high great wing, and occiput – the great wing being in external rotation, the occiput in internal rotation. (The low side has the great wing internally rotated, the occiput externally rotated).

The opposite obtains, of course, in a side-bending rotation with a concavity

ESSENTIALS OF CRANIO-SACRAL OSTEOPATHY

51 QUADRANT ANALYSIS

SPHENO-BASILAR SYMPHYSIS

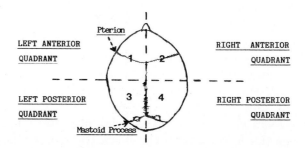

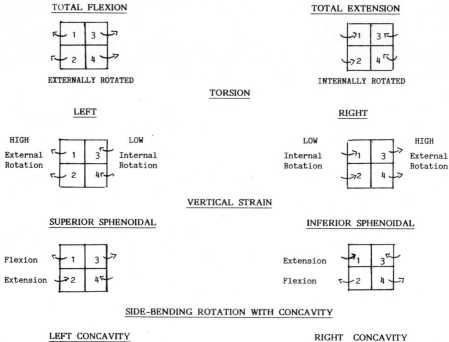

LESIONS – VAULT & BASE

to the right. Although seemingly complicated to understand, this will become much clearer by studying Plate 51 (on page 142), and by examining a skull.

When you have found the 'key' and seen to that first, try your original inclination again, you will often find that now the restriction gently undoes under your fingers.

REBECCA C LIPPINCOTT

'The mighty oak with sap running sways and bends to the elemental forces of wind, sleet and snow, or it twists and becomes distorted as it grows upward around obstacles which obstruct its normal development. So with the living bones of the cranium.'

'... every obstetrician and pediatrician should be a cranial technician, so that infants with either minute or gross cranial lesions may have them corrected promptly. Institutions are filled with spastics, Mongolians, and mental and physical deficients which are the result of cranial injury received before, during or after birth.'

CHAPTER ELEVEN

The Facial Complex

The structure of the facial part of the skull is very complex and consists of six paired bones and three single (although the ethmoid can be said to be part of the base functionally). They are not all easily accessible – ethmoid, vomer, etc – but access can be gained via the roof of the mouth, not only to the individual bones, but also to the base of the skull – e.g. sphenobasilar symphysis.

By far the greater part of the hard palate is formed by the maxillae, while the palatines quite often appear as relatively small bridges between the lateral pterygoid plates of the sphenoid and the maxillae.

Because of its numerous articular contacts with so many other cranial bones, normal maxillary function is an imperative to the mobility of the facial complex. Examine Plate 79. There you will be able to confirm these relationships: frontal, zygoma, nasal, lacrimal, inferior nasal conchae, ethmoid, vomer, palatine, and, of course, do not overlook the articulation between the two maxillae themselves.

So now let us take a further look at that high palate (Chapter 2). This is a lesioned state; the maxillae can be, and often are, locked in internal rotation, creating the appearance of the inside of a bird's beak. This is not of itself a painful condition, or one of which patients are aware. If they have noticed it at all they may tell you that their parents (or perhaps their children) are the same; and that they have all had 'troubles with their teeth,' or that 'all our family have constant colds, etc.'

The condition is not truly familial but often has hereditary characteristics; or is evidence of a forceps delivery or a prolonged birth. There will be a history of local toxic states, breathing difficulties, sinusitus, frequent colds, post-nasal drip, catarrh; allergies, hay fever; lack of visual acuity; anosmia; crowded/ irregular teeth, etc. In children the teeth will be overcrowded and this internal locking may well prevent secondary dentitional placement – the permanent teeth will have great difficulty erupting, as the first teeth have little room to be shed. So some children even present with two rows of teeth, one above the other. This is the child who breathes through his mouth; sucks his thumb; has

ESSENTIALS OF CRANIO-SACRAL OSTEOPATHY

52 FLARING THE MAXILLAE

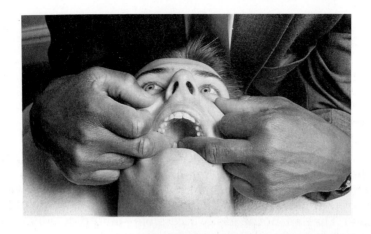

First Position
(At the Palatines)

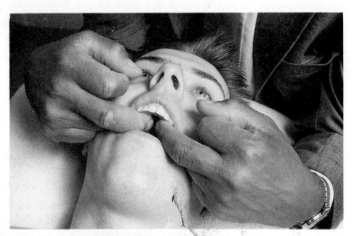

Second Position
(Incisive fossa)

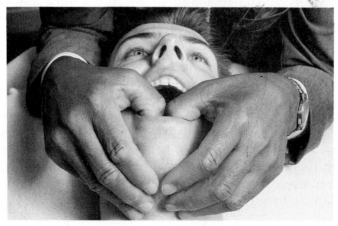

Mandibular flare

braces on his teeth; or has his baby teeth removed by the dentist to aid that secondary dentition.

In these cases (and you will see the results of this in adults, as well as children), it is necessary for the cranial practitioner to check, and often treat, the mandible as well as the hard palate. The child is not sucking his thumb, or a blanket, etc. due to bad habits, naughtiness, or because it's right for him to do so: he is unknowingly elevating the palate to create the requisite airway. Hence he's often lethargic, sleepy, and uncaring, as the intake of oxygen to the brain is reduced. Treat him and see the change to an aware, energetic, 'normal' youngster.

What is suggested by these anomalies is lack of proper drainage throughout the facial areas. The nasal fossa and sphenopalatine ganglia will be crowded, and the undue pressure in the area is a haven for disease, especially allergic conditions. There is congestion, stasis – but we can offer help to these patients.

Because the maxillae are crowded the tongue is not seated properly in the mouth, so it hangs outside – keeping the mouth open. Spread the maxillae in order for the tongue to have sufficient room, and flare the palate, and you will doubtless not only improve the child's breathing ability and general health, but think of the added cosmetic benefit. (It should be said here that similar results can be achieved on adults with like problems). The grateful patient will not only breathe normally but experience relief from the host of bothersome complaints to which he had probably become accustomed.

How do we identify this internally rotated maxilla as we cannot actually see the bone? With the patient supine abserve the stark facial asymmetry. Is there a unilateral exaggeration of the facial folds – naso-labial and supranasal? Is the nasal septum deviated? Look into the mouth; is the dentition crowded, especially at the canines and incisors? Is there an obvious concavity/convexity in the roof of the mouth (remembering that the concavity you see here will match the spheno-basilar concavity visible externally)? Is there a torus palatinus – a ridge or bulge at the inter-maxillary, inter-palatine suture line, where the vomer has been 'forced' inferoposteriorly with the hard palate, by the action of the lesioned maxillae, etc. – vomeric depression. This is to say that the vomer is displaced inferiorly, and has become a wedge keeping the maxillae in that locked position.

The vomer being a highly pliant, thin, flat sheet of bone, torsions easily, and due to its articular ramifications must be considered along with the maxillary lesion. Realise this complexity is not the norm, but rather an adaptation to compensate for earlier irregularities.

Check for motion by palpation. There is more than one way of palpating, and of treating this case. Sutherland, Magoun, Lippincot, Brookes, and Upledger, all favour slightly different methods, but they all aim at assessing the motion/restriction present and returning the area to full mobility . . . that's what really matters.

53 VOMER & ZYGOMA

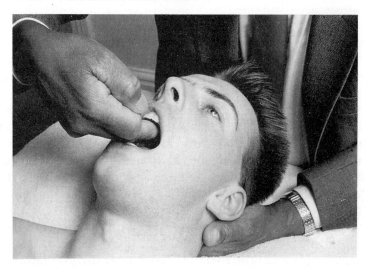

One finger method of elevating the Vomer

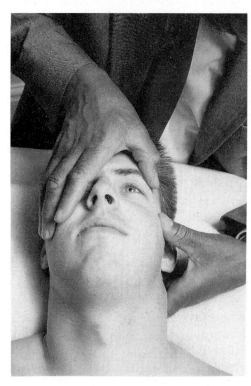

Opening the fronto-zygomatic suture

As is axiomatic in osteopathic practice, you are going to increase the lesion to effect a helpful change. The pressure you use in this endeavour must be minimal, as the inherent physiological forces will be 'on duty' as it were, to effect the desired change.

The method we have found most satisfactory is to place the pads of the middle fingers of your hands beside each other in the patient's mouth, with the tips just behind the transverse palatine suture on the horizontal plates of the palatine bones. (As you will realise by now the palatine plates and the palatine processes of the maxillae work together). Sense the motion. One side may well feel rigid, unyielding; and the other free, with pulsatile sensation. It is usually the side of the convexity that will be rigid. (You may now, if you wish, check your findings by moving to the maxillary palatine processes and repeating the above).

Now that you have assessed the situation it is possible to treat locally. Approximate the middle fingers and again contact the palatines with the pads. The patient can close his mouth until he is comfortable. Give a little upward pressure to increase the lesion with a slight lateral inclination, and wait. In a minute or two you will detect a marked pulsation under both fingers, denoting sutural release.

Hold the position until you sense an evenness of pulsation on both sides. Slowly and delicately withdraw your fingers from the mouth momentarily (this gives a little respite for the patient to swallow, etc.). Repeat the procedure with the same finesse only this time the pads of your fingers should be a little behind the incisive fossa – behind each upper incisor – in the centre of the palatine process of the maxillae. It is possible to use the teeth at the fossa to give added leverage – carefully! Undue pressure may well rupture the veins of Galen, with greatly undesirable consequences.

It is possible that the difference created in the position of the maxillae through your intervention is imperceptible at first, but do not be anxious. Often this treatment will need to be repeated a few times at weekly intervals, but the desired results will certainly present themselves. That abnormally high palate will begin to flare, and the torus palatinus will disappear.

If you are dealing with the mandible as well, the action is repeated with the thumbs either side of the symphysis menti internally – the rest of the fingers can be around the outside of the jaw for the practitioner's ease of working.

This may also take a few repeated treatments to secure the desired release. For the moment these procedures are all that are required locally; but there is still the underlying spheno-basilar lesion to rectify. You will not secure the mobility of the facial fields without involving the sphenoid. Any articular malposition or malfunction of this bone will not only affect cosmetic facial symmetry, but will also be significant in orbital function.

The sphenoid also influences the ethmoid through articular contact at the lateral masses, crista galli, and cribriform plates. In turn the ethmoid manifests

ESSENTIALS OF CRANIO-SACRAL OSTEOPATHY

54 INCREASING THE DIAMETER OF THE ORBIT

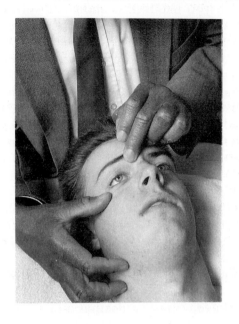

Oblique diameter

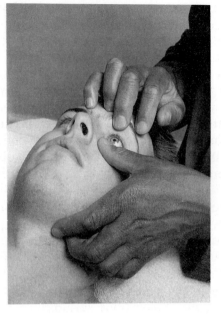

Vertical diameter

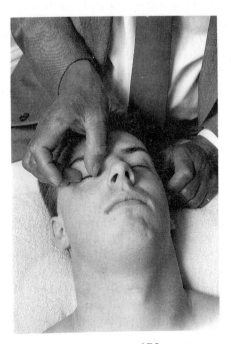

Moving the eyeball

THE FACIAL COMPLEX

articular contact with the vomer at the ala, through the rostrum of the sphenoid. To achieve mobilisation of the ethmoidal notch and frontal, think of these as a complex including the maxilla. Begin by distraining the nasals as previously described. This technique has the capacity to liberate the frontal processes of the maxillae and ethmoid by separation using the nasal bones as a lever.

In freeing these you create a 'knock-on' effect to these apparently inaccessible structures within the cranium. Therefore the lack of accessibility of a particular articulation should never be a deterrent to its mobilization if you continue to visualize the unit character of the mechanism.

Particular care must be given to the study of the bevels of all these bones and their articular facets, in order to obtain a heightened appreciation of the complexity of cranial mobility, especially in the facial fields.

Note again the description of the 'banana head' in Chapter 2. Basically the treatment entails increasing the lesion and waiting for the release. But, before proceeding with this, it is beneficial to spread the zygomae which, as we have seen, will also be in lesion.

Place your thumbs on the anterior angle of the zygoma – at the inferior orbital border. Gently 'spread' laterally, you will feel a resilience that 'gives' under your thumbs (probably more one side than the other) as the sutural restrictions are freed.

We are now ready to deal with the sphenobasilar concavity. Span the patient's forehead with your right hand so that the thumb and middle fingers are engaged with the great wings of the sphenoid – in front of the Pterion (the other fingers are merely resting lightly on the forehead). Exaggerate the middle of the arc of the concavity by applying minimal inclination laterally. Hold until there is that subtle yielding, whereupon you will deem that aspect of the procedure to be complete. (See Plate 45, p. 124).

Now let us consider further that very particular portion of the facial complex, the orbit and its contents.

In treatment of the eye the most important thing is to achieve proper drainage. Success depends on the release and mobilization of all local and peripheral restriction – thus restoring proper dimensional integrity to the orbit and its contents.

For the eye – as for the ear, nose, and throat – treatment of the Palatine bones must not be neglected. Stimulate the sphenopalatine ganglia by getting the patient to open his mouth and contacting the ganglia at the pterygopalatine fossa with your index finger. The perpendicular plate of the palatine forms the fossa's medial wall. The positioning of the body of the sphenoid turns the sphenopalatine notch into a foramen at this juncture. The other parts of the fossa are formed by the infratemporal maxilla and the pterygoid process of the sphenoid.

In order to stimulate the mass of soft tissue encountered, the practitioner

ESSENTIALS OF CRANIO-SACRAL OSTEOPATHY

55 NASALS & LACRIMALS

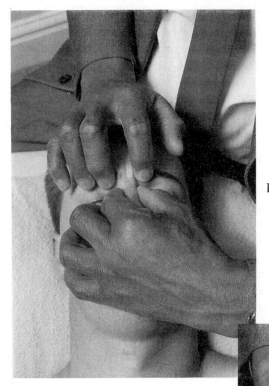

Distraining the nasals

Draining the Lacrimals

either increases the pressure of his finger with a slight pumping action, or enlists the patient's co-operation by having him turn his head medio-anteriorly. Within a minute or so you should feel the tissues relax. Lacrimal watering often occurs with this procedure.

The epithelia and glands of the roof of the pharynx, mouth and eustachion tubes, sphenoidal sinuses, nasal cavity, lacrimal nerves and glands are some of the structures supplied by the sphenopalatine ganglia.

The osseous components of the orbit must be freely movable – thus giving freedom to the extrinsic muscles. There must be unrestricted internal and external rotation. Recall that the inferior border of the frontal, the orbital border of the zygoma and the superior border of the maxilla form the rim of the orbit. As we shall see you can widen these and increase the whole dimension of the osseous bowl. Please note that before attempting any of the procedures in this Chapter, it is as well to apply 4VC in order to provide free drainage to the venous sinuses via the emissary vein.

Of course, the best results will always be obtained through treatment of the entire cranium. You may drain the eye and other aspects of the face to great advantage, but there is no reason to stop at that. Check the occipito-mastoid area for lesions. If present these can be crucial; and do not forget the rest of the frontal bone and the temporal – in fact the whole vault and base. Lesions in these regions can be very limiting to proper drainage. Sometimes they may even negate all your efforts. Remember the functional unison of the cranio-sacral mechanism and you will not be deterred by any apparent local lesion of the eye, etc. Drainage is by way of the opthalmic veins, the cavernous sinus, and the petrosal sinus. Hence the over-riding necessity to investigate the articulations which might harbour lesions that infringe the integrity of the drainage system.

So observation of the whole head and the facial and orbital symmetry in particular is the first priority. Does one orbit appear more crowded than the other? Do they lie in the same plane, or is one higher or more prominent than the other? Does the colour of the sclera and iris of each eye appear the same?

Test for intra-orbital pressure by first asking the patient to close his eyes. Then gently palpate over the centre of each eyeball with the third finger of one hand, and discern the resilience. The side that shows least 'bounce' denotes a crowding, a congestion of that orbit.

Widen the oblique axis of the eye by gentle digital traction (separation) with the thumbs at the frontal notch and zygomatic process.

Wait for the registration of a directional slackening of the tissues under your thumbs. Do not oppose this, for this is significant of a necessary change of fluid pressure. Just hold and wait for the motion of these fluids to abate.

Drain the lacrimals by digital pressure (20 secs) on the medial aspect (inner canthus) of the eye, at the Alar grooves, and at the symphysis menti. Distrain the nasals by holding the bridge of the nose with the thumb and index finger of one hand, whilst the index and middle fingers of the other hand are 'hooked' under the medial angles of the frontal – either side of the glabella. Apply opposing force until there is a slackening as previously described. This affects the sphenoid, ethmoid – as far as the lamina papyracea of the ethmoidal labyrinth.

Next, further widen the diameter of the orbit, this time vertically, by gentle digital pressure using the index fingers, under the supra-orbital foramen of the superciliary arch, and the infra-orbital margin of the maxilla. Distrain as before described.

Now with great care and extreme gentleness move the eyeball with your thumb and first finger. First from side to side. Find a point of balance and hold for a few moments. This will aid decongestion. Holding it at the point of balance you will sense the movement of fluids within. Then adopt the same procedure with an up and down movement of the eyeball.

To complete the treatment gently rest the thumbs on the frontal eminences (ossification points) for a minute or two. This 'settles' the tissues. You may find there is a change in the complexion of the patient. But if this does not occur within two minutes do not continue holding as the patient will then be left with a 'heaviness' – the opposite of what you are aiming at.

Now with a feather-light touch of your thumbs stroke over the superciliary arch (the eyebrows) from the frontal notch laterally several times. This enhances the patient's feeling of well-being.

The procedure described can be of great benefit in cataract, glaucoma, diplopia, nystagmus, astigmatism, etc. With practice the cranial practitioner will find variations in this routine to suit his individual patient's needs.

Another familiar facial area of concern is the temporomandibular joint. Maladjustment of this is a lesion of common occurrence. The aetiology is varied, but the most prevalent – other than direct trauma to the jaw anteriorly or laterally – is attributable to injudicious dental treatment occasioning a malocclusion.

Contributory factors can result from a strain at the sphenosquamous pivot – a shift of one pterygoid process causing congestion of the coronoid process; unilateral temporal rotation (internal or external) – there are no T.M.J. lesions without temporal repercussions.

The patient usually presents with pain and/or soreness at the T.M.J., especially felt when talking, laughing, or yawning; and with difficulty chewing food. There can also be the added nuisance of a disturbing clicking or grating whenever he moves his jaw. The diagnosis is usually obvious and simple. Have the patient supine and sit behind his head. Place your middle fingers on each of his mandibular fossae, then ask the patient to open his mouth wide and close slowly. You will find that the lower jaw will close with a little lateral 'jump' to the lesioned side. The symphysis menti will also be inclined to that side.

THE FACIAL COMPLEX

Here we must digress. Occasionally there is a fixation in either the closed or open position of the jaw – a dislocation in fact. Sometimes you will find a chronic condition where there is now no pain, etc. but the patient has been left with a jaw that will only open 2 or 3 fingers breadth. This condition is often described as 'arthritis of the jaw' but it is actually where fluid has infiltrated the joint space and subsequently hardened/calcified. This does not have to be a permanent state. In our experience 4VC repeated over a few weeks will secure the necessary resolution.

Returning to the more usual conditions that you will encounter, there are several techniques available for tackling this problem both externally and internally, and all of them to some degree are valuable – effecting a quick local resolution.

The shot-gun method most often used osteopathically is to turn the patient's head ¾'s away from the lesioned side, angle the hypothenar edge of your hand along the line of the jaw and as the patient takes a deep breath and then exhales, give a little thrust medially – towards the symphysis menti. An audible 'click' will usually be heard as the head of the mandible reseats into the T.M.J. fossa.

A.T. Still's method was to sit behind the patient and span the angles of the jaw with one hand (from below) and ask the patient to open his mouth. Then he cradled the occiput with the other hand, aligning the thumb on the T.M.J. A firm forward, somewhat rotary movement, replaced the mandible. To stabilize this correction he placed thumb and forefinger at the internal angle of the jaw (at the level of the 3rd molar) and the other hand on the outside of the same and pressed medially.

But here we are concerned with the 'knock-on' effect cranially, of this seemingly local problem. What you see may, as we have indicated, suggest that you further disarticulate the joint in order to effect a resolution. But in reality this is like putting the cart in front of the horse. You will find a better result obtains if a gentle cephaladly directed traction is given to the mandibular ramii. The middle finger can be 'hooked' under the angles of the jaw. This is little more than a stretching of the skin, you are not grasping. As this force reaches its maximum efficiency there will be an automatic impaction of the T.M.J. – you will begin to feel something happening. It may be a lateral or A.P. movement. Follow this. It is the precursor to the impending balanced state.

You will soon be aware of some degree of movement higher up in the temporoparietal sutures. This will register in the palms of your hands on either side of the patient's head, as the parietals are obliged to move into external rotation and the angles of the temporals change. At the same time this movement is effecting a stretching of the dura acting as a diaphragm, changing the fluid pressure in the cranium. As soon as you perceive a cessation of activity realise that it is time to stop this aspect of the treatment.

Now you are in the position to do as your inclination would have been in the first place, had you not been thinking cranially. Apply caudal traction to the mandible without attempting to manipulate it.

The T.M.J. will be amenable to balance as you continue the traction; the temporals, parietals and C.S.F. will harmonize physiologically. The treatment is complete when movement ceases, but it is as well to instruct the patient not to take 'large bites out of large apples' as we say to patients in our Clinic, for at least 48 hours.

Before we leave this subject it is worth mentioning that for many unstable shoulder conditions it is necessary to examine the T.M.J. and Temporal bone. Despite lack of any symptomology these areas are often the hidden cause preventing desirable resolution at site.

CLAUDE BERNARD

'A dextrous hand without a head to guide it is a blind tool. A head with a hand to realize its wishes is an impotent nothing.'

'Milieu intérieur, the constancy of the inner state in the higher forms of life.' (As the 'founder' of endocrinology and the term 'internal secretion' Bernard paved the way for recognising the state of homeostasis).

'Scientific medicine, gentlemen, which it ought to be my duty to teach here, does not exist.' (From first lecture in physiology to students).

'That which we know is a great hindrance to our learning that which is as yet unknown.'

CHAPTER TWELVE

Special Techniques

E.T.T. ENERGY TRANSFERENCE TECHNIQUES

This application of tactile capacity is primarily devised to harmonize sutural articular behaviour, and facilitate intracranial membraneous activity. It is useful for evaluation as well as treatment, and is a therapeutic means of transferring energy from one part of the body to another.

Some aspects of E.T.T. (as we shall now refer to it) are known as 'V-spread.' It can be used in a specialized way to free restricted sutures; restoring their integrity.

E.T.T. can be used somatically, but always with one finger, or hand, on the head, and the other on the area needing 'release.'

It must be borne in mind that cranial restriction means lesioning, and lesioning means imbalance; not only to the local area, but also of the entire human structure, which, in the final analysis is jeopardizing to health. This is particularly important in the case of tension in the soft tissues with their osseous anchorings, at the nuchal/cervical area. This area is continually at risk from such restrictions via the dural/fascial relationship.

With E.T.T. the energy will transfer from the directing fingers to the restricted area and the mobilization will be manifest. So let us see how we would approach a patient to free a sutural imbalance.

Start by working over the whole scalp, palpating gently with one or two fingers to find any sore or 'hot' spot. You may find more than one, or a line of soreness. Take a 'V-spread' of two fingers of one hand so that they are angled to the farthest point of the scalp contralaterally, and that is where you place the middle finger of the other hand. Wait – you will most likely feel a softening or relaxation under one or both hands or be aware of an initial throbbing at the site of restriction that then abates.

With practice you will know the moment to release – when the 'still-point' has been reached, all pulsation ceases and the area appears to settle. This might be heralded by the patient's body language (a sudden visible relaxation) as an obvious relief from undue pressure, whereupon the patient sighs, twitches pleasurably or simply relaxes deeply. Deal with each area as necessary. It is sometimes necessary to complete the above procedure and then take another

SPECIAL TECHNIQUES
56 E.T.T. FOUR FINGER TECHNIQUE

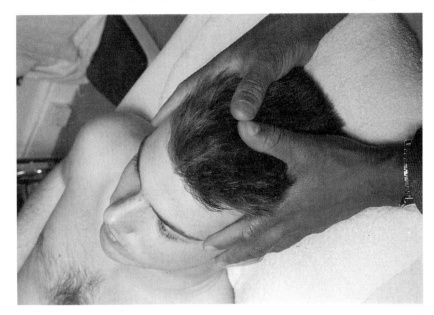

Four finger Hold

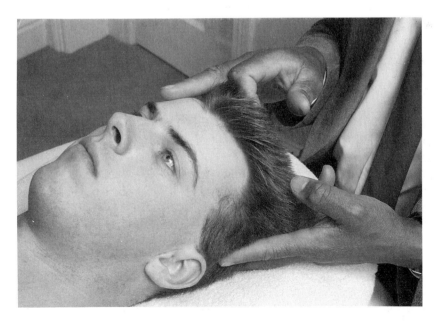

'V'-spread

57 ENERGY TRANSFERANCE TECHNIQUES
FOUR FINGER TECHNIQUE

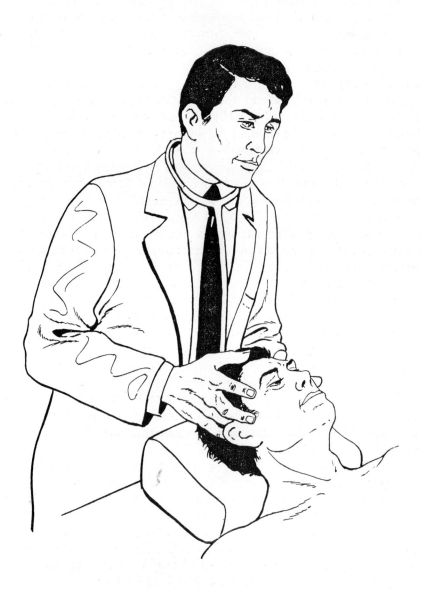

angle with the V-spread to complete the treatment (almost as if to surround the area).

Again palpate the scalp (using your fingers over a small area at a time as before) and you will find the soreness and heat have gone, and the patient often expresses a feeling of being 'much improved' and often symptoms that have remained from a particular condition, despite perfectly competant previous treatment, will have disappeared.

Basically the same technique is used when working from any other area of the body. It is obviously easier to work on the trunk and upper limbs as the practitioner would find it physically difficult to have one hand on the patient's foot and the other on the head at the same time (although the distance can be reduced by having the patient sitting down).

Again a contra-lateral V-spread is used, but one can use the whole hand on the head if so desired. When working on the trunk in particular a unique phenomenon is often observed. The head and neck will go through a series of movements/contortions as if winding and unwinding itself. As with all cranial procedures go with what is happening do not attempt to restrict these movements. They may last a few seconds or as long as thirty minutes, but again there will come a still-point where all motion ceases, and after holding a little longer to stabilize the effect, the treatment is finished. The sore spot will be gone and the patient will usually say he feels better.

The movements are almost certainly dural, and often appear to be a recurrence of certain actions/restrictions the patient experienced at an earlier time, even years ago, in other words, not just related to the present complaint.

This is particularly so in dorsal hot-spots associated with cervical tissue states.

Particular attention should be paid to not allowing the head and neck to 'return' in the same direction as it described. Put another way the practitioner should guide the head and neck in a direction he has not seen it take in winding and unwinding.

Although a V-spread of two fingers on one hand and the middle finger of the other is the most usual approach, it can be, as just mentioned, the whole hand either end (but not both) when you are well practiced in using this technique and can accurately evaluate its potential effects.

This technique is also effective for mobilization of the Falx Cerebri. Place the palmer surface of one hand over the patient's forehead sagittaly, so that the tip of the middle finger abuts the nasion. With the other hand under the patient's head, position that middle finger at the inion. Slightly incline the superior hand cephaldly and wait. You will become aware of a 'lifting' or freeing sensation under the upper hand as you mobilize the anterior poles of attachment at the dorsum sellae and sella turcica.

The middle finger of the lower hand is, of course, adjacent to the confluence of sinuses and therefore to the division of the falx cerebri to form the tentorium cerebelli and the falx cerebelli.

When there is a resignation – a relaxation of surrounding tissues you may gently remove both hands. You will observe that the patient's eyes are less heavy – wider open and clear; that the complexion has changed; and the patient appears to be much brighter and livelier.

There are occasions when E.T.T. will be helpful in our next subject.

MIGRAINE

'Headaches' and 'Migraine' are perhaps the most frequent ailments affecting patients arriving at our Clinic, and we should be careful to distinguish between these two labels.

The layman's idea of migraine is any recurrent head pain beyond the bearable 'ordinary' headache, and one which is accompanied by one or all of the following: sensitivity to light (photophobia), blinding flashes of light, nausea, vomiting – and consequent loss of appetite – dizziness, vertigo, etc. all of which may last one day or a week. They will often say that they 'know' it's a migraine because certain indications (known as aura) precede onset of head pain.

Now, in our understanding as practitioners, we would classify a headache as a symptom – most probably of extracranial origin, and due to a variety of primary or secondary factors, sometimes of non-specific derivation. Generally these can be said to emanate 'from the shoulders upward' – cranial and cervical nerve irritation, emotional and mental stress, toxic states, referrals from eye, ear, nose, and throat conditions, etc. Other causes may be referrals from gastric and abdominal disturbances, lumbar and sacral or other musculoskeletal anomalies, and, of course, do not forget to include fascial restriction. Congestion and immobility in (or under) old scar tissue is a notable 'hiccup' (interruption) to effectiveness of treatment in many conditions; remember fascia and dura interact – stasis in peripheral fascia therefore can mean dural instability.

It is obvious, then, that many of these headaches respond well to soft-tissue and manipulative procedures, which reduce the tension and congestion, lessen the stress factors, and thereby have an effect not only on the symptoms, but also on some of the underlying causes.

Migraine on the other hand is a clinical entity. It often seems to run in families or be hereditary; usually affects highly intelligent, well educated people; has an element of neurosis (especially in female sufferers) and may be linked with an allergic tendency (i.e. eating chocolate, cheese, bananas, red meat; or drinking coffee, etc. can precipitate an attack). It almost always exhibits as pain on one side of the head only (Migra – Gk: hemicrania) and tends to begin in adolescence and gradually disappear before the age of retirement.

It is accompanied by one or all of the symptoms previously listed and may also occasion diarrhoea or constipation, irritability or depression, amylopia (disturbances of vision without detectable organic lesions) and teichopsia ('fortification figures' – a characteristic zig-zag of brilliant light seen at onset of migraine). Attacks are periodic (in women they are often associated with the menstrual cycle) and can herald onset of pathological conditions such as hypertension, arterosclerosis, and intracranial aneurysm. Migraine is often described as opthalmic, abdominal or gastric depending on the area most affected.

So what is this disabling condition that results in the loss of so many working-man hours? It is congestion – fluid stasis – most often synonomous with a cranial (sutural) lesion (or restriction), and/or an upper cervical lesion – constriction of cranial arteries appears to be the trigger to these attacks, then dilation of the venous vessels ensues, accompanied by cranial oedema.

Transmitted generally by the 5th (trigeminal) cranial nerve, the pain is often excruciating – of a very high threshold – blocking out all other sensations and leaving the patient totally exhausted afterward.

This nerve (along with the 10th (Vagus) cranial nerve) supplies the fibres of the meningeal coats, hence the asthenia and loss of reflexes, trophic and sensory disturbance in the area of distribution, etc, and the pain in those highly sensitive parts of the head – the sutures and foramina.

Pain-killers, ergotamine (an oxytoxic) alpha blockers (which depress sympathetic activity), vaso-constrictors, etc. are often prescribed, but these are merely suppressants/alleviators, they do not prevent the re-occurrence of migraine (though they may reduce the incidence of attacks) nor do they restore functional integrity as do adjustive therapeutic techniques which affect the sympathetic cervical chain, upper thoracic ganglia, etc.

It is necessary to understand a little more of what is happening to the meninges and craniovascular system here. Whether we sit or stand, move or lie down, the pressure in the veins of the body varies, being subject to gravitational pull, hence there is a part of the cervical area where zero pressure is observable when a body is standing – the neck veins collapse, and so on. is why you sit a person down with his head between his knees when he feels faint, or you raise the feet and legs above the level of the heart in traumatic shock – to heighten venous integrity in the head and thorax – increasing blood supply to the vital organs. But the meningeal venous sinuses cannot reduce pressure in this way. They do not have 'collapsible' walls but firm, inelastic walls, which do not 'give' to reduce pressure within.

This pressure is 'sub-atmospheric' (below negative pressure) so much so that if a sinus is exposed to the outside air – from trauma or surgery, say, it will 'suck-in' air and create an embolism in the venous lumen.

Taking a case history from a patient complaining of migraine is not easy. Often no one event appears to have precipitated the onset of symptoms, or any traumatic event that did occur seemed so insignificant at the time that it has been ignored. It is highly probable, however, that trauma is a prime causative factor in the production of the precipitating cranial lesion. A blow on the head, perhaps, even years before the onset of symptoms, that (as we have said) neither the patient himself nor his parents or friends thought significant, can produce these pernicious results. In fact, all injuries to the head, even relatively slight ones, can, in course of time, be serious in their effects. Of course, if there is a clear history of injury involved – however long ago – that is obviously the place to start.

Sphenobasilar lesions are commonplace in headaches and migraine, as well as in facial paralysis, myopic astigmatism, vertigo, hypertension, influenza, sinusitis, hay fever, mental stress, and they often follow from dental work, extractions, etc. The greater wing of the sphenoid is often elevated on the side where the pain occurs. This creates dural tension, due to constriction in the basal area generally.

Treatment therefore will depend on the results of your evaluation. Often 4VC and/or Frontal lift is enough to ensure amelioration. The headache or migraine will abate almost immediately – even while you are carrying out these techniques at the first visit.

If it does not, there is most likely an underlying structural fault – a spheno-basilar side-bending or torsion lesion is the most likely, or an externally/internally rotated temporal. If it is possible to mobilize all the bevels of this bone (and it is not always easy to achieve this) great relief will be afforded. Many neuralgic conditions, temporomandibular joint dysfunctions, and facial palsies, as well as ear problems, will also respond favourably to temporal techniques. Freeing the parietal bones may also prove beneficial in migraine conditions. As with all other cranial procedures the aim is to achieve homeostasis and reverse pathology however long it has been present.

EAR PROBLEMS

Let us now consider what help we can give to patients complaining of ear problems. Many of these people come to us with diagnoses such as middle ear infection (otitis media) tinnitus, vertigo...

Tinnitus is, perhaps, the most prevalent. Patient's present with noises in the ear, often accompanied by persistent headaches, eye problems, catarrh, sinusitis, etc. These noises can range from a disturbing low roar to a high pitched whistle.

In severe cases this can affect the patient's entire life-style. They can be irritable, depressed, withdrawn; not being able to hear well and therefore being unsure of themselves.

Despite much research in recent times, many books being written on the subject, and the use of devices such as sound maskers there still does not appear to be any genuine popular solution to the cause of this disabling condition.

If you examine the ear itself there is usually nothing anomalous to be found. The answer lies in examining the temporal bone in which the ear is housed, and the surrounding osseous, cartilaginous, and soft tissue structures. The first thing that you ought to suspect is that the Eustachion tube is in dysfunction.

A little over two inches in length this tube is partly cartilaginous and fibrous; and partly osseous and has a mucosal lining. It begins at the middle ear and extends anteromedially (and slightly inferiorly) to the nasopharynx. The bony one third is in the petrous portion of the temporal bone and normally remains open, and the remainder projects from its inferior border via a groove at the lower edge of the medial pterygoid plate of the sphenoid's inferior surface.

This auditory tube helps to equalize pressure on either side of the ear drum. This equality of pressure allows the drum (tympanic membrane) to vibrate and conduct sound. In infections of the nasopharynx the mucous membrane at the lower end of this tube becomes inflamed (swollen) closing the orifice, and thus any attempt to open this mechanically by 'blowing,' swallowing, etc. can transfer such infection to the middle ear.

However, clearing the tube mechanically is of benefit when the pressure outside and inside are temporarily unequal, such as during rapid descent when travelling in an aeroplane. This clearing by swallowing or chewing tends to obviate internal bulging of the tympanic membrane and subsequent rupture.

In health the movement of the temporal bone controls the opening and closing of the orifice of the Eustachion tube. In inspiration, the petrous portion of the temporal rotates externally opening the tubal orifice, and in exhalation the opposite occurs. (The petrous portion internally rotates closing the orifice). Therefore, fixation of the petrous portion in either direction will keep the orifice artificially open/closed. If fixed in the wide open position the patient will complain of noises such as roaring, ringing, or blowing.

If the noises produced are described as whistling, hissing, or buzzing, this indicates that the tube is sagging and is held in the closed position.

As has already been indicated yawning, chewing, sneezing and swallowing also affect the function of the auditory tube. These noises are thought to be from the passage of blood in the surrounding vessels – internal carotid artery, jugular vein, etc.

It should be noted that the two levator veli palatini attach to the cartilaginous

ESSENTIALS OF CRANIO-SACRAL OSTEOPATHY

58 SPECIAL TECHNIQUES

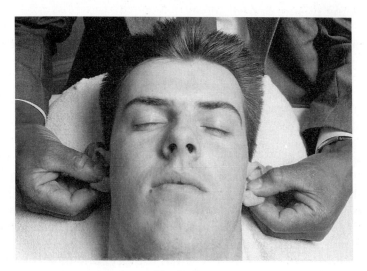

Ear Pull

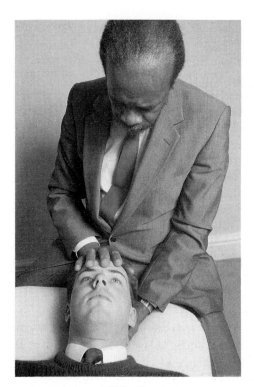

Falx Cerebri

SPECIAL TECHNIQUES

portion of the auditory tube, and the petrous portion of the temporal; controlling the position of both structures. The tensor veli palatini extends from the sphenoid and the Eustachion tube to the palatine's horizontal plate, and controls pterygoidal function. The palatopharyngeus aids opening of the Eustachion tube; sphenobasilar torsion and sidebending rotation can irritate the tubal mucous membrane causing tinnitus and hearing loss.

The petrous portion technique for adjusting an external rotation of the temporal bone is to loosely interlace your fingers and slip your hands beneath the patient's occipital squama, making sure your thumbs are relaxed, but extended along the mastoid portions of the temporal bone. Incline the head slightly to the lesioned side. Find the point of balanced membraneous tension in accordance with the rotation. Holding the occiput slightly posteriorly while holding the tips of the mastoid process anterolaterally might prove an added advantage in securing the best results. Have the patient take a deep breath holding it to the limit. This brings the body's corrective forces into operation, as the lesion is exaggerated.

For an internal rotation lesion of the temporal the correction is almost opposite – the difference is that you hold the occiput slightly anteriorly with the tips of the mastoid posteromedially. Have the patient exhale to the limit for inherent corrective co-operation.

Another reliable technique for temporal dysfunction, which we have proven in our Clinic, is this. With your forearms resting on the couch, lightly take hold of the patient's external ears (pinna) making sure that your thumbs are securely nestled on the inside in a firm, delicate hold, together with the index, second, and third fingers on the outside. Incline posterolaterally (down and out) in a sustained balanced fashion well within the patient's pain tolerance. You may quite safely persist with this hold on the ear for several minutes.

Incidentally, this is not usually painful, nor uncomfortable, but it is imperative the patient must feel secure in order for the requisite response to be elicited. Therefore it is vital for you to establish a good working rapport. Your fingernails must be short, that there be no scratching nor pinching.

In a little while a discernable slackening of the tension of the hold will be manifest. This is the sign that the treatment has had its effect. Ask the patient to take a deep breath and then exhale to the limit, and hold without breathing in for as long as possible. You may now gently remove your hands from the ears, for the treatment is complete. This technique is probably the most innocuous of these listed.

There is also a correlation between this condition and restrictions/dysfunctions of the cervical vertebrae in general, and C2/3 in particular. When any lesion at this level has been treated, there is often a marked reduction in the level of noise, or it may disappear altogether.

The efficacy of any treatment of the ear may be greatly augmented by reducing any undue tension of the nuchal tissues at the base of the skull. It is advisable before commencing any temporal techniques to check the temporomandibular joint and the tone of the sternocleidomastoid.

It may be necessary to repeat these procedures for the desired results to be achieved. Persistence will prevail.

VERTIGO

As far as torment/torture is concerned there is possibly not much to choose between tinnitus and vertigo save that the effects of the latter are more strident and spectacular – a health disturbance of some magnitude – this falls into two categories, objective and subjective. Both are concerned with movement – a feeling of movement.

The objective type is found in the patient who suffers the illusion that his environment is in rotation. This is to say he is the object. He has the sensation that the world is revolving around him.

The subjective type is the one who has the illusion that he is revolving in space. He is the subject.

Neither of these conditions is to be confused with dizziness, which is concerned with unsteadiness, confusion; as they are not one and the same thing. Suffice it to say the aetiology is unclear, but the question is: as a cranial osteopath can you offer the sufferer any help? I believe you can. Firstly you must know what the lesion is. Begin by evaluating the integrity of the neck muscles. In these circumstances they are usually found to be in sustained contraction.

This offers you the first clue to what may be expected cranially, a temporal bone lesion, perhaps? This could, of course, be unilateral or bilateral, but essentially this lesion is associated with the cervical constriction.

The history may reveal a blow on the head, a neck jolt, or some toxicity, occasioning tissue imbalance. Disharmony within the delicate tissue arrangement concerned in these structures may well have some such aetiological bearing. However, the temporal being locked impinges on the integrity of the rest of the cranio-sacral system. Hence the nervous system is also in disarray producing this specific result – vertigo – illusion.

These symptoms may be accompanied by sinusitus and dizziness – often called Meniere's Disease.

In your analysis of this complaint let this dictum be your guide. Any restriction perverting normal cranial articular activity is a blatant evidence of dysfunction in the cranio-sacral mechanism. Having given this due consideration, your technique for alleviating the burden of vertigo may follow the same pattern as for tinnitus. Special attention must be given to balancing

SPECIAL TECHNIQUES

the temporals, and you will have a very grateful patient. Now we'll look at problems a little further afield.

THE COCCYX

This is largely neglected by practitioner's as a significant site of lesion possibilities. In fact any osseous structure that has as many muscular attachments as this unit must perforce be very important to cranio-sacral considerations of respiratory excursion.

In health this unit can be found occupying various positions. In some people it is greatly anteriorly curved, in others less so.˙ Some are slightly torsive/twisted. In any event homeostatically this osseous complex must be mobile.

59 SPECIAL TECHNIQUES

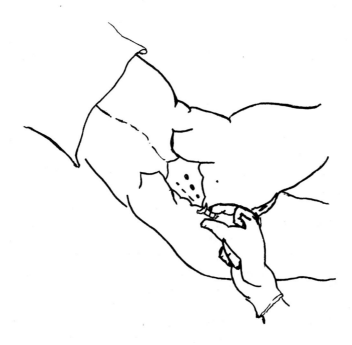

COCCYGEAL ADJUSTMENT

Pain from coccygeal lesions can be very severe (coccydynia, coccygalgia). This is partly due to the close proximity of the Ganglion of Impar which is the most inferior part of the sympathetic branch of the autonomic nervous system's chain of ganglia, to the anterior surface of the coccyx.

Because of its location, injury here can cause pelvic disturbances such as uterine and prostatic malfunction, bowel movement and elimination impediment, etc. It is not unusual to find that despite symptomology being absent, reflexes from the coccygeal area are responsible for severity of pain and dysfunction being maintained in lumbar, lumbosacral conditions. The patient who does not appear to adequately respond to treatment that would normally be effective may well have a 'silent' coccygeal lesion, with jamming of the sacrum between the ilia. This complex lesioning is usually the result of trauma. It is the type of thing that occurs in childhood games. The child is playfully induced by another to sit on a chair and just as he is about to do so, the chair is pulled out from underneath him. The result is that he falls heavily on the base of his spine. He may of course jump up and appear to think little or nothing of this prank, and that it is no more than a big joke. To the young and energetic this injury may not be considered to present more than a passing problem as the pain or particular discomfort does not seem to be sustained. Unhappily, however, it is not always so simple. Nature's memory is not so deficient. The joke of today may well result in the horror of tomorrow. As the individual matures, so does the effect of that injury.

But this injury is not confined to the young. It is also the injury that occurs in the 'banana skin' slip. The person falls heavily on the base of the spine causing not only local trauma but, of course, sending shock waves to the atlanto-occipital area, etc. The sacrum can and often does wedge itself caudally between the ilia, and the distal aspect of the coccyx suffers injury, being dislodged and driven anterolaterally.

Think of what happened to the coccyx. The position it assumed by force may be accommodative, and it is then fixed in that state. It no longer shares in the respiratory phenomenon of flexion and extension of the sphenobasilar symphysis.

The patient/parent, and sometimes even the doctor, would never associate the results of this injury with a child's subsequent asthmatic condition. They would never attribute the shortness of breath from which he is now suffering to anything like that. His lack of energy or alteration in his general standard of health – due to the lack of available air, etc. is not deemed to be significant. Nor would they look to this cause for the child, or adult, who fidgets and is never comfortable sitting down for any length of time. Yet you and I know that, in health, the coccyx must move in correspondence with the laws of the primary respiratory mechanism (which will maintain the vital capacity reading), so that now that young person is consigned, as a consequence, to a substandard liftstyle.

Hence this can be serious, occasioning at the least headaches, and/or nausea because of the resultant abnormal tension conveyed by shock waves through the dural tube to the intracranial mechanism (falx cerebri, etc).

What can the cranial practitioner do for these anomalies? With tactile finesse he can reverse the entire handicap. If it is a compound lesion, that is to say one involving both coccyx and sacrum both may be treated at the same time. The patient lies on his side with his back to the osteopath, his knees comfortably flexed. With a gloved hand the osteopath then inserts his lubricated middle finger gently into the patient's rectum. He now grasps the sacrum between the inserted finger and the thumb and skilfully articulates/mobilizes that structure by working it free with an A.P. (anteroposterior) movement, and laterally. If the thumb and finger do not appear to harmonize in facilitating the desired freedom, the practitioner may choose to involve his other hand, working over the sacrum in unison with the finger inside, to induce relaxation of the sacral and coccygeal muscles and ligaments. In no more than one or two minutes he will have achieved his aim by utilizing the same technique for the coccyx. Relief is often immediate. Pain will disappear, the patient will be able to sit comfortably – though should be advised to sit down gently for the next forty-eight hours to allow the area to stabilize.

The fact that you can increase or decrease a headache by judicious movement of the coccyx should confirm your diagnostic evaluation. Patients who have suffered from respiratory conditions often are seen to take a deep breath or sigh almost immediately after treatment as the whole mechanism is freed. Respiratory excursion can be used during this procedure to assist the practitioner.

Most often one treatment is enough to bring the coccyx into full function.

However, there are some occasions when this manoeuvre has to be repeated after an interval before full resolution can be achieved.

Of course, there is always more than one technique for effecting mobilization of any structure. The patient may be prone with a pillow underneath his lower abdomen and upper thighs, and the practitioner may follow the same procedure as previously described, but, however it is effected the results are often so dramatic in improved health and well being that consideration of the coccyx should never be left out of our therapeutic armoury.

MOULDING

Moulding is an often neglected technique. It was devised for reversing abnormalities in the contours of any osseous structure which, by the very nature of its contiguity will not permit normal development and physiological

ESSENTIALS OF CRANIO-SACRAL OSTEOPATHY

60 MOULDING

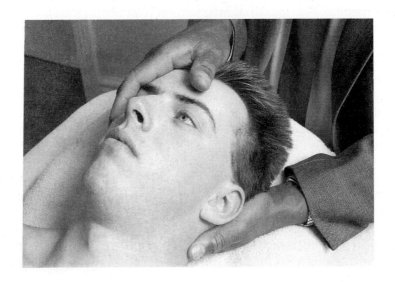

Vault

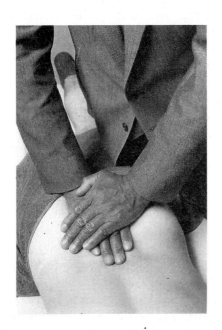
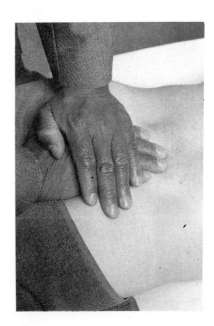

Sacral

function. This is observable when certain bones are anatomically out of balance with their neighbours due to the imposition of abnormal or restrictive forces pre or post natally, predisposing to cranial malfunction.

In the young child moulding is particularly indicated. The skull may be resistant to change such as should normally have taken place at the earliest crying. There will be obvious warping – the result of faulty arrangements of the bones at the base of the skull. Left unattended over a relatively short time – a week or so, perhaps – that individual may well be consigned to some of the most distressing maladies imaginable – allergies, postural imbalance, gastritis, nervous disorders, deglutitional stress, depression, meloncholia, obesity, dysplasia, lack of coordination. . . He or she may never be able to compete with others on an equal footing in a world already rife with so many injustices.

In our clinics inquiry into the birth pattern of our patients should always form part of our investigation – and here I must digress to bring in the importance of the patient's history and hereditary background.

Pathological osseous changes manifested in the spine have their counterpart in the skull. The clearest example of this is spinal scoliosis. Contrary to many practitioners thinking, this does not only correlate to the cranium but most often originates there.

The history of this is usually traceable. Great pains must be taken in eliciting all the relevant facts – even those which have passed into antiquity through ignorance or forgetfulness must be brought to bear on the more obvious findings. In the final analysis they have their place and may well be the vital trigger to the urgently needed solution. It is therefore essential to base the history on the broadest possible plane, maintaining due regard for the entire human organism, as an integrated physiological unit.

From this history you will be able to evaluate and classify abnormalities; whether hereditary, dietary, endocrine, environmental or whatever; not forgetting that in many cases it will be a combination of such elements. A correct diagnosis demands this and will automatically lead to the right conclusions and therefore the right treatment, given that you possess the required finesse.

I would put heredity at the top of the list for investigation.

We need to be aware that if our parents are not healthy we are hardly likely to have inherited good health. The health of the genetic cell is all important. A healthy apple tree will normally produce perfect apples; of the right size, colour and shape, and according to its variety. Human beings are similar. If the parents are healthy and from a healthy stock, their children will inherit those good traits – subject to certain provisos.

If the parents have an endocrine or nutritional imbalance, it will always be reflected (even if latently) in their offspring. Therefore, it is often blind, foolhardy, and even a matter of hope rather than educated judgement, to attempt treating your patients without some enquiry into their parental background.

So with the birth pattern that we have been discussing – the nature of it should be recorded at the initial consultation and examination. The pity is that so many people have gone from birth to the time that they walk into our clinics perhaps ten, twenty or even forty years later without this assessment ever having been made. It is worth emphasizing that many a tragic condition might well have been avoided if proper moulding had taken place during the birth process and where this did not occur naturally, a cranial practitioner could have offered lasting help if that had been obtained early enough – Magoun would say immediately after the birth. However, we can still effectively deal with the problem even years afterward.

Despite what we have said in Chapter 10 (Lesions – vault & base) it must be understood that the first cries of the infant are not guaranteed to alter the shape/contours of the skull to that which it should be in every case. There are certain occasions where extreme moulding occurs and this will result in pathology.

It should be discernable on examination that this 'over-moulding' is the cause.

Now that we have very briefly examined the effects of the infant's first cries, let us remember that this happens when he takes his first breath. This breath is epic, in the sense that it inaugurates pulmonary activity as a substitute for foetal gasiform placental procedure. Normally this phenomenon of the first breath and cry occurs immediately after birth – sometimes as the head emerges from the birth canal, but a good many births in our so-called sophisticated society are neither normal nor natural. The advent of injudiciously applied anaesthesia and analgesics for the mother make the difference. They are often responsible for protracted contractions and subsequent maternal difficulties, suffered even months after the birth. Drug intervention may offset the immediacy of that baby's urgent first breath by slowing down normal physiological responses, thus facilitating mechanical trauma/restrictions and cranio-sacral locking.

Moulding techniques are not restricted to infants and children, and may be equally applied to cranium, sacrum, or any other part of the body, wherever indicated. Bones form and reform according to the pressures that are imposed upon them, and resultant pathological deformation is not unusual.

In considering treatment let us take an infant skull for an example and deal with a very familiar problem. We will look at the baby that has predominately been laid on one side in his cot and now presents with a rounded, even skull on one side and an extremely flattened one on the other. It has been said that the child 'will grow out of this' and it may well be that the bony contour will become more rounded with time but the internal damage caused by such pressure will have already taken place.

SPECIAL TECHNIQUES

That pressure will not only impinge on the cerebral structures themselves and the glands, ventricles, and vessels, but also on the meningeal 'tent' – thus transmitting imbalance/restriction to the matal coats of the spine, the body fascia, and so on.

For the particular condition we are considering, sit at the head of the couch cradling the infant's head in one hand in the sagittal plane – that is, with the fingers abutting the foramen magnum and the heel of the hand at the parietals, the other hand will be on the frontal (on the lesioned side). The palms of the hands are the part that will now gently mould, inclining toward approximation.

A very small amount of pressure is all that is necessary. You are aiming to 're-shape' the skull, so you will move your hands from place to place to achieve this. It may be necessary to treat on several occasions until the desired effect is obtained.

In the adult a slightly different method is employed. Where there is obvious bulging of the right frontal, let us say, take a contra-lateral line (as explained in V-spread) and place one finger, or the flat of the hand on the bulbous area; the finger or palm of the other hand at the contralateral site. Gently incline as before and wait until a reaction is perceived. It is by persuasion, not force, that you will achieve your object.

At the sacrum, have the patient prone, and use one hand on top of the other, to mould from various angles (Plate 60). It is a similar procedure when moulding a foot, leg, or hand – the aim is always to restore optimum function and physiological balance (not necessarily to obtain cosmetic symmetry). As with a patient with a scoliosis, or kyphosis, etc. the discerning practitioner would not attempt to alter asymmetry, if there are no pathological indications to warrant it. Diagnosis and correct evaluation, therefore, are of the utmost importance.

HAROLD IVES MAGOUN

'Every organ in the body exhibits the phenomenon of pulsation or rhythmic action, and the brain is no exception.'

'The cranial picture, in so far as it influences the central nervous system, dictates the structure and function of the entire body.'

(Cranial) 'lesion correction is not manifested by a "chug" but as a soft slippage of the membraneous, cartilaginous or bony element within its dural envelope in relation to its fellow, when the natural motive forces of cerebrospinal fluid fluctuation and membraneous pull are put into operation.'

CHAPTER THIRTEEN

Gynaecology

Gynaecology does not appear to be high on the list of priorities in some osteopathic Clinics. Many reasons may be advanced for this omission, but lack of knowledge of the subject is probably the chief cause. Therefore a brief survey of what is involved (the consequences of gynaecological disorders and the benefits of proper evaluation and treatment) will doubtless be of great value to some of us. At least, it is hoped, we may be provided a good working knowledge. To begin with we need to know the anatomy and physiology of the female genitalia.

We are not only concerned with inherent abnormalities that interfere with the functional efficiency of the female reproductive system itself. Nor are we only discussing the pain, discomfort, and misery that so often afflicts females in these areas. Attention is focused on the patient who presents with period problems – too long, too short, too heavy, none at all; infertility, prolapse, fibroids, malignancy; the menopause – hot flushes, vaginal dryness, irritability, depression; as well as intransigent low back pain, headache, pain in abdomen, gluteals, thighs (especially on the inside surface), which are maintained reflexly by disorders in the genitalia.

Contrary to popular (and some medical) opinion, menstrual and menopausal problems are not 'normal.' Time and time again patients coming to the Clinic say that they have been informed that 'all women suffer like this,' 'you'll have to learn to put up with it – until the menopause' or 'it's normal.' This is just not true. Pain, discomfort, dysfunction, etc. should always be investigated with a view to effecting a solution to the underlying cause.

The menstrual cycle is controlled by both the endocrine and the autonomic nervous systems and therefore any dysfunction of either (such as an undersecretion of the pituitary) has to be taken into consideration and may need to be treated initially.

The whole of the pelvic structure – osseous, muscular, ligamentous, and fascial – monitors reproductive function, often by reflex stresses.

The 10th and 11th Dorsal vertebrae carry the sympathetic nerve supply to the ovaries and these together with D12, L1 & L2, supply the uterus. The cervix, however, receives innervation from the parasympathetic chain via the 2nd, 3rd, and 4th sacral vertebrae. Hence the need to examine carefully, not only the pelvic bowl itself, but the lumbar and sacral spine.

Most young women's menstrual problems appear to be structural (and can be 'familial') usually associated with congenital hip disorders, sacro-iliac and low back strain, arising from sacro-occipital anomalies. So treatment of the purely 'local' findings will not suffice. It is always necessary to examine the cranium as well. More often than not a cranial base lesion/restriction will be found.

Examination will reveal one side of the occiput (and therefore the sacrum) to be elevated. It is obvious therefore, in such a case that the best solution will be achieved by treating both sacrum and occiput. When harmony is established between these two structures (and that means to the rest of the cranio-sacral system) the menstrual cycle should become normal.

It is as well to remember – especially in young women – that the emotions play a large part in gynaecological disturbances. The soma and psyche are inextricably linked and emotional disturbances at home, school, work, etc. or difficulties with boy-friends, exams, and so on, can greatly disturb the menstrual cycle and intensify symptoms.

In older women of child-bearing age these same findings may apply, but other factors come into play. Let us first discuss infertility. It should be noted that as the woman reaches her late thirties the fertilization level drops (especially in nullipara women – those who have not borne children) and, incidentally, the risks of pregnancy increase.

Sterility is usually from three main causes. Absolute, Functional, or Acquired. Absolute sterility is a lack of, or serious defects in, those factors that make up the female reproductive system (genitalia, endocrine. . .). Functional is a treatable defect in the organs themselves, the nutritional needs necessary for successful pregnancy, or other related functions – of the endocrine glands in particular. Ignorance of reproductive behaviour, unruptured hymen, and vaginismus come into this category.

Acquired infertility is any factor preventing or impeding conception or gestation that is the result of pathology or trauma (infection, accident, malignancy, new growth, displacements) surgical sterilization (often after normal births have taken place), use of family planning devices such as the contraceptive pill and interuterine coils, etc. Obesity can also be part of this acquired infertility.

It should not, of course, be forgotten, that one of the causes of a woman not becoming pregnant is infertility in the husband.

Often infertility does not exist because of some endocrine or even cranial abnormality – although these will be present. These women are infertile because their posture is wrong, and this is very significant, for there is no likelihood of change for the better until this is altered.

GYNAECOLOGY

The pelvis is 'frozen.' Like the 'frozen shoulder' which is not an unusual sight in any osteopathic Clinic, it's rigid. According to Tidy, neglect the frozen shoulder and movement will become permanently limited.

Well, the same description as applied to many a woman's pelvis doesn't mean 'permanent.' It is a functional disturbance. The saving grace is that you can undo that malfunction which, incidentally, is usually a pointer to a host of other bothersome anomalies. Physiologically you can mobilize that pelvis, and depending on the prevailing family circumstances the population will be increasing!

How will you do this? The technique is not the most important thing, as there are several of these in common usage throughout the profession. It is more important to be able to identify the problem in the patient. The symptoms are usually obvious. An anteriorly locked sacrum, so the stance is forward but the back is straight, the feet are everted, the hips swing – viewed posteriorly this walk may appear pleasing, attractive, but it is anomalous. Please note however that the ilia will appear mobile, but the coccyx will often be immobile (in partnership with the sacrum, of course). This patient is the one who often appears jovial, happy, confident; but in reality is more likely to be depressive and suicidal. Because of the coccygeal restriction, respiratory distress or incompetence is frequent, the patient being unable to take a deep breath.

Occasionally you may find a bi-laterally anterior sacrum maintaining an antalgic stance (an increased lumbar lordosis) an upward and backward rotation of the sacral apex resulting in an extension lesion of the sacrum.

For the majority of cases lesions such as we have already touched on make up the multiple causes of infertility:

- Hormonal imbalance (most often between (pineal) pituitary, thyroid and ovarian function) which governs circulation and is supplied by the sympathetic nervous system;
- Other musculo-skeletal disturbances – vertebral lesions which impinge on nerve roots and inhibit blood supply to fallopian tubes and endometrium – that is, vascular incompetence;
- The state of the cervix (with reference to the sympathetic and sacral nerves).

Restore functional balance generally and that frozen pelvis in particular, and the infertile woman becomes fertile, and the woman who has had several spontaneous abortions, or miscarriages, carries to full term.

Many of the period difficulties in the older adult – especially in those who have borne children, result from uterine inflexion and mismanagement in care during labour. This latter may produce sacro-iliac strain, cervical and occipital inconsistencies (sometimes from the administration of general anaesthetics).

61 GYNAECOLOGY

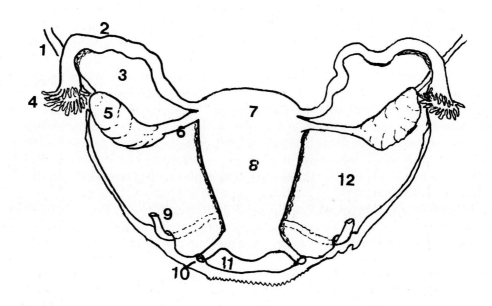

FEMALE REPRODUCTIVE ORGANS

1. Ovarian Suspensory Ligament
2. Fallopian Tube
3. Mesosalpinx
4. Fimbria
5. Ovary
6. Ovarian Ligament
7. Uterine Fundus
8. Uterine Body
9. Ureter
10. Uterosacral Ligament
11. Pouch of Douglas
12. Broad Ligament

Many problems are also as a result of epidural injections, which can, in severe cases, cause long-lasting paralysis of the lower limbs, and coccygeal innervatory disturbances, which will cause extreme pain. The pelvis is disturbed. When the ligaments between the sacrum and coccyx, and those at the symphysis pubis open (stretch) during labour they do not always return exactly to the norm – putting unequal strain on the sacro-iliac joints. Nerve impingement and circulatory disturbances are common – giving pain in back and legs and a propensity to varicosity later in life. Merely examining/treating posteriorly (at the lumbar and sacral spine) then is not sufficient. This patient may also present with unequal leg length, recurrent back pain, an inability to sit comfortably for more than a few minutes, period pains, heavy bleeding, etc. Later in life, fibroids, or uterine or pelvic floor prolapse, are the most common symptoms.

Of course, the first step is to examine the patient thoroughly from head to feet. Having noted musculo-skeletal disturbances, etc. you may procede to examine with one or two fingers of a gloved hand intra-vaginally – with the patient in the lithotomy position.

(It is more convenient to examine if both bladder and bowel are empty). Note the condition of the external genitalia, the shape of the pelvic bowl, the width of the hips, symphysis pubis, and so on. Is there any swelling or inflammation, or discharge such as blood, pus, leucorrhea? Is there any local tenderness? Does the pelvic floor seem firm and elastic? Note any evidence of perineal tears or repair; scars or rashes. Are the vaginal walls smooth or corrugated, dry or moist? The cervix (or uterine neck) can be felt as a half-inch long circular band of tissue at the mouth (os) of the body of the uterus. It should be in the mid-line and show no evidence of swelling or cysts. The os of the uterus should be closed but may bear scars of lacerations received during childbirth (in partous females). The cervix is usually hard, but in pregnancy becomes soft and flattened.

The vagina can be roughly divided into four areas (fornices) and the uterus should be found centrally, towards the anterior fornix, which may also show evidence of oedema, fibroids, or tenderness. Distension or tumours of the bladder can also be discerned.

The uterus itself is almost three inches long (with the cervix) pear shaped, the upper ⅔rds being the body (fundus). It is hollow and muscular and lined with endometrium. It lies in the pelvis just below the pelvic brim, but may be offset or pushed aside in the presence of tumours, fibroids, or adhesions. It is maintained in its position by six ligaments (anterior, posterior, two broad and two round ligaments) which attach to the walls of pelvis, rectum, and bladder. The broad ligaments are said to cover the uterus, fallopian tubes and ovaries 'like a blanket' (with the aid of the suspensory ligaments). The cardinal ligaments attach at vagina, cervix, and pelvic lateral wall. The cervix also has utero-sacral ligaments (which insert at the sacrum). The uterus' position is also

62 GYNAECOLOGY

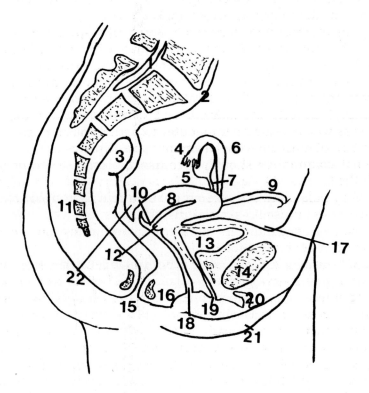

LATERAL VIEW OF PELVIC BOWL

1. Sub-arachnoid Space
2. Sacral Promontory
3. Rectum
4. Fimbria
5. Ovary
6. Fallopian Tube
7. Ovarian Ligament
8. Body of Uterus
9. Round Ligament
10. Os
11. Coccyx
12. Cervix
13. Bladder
14. Symphysis Pubis
15. Anus
16. Perineal Body
17. Perineum
18. Vagina
19. Urethra
20. Clitorus
21. Major Labium
22. Pouch of Douglas (Rectouterine Pouch)

maintained by the muscles of the pelvic floor – the eight perineal muscles which meet at the perineal body being the most important. Weakness of these is responsible for uterine prolapse (prolapsis uteri).

Lateral or posterior (and to some extent anterior) displacements can be the cause of sterility, infertility, dysmenorrhea, backache, headaches, constipation. Retroflexion describes the fundus of the uterus being displaced backwards – but not the cervix. In retroversion both are displaced posteriorly. In either case the uterus will be located in the posterior fornix (which is normally empty) close to the anterior wall of the rectum in the pouch of Douglas. It is as well to remember that uterine inflexions often go undetected as a concomitant of musculo-skeletal and postural disorders.

This internal examination should, of course, be conducted very gently but firmly, with the free hand being used to be supportive over the pubes, and to aid diagnosis by palpation. This should not be a painful exploration – pain or extreme discomfort indicates abnormality.

If the free hand is engaged whilst examining the uterus you should not be able to detect its lower border externally.

In the lateral fornices lie the fallopian tubes and ovaries. It is sometimes possible to ascertain an irregularity here. One ovary may be barely palpable (the norm) the other swollen or tender – perhaps indicating an ovarian tumour, fibroid, or inflammation. (An enlarged ovary could also indicate an imminent period as ovulation occurs, or an early stage of pregnancy). Fibroids are usually hard, solid material, whereas malignancy is felt as a mass of wet sand or seed.

It should not be possible to feel the fallopian tubes either. These end at the ovaries in funnels which have fimbria – finger-like fronds which waft ovum into the tube. If one is blocked it may appear very swollen or tender medially, but if it is very painful, it usually indicates an ectopic pregnancy – which is a medical emergency.

Externally, examine the abdomen with a palpating (flat) hand for any tenderness midline (just below the umbilicus) which suggests uterine inflexion; tenderness or swelling along the internal border of the anterior superior iliac spine – indicating ovarian/fallopian involvement. (Pain described as being every other month may indicate which ovary/tube is involved).

As with most other physical examinations it is the practitioner's eyes, nose, and hands, which are the most sensitive diagnostic tools. No mechanical device or test has yet been invented to replace observation, palpation and smell. We should develop these abilities to the full. Keeping accurate records is another good habit to cultivate. It is as well to chart any anomalies found – their position, size, shape, consistency, the amount of pain present, for example, so that progress can be monitored at subsequent visits.

Referred pain can give very precise clues to lesioned areas. Pain at sacro-iliac joints and S2, 3, & 4, can indicate disorders of the cervix. Pain at D10, 11, 12, &

63 FASCIAL PLANES

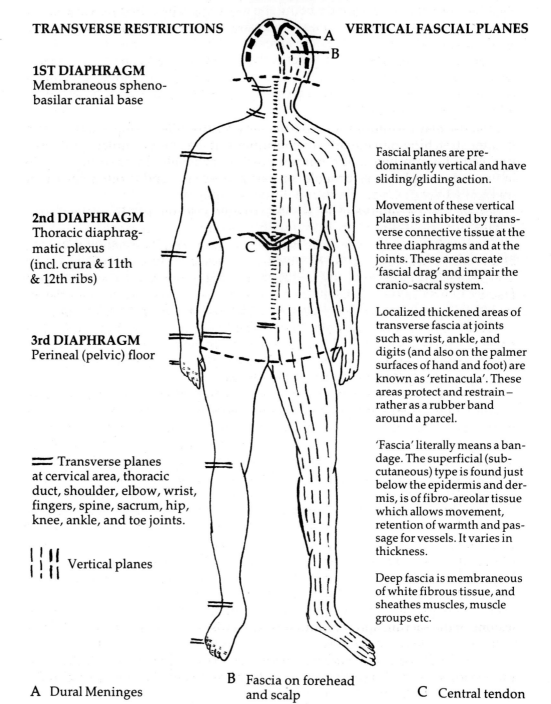

TRANSVERSE RESTRICTIONS

1ST DIAPHRAGM
Membraneous spheno-basilar cranial base

2nd DIAPHRAGM
Thoracic diaphragmatic plexus
(incl. crura & 11th & 12th ribs)

3rd DIAPHRAGM
Perineal (pelvic) floor

= Transverse planes at cervical area, thoracic duct, shoulder, elbow, wrist, fingers, spine, sacrum, hip, knee, ankle, and toe joints.

||| Vertical planes

VERTICAL FASCIAL PLANES

Fascial planes are predominantly vertical and have sliding/gliding action.

Movement of these vertical planes is inhibited by transverse connective tissue at the three diaphragms and at the joints. These areas create 'fascial drag' and impair the cranio-sacral system.

Localized thickened areas of transverse fascia at joints such as wrist, ankle, and digits (and also on the palmer surfaces of hand and foot) are known as 'retinacula'. These areas protect and restrain – rather as a rubber band around a parcel.

'Fascia' literally means a bandage. The superficial (subcutaneous) type is found just below the epidermis and dermis, is of fibro-areolar tissue which allows movement, retention of warmth and passage for vessels. It varies in thickness.

Deep fascia is membraneous of white fibrous tissue, and sheathes muscles, muscle groups etc.

A Dural Meninges
B Fascia on forehead and scalp
C Central tendon

L1, uterine complications; D11, 12, fallopian; D10, ovarian. Needless to say dealing with the 'guy ropes and canvas' (musculo-ligamentous and fascial restrictions) and not just the 'tent pole' (vertebral column) will alleviate many pelvic disorders.

Uterine or pelvic floor prolapse is characterized by a heavy, full, 'bearing down' sensation in the vaginal area. It is found mainly in multipara women (those who have had several children – often in quick succession) or in advancing age as tonus is lost.

Prolapse may be intermittent (particularly noticed after lifting heavy objects, or after stretching movements) or continuous. It may be a complete prolapse – unable to be returned to the normal position or totally dropped beyond the labia; or incomplete – returnable, or partial descent – and is often dealt with medically by suspensory devices or surgical repair.

But by cranial intervention we can trigger visceral somatic reflex. (It is advisable to replace the uterus, if possible, before treating cranially).

By treating the head on a fascial plane (releasing occipital/scalp aponeurosis and cervical fascia) it is possible to resolve over one-third of gynaecological conditions. The head is the suspension point for all body fascia and this 'cap' of fascia extends to C7/D1. Peritoneal collapse is secondary to spheno-basilar fascial collapse (via the central tendon) which can be thought of as a sling.

Visualize the old-fashioned sling held at the two thin ends (the spheno-basilar fascia and C7/D1) and the wider rounded middle section (3rd diaphragm) containing the stone or sling-shot (the uterus). As the sling moves anteroposteriorly it alters the tilt of the uterus.

C7/D1 is a most important part of cranial osteopathic study. Because of the division of the Vagus at this point different effects can be obtained by treating on the left, or the right-hand side. C7 is the control point for coccygeal lesions, rectal problems, uterine displacement, and non-malignant tumours, hiatus hernia, and so on. Any aberration in this area will irritate the thyroid and produce inhibition or stimulation of these areas. Tumours can be the result of thyroid inhibition, causing acceleration of gonadotrophic function.

The right side of this cervical prominence is where to look for the answer to constipation, appendicitis, haemorrhoids, and bladder disturbances. The left side often provides the solution to diarrhoea, persistent heavy menstrual bleeding (especially when combined with the administration of homoeopathic iron), miscarriages, abdominal ptosis, irritable bowel syndrome, impotence and prostatic disorders.

D9 is the genito-urinary reflex, and although L5 'makes and controls all lesions of the sacrum and innominates' as Denis Brookes used to remark – you will not find a lesion at that point.

And if C7/D1 does not evidence tenderness, restriction or lesion? Then find the minimal lesion – remember, it will almost always have a visceral reflex action (see Chapter 15).

A direct correction for a retroflexed/retroverted uterus can be made by pressing the end of the gloved middle finger against the flexed fundus of the uterus, attempting to free it from its adhesions – this can be aided by the index finger on the anterior aspect of the cervix inclining posterosuperiorly. (There is some evidence that maintaining a 'knee-chest' position for a few minutes after this treatment helps to stabilize the corrected position.

Alternatively – and this is to be preferred – whilst the patient remains in the supine position raise both legs above the vertical until the buttocks are just clear of the couch. With the other hand stroke gently but firmly from symphysis pubis to umbilicus several times. Repeat this procedure two to three times.

An anteflexion/anteversion is treated similarly, the inclination of the middle finger being directed superoposteriorly (anteroinferiorly at the cervix). Anteflexion/anteversion is normal in the nullipara (women who have not been pregnant) when the bladder is empty. The round ligaments (in the broad ligament) maintain this position, attaching at the symphysis pubis anteriorly.

However, one of the most successful ways we have found to treat these female structures locally is per rectum. The patient may be prone over a pillow or lying laterally (Sim's semi-prone position) and facing the practitioner.

Insert a lubricated gloved finger into the rectum keeping close to the anterior wall. Sustain pressure on the anterior wall with the pad of the finger (the finger is therefore slightly flexed). This can be very uncomfortable, but after a minute or two there will be a perceptible slackation and, as a consequence, the patient will relax.

If this slackation does not occur within a minute or two ask the patient to take a deep breath and hold – then breathe out slowly. On exhalation take up the slack (that is, give a little added pressure). Withdraw the finger slowly. Insertion and withdrawal are made much easier by the patient's respiratory co-operation. Now check all four walls of the rectum for tenderness – there should not be any discomfort here.

We usually find that one treatment is sufficient, though in a few cases a repeat may be necessary. The best time to treat any gynaecological condition is four to five days after the end of a menstrual period. This procedure has been found to be most effective, not only for retroversion/retroflexion, but for most gynaecological disorders.

Uterine inertia in labour is overcome by 4VC. It helps the uterine centres at the base of the spine to release their accumulated spurious and toxic matter. The level of Pituitrin (from the neuro-hypophysis) is increased, and the uterine contractions return to complete the labour.

Pituitary function is most important in gynaecological considerations. Any encroachment at the borders of the gland – especially at the cavernous sinus – can inhibit growth, disturb the menstrual cycle, or repress the menopause.

A most effective treatment that we use, especially for P.P.P.D. (post-partum pelvic displacements) is to have the patient supine with the practitioner standing at the opposite side of the couch to the pain. Fully flex the knee and hip. Place one hand on the outer surface of the thigh, just anterior to the trochanter of the femur. (The practitioner's forearm may support the outer thigh). The other hand rests firmly on the knee, whilst the practitioner's chest helps to support the foreleg. A quick thrust towards the trochanter usually results in an audible 'clunk', whereupon there is an immediate relaxation, and relief from pain.

Primarily, however, we must think holistically and look to the cranio-sacral mechanism for the overall solution to gynaecological disorders.

IAGO GLADSTON

'The competent clinician will inquire into the patient's diet, work, and recreation, and may venture to inquire into his more intimate life.'

'The endocrines appear to be the regulators of the body's inner relations, even as the nervous system mediates between man and his external world.'

'Time and greater knowledge brought to our notice the 'enemies within,' the diseases due to malnutrition, those due to disturbances in the glands of interaal secretion, and more recently those due to psychological malfunction, the so-called mental illnesses.'

'Treatment of the whole patient is the ideal taught by the leaders in medicine, and practised by an increasing number of medical men.'

'The fact remains, however, that he' (the average man) 'thinks of health only in terms of freedom from disease.'

'It is my conviction that the ultimate destiny of medicine is to devote its energies to the development and realization of the individual's potentialities for growth, achievement, and well-being. I have termed this the practice of personal preventive medicine, to distinguish it from the medical practice of today, which is primarily concerned with the treatment and prevention of disease.'

CHAPTER FOURTEEN

Extracranial Considerations

Outside the cranium the Psoas is arguably the most lesion prone structure of the human anatomy, affecting the spinal complex and consequently the entire organism. Situated between the crura and diaphragm the psoas mediates internal and external rotation of various long bones including the ribs during sphenobasilar flexion and extension. It collects toxins from all over the body and therefore we cannot afford to be localized in our thinking during our clinical investigation of this muscle. We must begin to search for the constitutional causes of the toxicity. Many a low back condition with psoas involvement needs to be looked at very seriously.

Acute psoas spasms are readily recognisable. The patient usually presents in spasm, maintaining guarded restricted posture and gait, being bent forwards and sideways. When there is great concavity to one side you would not normally expect both psoas to be involved. What you will find is that the lumbars are bent anteriorly, but resist posterior bending, and the apex of the posterior concavity denotes the area of greatest concern. These lesions usually correlate to sphenobasilar extension and often treatment of the one, or the other, will suffice to produce the requisite balance and be the solution to a host of bothersome toxic complaints, vague or otherwise. These can be catarrhal states, decayed or 'dead' teeth, post nasal drip, chronic sinusitis, otitis media, eye strains, occipito-mastoid conditions, neurocirculatory asthenia, bowel disorders, undiagnosed abdominal pain (often mistaken for appendicitis) and so on. Why should this be? Because of the fascial relationship between the structures at the base of the cranium, the anterior respiratory structures, diaphragm, abdominal 'guy ropes' (iliopsoas, piriformis, etc.) and the pelvis. These structures have a reciprocating fluid rhythmic excursion – both down and up – which maintains postural and respiratory balance in the body. (There is not room here to go into greater details on this very rewarding study; suffice it to say that here we are concerned to highlight the relationship of the states described, with psoas lesions).

There is something else that must not be overlooked, the Psyche. Is the patient confused? Many a Psoas condition associated with low back pain produces psychological states. So the patient may well have difficulty remembering details, seems vague, or, one may even be tempted to think, is stupid, when really there is a pathological state underlying his entire behavioural pattern.

If the Psoas contracture is allowed to persist the natural concomitant-oedema ensues, as at any lesioned site, crowding the vessels. They being delicate and unable to withstand the undue compression are easily 'kinked,' then the 'back pressure' invades the kidney, and if left consolidates, precipitating renal calculus, bladder stones, etc. these are soon manifested as parenchymal infiltration takes place.

Poor descent of the diaphragm is attributable to psoas contraction, and any pernicious activity limiting diaphragmatic excursion is of tremendous significance. This is borne out by the quality of change that takes place once the structural integrity of the psoas is restored.

Often this is all that is required to mobilize the defence mechanism of the body, and may be the only assistance indicated.

What is the procedure for normalization? Note again the level of the psoas. Locate its origins, 11th and 12th dorsal, 1st, 2nd, 3rd, and 4th lumbar (but not the 5th, it has no origin there) and the iliac fossa at the crest. Note the insertion at the lesser trochanter of the femur – thus it flexes the thigh and trunk. It is innervated by the femoral and 2nd and 3rd lumbar nerves.

It should be said here that when we are talking of the 'psoas' in this instance we are including the iliacus as part of the iliopsoas function – for these purposes they are inseparable. The iliacus' are triangular sheets of muscle that arise from the interior aspect of the iliac crests, the base of the sacrum, and the iliolumbar and sacroiliac ligaments. Their fibres converge with the psoas major on its lateral aspect and also insert into the lesser trochanter. The nerve supply is also the Femoral and the iliacus aids forward flexion of the pelvis and thigh.

Hypercontracted bilaterally, the iliacus will lock the sacrum in cranio-sacral extension – and therefore the cranio-sacral system. Unilaterally hypercontracted it will, of course, distort the sacrum laterally and therefore the occiput, and again the whole of the cranio-sacral system will be impaired.

The minor psoas is also part of this group and lies in front of the psoas major. It arises from the 12th dorsal and 1st lumbar vertebrae and inserts into the iliac fascia, iliopubic eminence and pectineal line. It is innervated by the 1st lumbar, and aids flexion of the trunk. However, as it is missing from well over a third of the population, it does not play a large part in our consideration of the iliopsoas complex.

The iliopsoas complex then, acts as a regulator between the pelvis and the dorsum. Anomalies occurring below the sacrum are adjusted by the psoas through the lumbar spine, with those above D12.

Returning to considerations of treatment, it is obvious that there is a choice

64 ILIOPSOAS & PIRIFORMIS MUSCLES

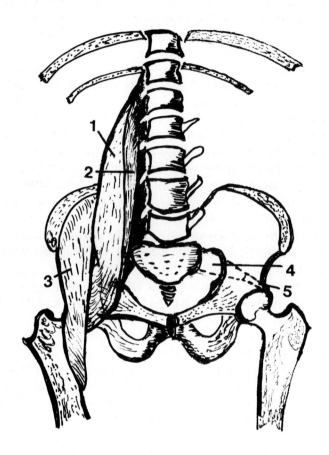

1. Psoas Major
2. Psoas Minor
3. Iliacus
4. Line taken by Piriformis muscle (behind pelvis)
5. Line taken by Piriformis tendon (behind pelvis)

N.B. – Branches of the lumbar plexus (arising from L1–L4) invade the posterior fibres of the psoas major – in 85% of people the sciatic nerve runs posterior to the piriformis. In 15% it 'bisects' the muscle by running between its consequent two bellies of position or direction from which adjustment may be effected. One way is to contact the transverse fibres of the Psoas, with the pads of the fingers of one hand placed on the abdomen. These fibres are found approximately '2 inches across and 2 inches down' from the umbilicus. Apply deep and even pressure while the patient cooperates by taking a few deep breaths. On each excursion let your fingers be carried right down into the triangle of the anterior sacral fossa. To enhance the effectiveness of this procedure you may use the leg on the same side as the lesion as a pump, either by flexing and stretching the leg rhythmically, or by enlisting the patient's co-operation in an isometric manoeuvre. This flexion of the thigh is necessary to relax the rectus abdominus and thus facilitate palpation of the iliopsoas. Of course, there are several variations on this, but whichever method is used one can normally feel – and sometimes hear – the restriction giving way under one's fingers.

Another technique may be effected by controlling the lower ribs – forcing the diaphragm into exhalation (the diaphragm contracts at the point of inhalation), or by inducing a long axial release on the crest of the ilium, and exerting pressure on the anterior sacral fossa. Have the patient sitting; stand behind him and clasp around his 10th, 11th, and 12th ribs bilaterally, forcing them deeper and deeper medially as he breathes out.

Maintain your hold on these ribs and during inhalation incline them forward in a stretching manner and the good results are soon at hand. That psoas lesion will relent.

Whatever technique you employ the prerequisite to homeostasis is that the psoas must be emptied of its toxic matter.

Thrust techniques can prove helpful. This is always provided the law of transverse functioning muscle stimulus is suitably applied. All this means is that if you sufficiently irritate a muscle across its fibres you will break its reflex. Apply this principle to the psoas as described and you will have a grateful patient.

You may wonder why the thrust produces such good results. It is simply a 'shot gun' method – one of hopefulness – rather than the definiteness and cognisance which should be our hallmark. Often by using the thrust a practitioner is of the opinion that he has corrected a disc lesion, but we know that he hasn't. He has by mere chance broken a psoas spasm. What we ought to find out is why the spasm occurred in the first place. This requires investigating a little beyond what we have already discovered.

Think of the psoas 'shelf.' Trace again the route it takes to invest D11 & D12; L1, 2, 3, & 4. By lateral transverse processes it procedes outwards only to turn later and again rotate outwards. There is a positive reason for this peculiarity. It facilitates breathing. In Chapter 2 we briefly surveyed the behaviour of long bones during P.R.M. excursion. The psoas does the same as they do, by following the axis of the femur. It is interesting to observe the vessels that run

ESSENTIALS OF CRANIO-SACRAL OSTEOPATHY

65 DRAINING THE PSOAS

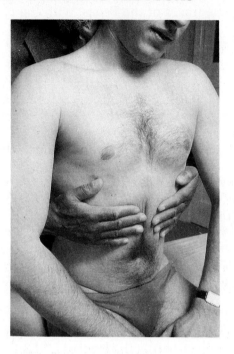

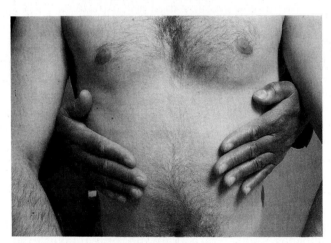

along the shelf; the mesenteric plexus, ureters, ovarian vessels, etc. It is within the area of these vessels that trouble often develops.

The question that remains, however, is in regard of the chronic psoas. How is it sustained? One thing is sure, it is aided by the fact that its antagonist, the piriformis, is also out of balance. It is worth emphasising that a chronic psoas condition (psoitis) is a serious clinical entity. The posture of the patient is often drastically altered. Due to its contraction unilaterally the spine assumes a scoliotic presentation – a side-slip. The pelvis is inclined to one side, and the trunk to the other. Any practitioner of even a short time will doubtless have already seen this, as the condition is so prevalent.

As we have indicated what we are saying about the Psoas can equally be said of the piriformis. Arising from the anterior foramen of the 1st, 2nd, 3rd, & 4th sacral vertebrae and the sacrotuberous ligaments, it passes through the greater sciatic foramen and inserts into the medial aspect of the femur's greater trochanter. It receives its nerve supply from the 2nd sacral nerve, and sometimes the 1st. It externally rotates and abducts the thigh and helps extend it.

It is therefore evident that many patients who present with 'sciatica' and 'backache' will be found to have a hypertonic contracted piriformis as a torsive side-bending of the sacrum occurs.

Remembering the see-saw effect of the pelvic girdle and the cranial structures via the dura it will be seen that this contracture will immediately be mirrored at the occiput – a torsive side-bend to the same side. It is not unusual unusual for this condition to recur due to instability of motion of either piriformis.

However, don't expect to find the piriformi contracted bilaterally, as this cannot be. What you may expect to find with unvarying regularity is that the apex of the spinal concavity is at the level of L2/L3.

Here let us digress a little to say that, depending on what school of thought you follow, or what literature you have read, the psoas, piriformis, or lumbar subluxation are blamed for the symptom picture we have been describing. But, as we can see, it is not possible to apportion the blame to any one element without regard to the rest. It is the relationship of them all to the whole clinical picture that we have to keep in mind.

So, faced with this condition you may also be tempted to think of a nucleur bulge, because of the scoliosis. Don't. In all probability it is neither that nor the so-called 'slipped disc.' It is most likely a decentralization of the nucleur polposis towards the convexity of the scoliosis. But why particularly at L2/L3? Opinions again vary, but I believe that this is the most vulnerable part of the entire column – it has just lost its rib support and has not yet gained the support of the sacrum.

Think of the action most people use to climb into a car, for example. One foot extends laterally forcing the upper part of the body to move the opposite way. Where is the cross-over part of this 'long axis'? At L2/L3. Hence the most sensible way to enter a car is to sit on the side, and then swing both legs in together, and the reverse for emerging.

Or again, when people are bending forward to retrieve something from the floor, and they twist to put it on another plane; again the cross-over point is L2/L3. There is no strutting of any kind in this area. Again we caution our

66 CROSS-OVER POINT
L2/3

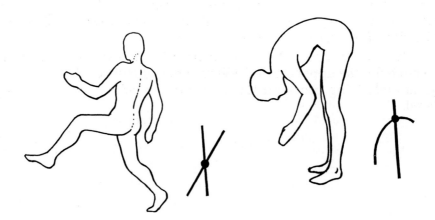

Getting into a car   Picking up from the floor

patients on lifting techniques, don't we?

Athletes and acrobats benefit from this free unrestricted portion of the spine. They are able to perform great feats of contortion which many of us envy. But one man's meat is another man's poison! We are not all so agile!

It is worth repeating that for many people the spinal complex is bedevilled by lesions involving the psoas. But, as practitioners, we must know how to differentiate between piriformis and psoas conditions.

One way is to take account of the pedic angulation with the patient supine. An externally rotated (everted) foot and an apparent *short* leg suggests piriformis. Also the patient often says he is best standing and has trouble sitting on his haunches, and you will find on palpation that there is pain in the opposite upper cervicals and the opposite sacroiliac joint. There is also likely to be pain at the superior border of the femoral triangle on the lesioned side, and sometimes as far as the knee. Occasionally D3 & 4, and D11 & 12 are also involved.

With a psoas lesion on the other hand, the knee and foot will be everted with an apparent posterior ilium, and usually an apparent *long* leg – the bodies of the lumbar vertebrae being rotated towards the convexity.

A psoas lesion can appear bilateral, if the original unilateral lesion becomes fibrosed (contracted), and the other then compensates by hypertrophizing; but a standing X-Ray shows unilateral bulging.

When in doubt do not experiment. X-ray will reveal that psoas outline with all its underlying malevolence. It may not always be found to be heavily laden, as we would expect. There are occasions when it might be seen as insubstantial. In fact, the patient may well have entered your clinic without any indication of trouble in this area.

But, the lumbar condition that will not stabilize; the sacro-iliac correction that will not hold; the upper cervical adjustment that will not abate; these may all have an underlying psoas/piriformis connection which you have not yet considered.

JOHN MARTIN LITTLEJOHN

'The foundation of pathology is congestion and inflammation. Here we have both a structural and functional abnormality.'

'The delicacy of structure, the finesse of adjustment and the elegance of contour form the basis of a perfect body organism.'

'Order is the law of life and harmony is the principle of body architecture and body activities.'

CHAPTER FIFTEEN

The Minimal Lesion

This 'lesion' is little known or understood despite the fact that it is prevalent and very frustrating to the unsuspecting practitioner. The trouble is that it is often obscure, non-strident and evasive. You can only detect it through minute analysis and even then you are not likely to find an adverse symptomatic clinical entity, but a restriction, a lack of normal mobility somewhere in the spinal column. All your cranial efforts can be in vain if you fail to take this into consideration.

The minimal lesion will always produce a visceral reflex. If it does not – it's not a minimal lesion. On questioning, you will discover the patient complains of indigestion, gastric discomfort, diarrhoea, irritable bowel, flatulence, or belching. It is irritation at the minimal lesion which produces this visceromotor reflex.

I recall giving a lecture at a certain college in the south of England where I made mention of the minimal lesion. It is sad to relate that none of the folk listening to me appeared to have any notion of what this meant. Why? According to my late tutor, little or nothing is taught about it even in well known Osteopathic Colleges. Isn't that amazing, and especially so when we realize the undermining influence such a lesion can have on even the best efforts of any practitioner.

As we were saying, this is not an integrated osteopathic lesion. It is one for which you will begin to look when you have used up all your options, and are at your wit's end. With opposing thumbs on the spinal facets of a patient (prone position) check the mobility of each aspect. Start at the top and investigate all articular facets down to the sacrum. Somewhere en route – usually dorsal – you will doubtless discover that subtle evasive restriction. Articulate that area and you will be delighted with the results. Lesion sites of possibly grave concern over which you might have been labouring without success suddenly become amenable. Even the most resistant osteopathic lesion will then begin to yield.

For example, Mrs Collier attended our clinic recently, complaining of severe pain in her low back, radiating down her left leg. On examination L1/2 was

TABLE G AN ADAPTATION OF MARTINDALE'S POSTULATION
(MINIMAL LESION)

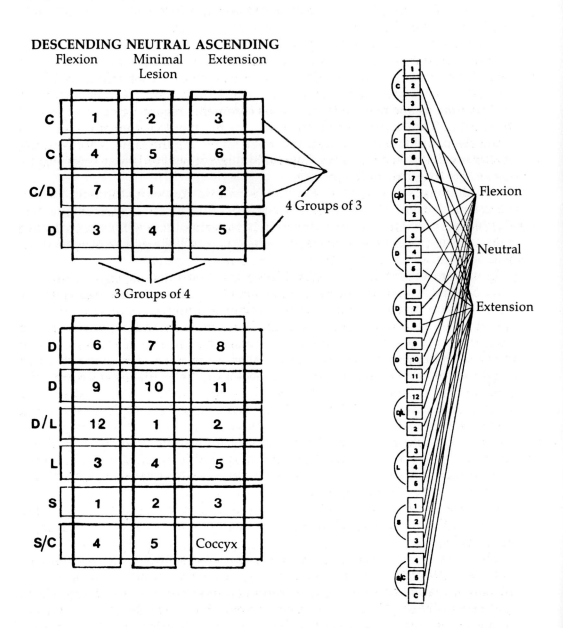

THE MINIMAL LESION

deemed the major offender, and the treatment we gave soon procured the necessary relief from pain. There was no fuss, nothing unusual, hers was just an every-day problem. We recommended further treatment to stabilize the condition. Two days later she telephoned asking whether she might return to the Clinic earlier than booked, as she was in pain again.

On her arrival this time we again examined her thoroughly only to discover that the findings were practically the same as they had been previously. If we were ignorant of the possibility of the minimal lesion we might well have treated the same area purely conventionally. However, she was more helpful to us this time as she made a few nervous comments regarding other aspects of her health. 'I am awfully tired' she said. 'It's not that I've done much or that I don't sleep, but I go to bed tired and wake up feeling the same. Another thing is that my throat is often sore.' Couched in those few words was a meaningful clue to the true state of the patient.

So where would we go now? This was the time to start searching for that elusive restriction. We examined the dorsal spine carefully. Remember, Mrs Collier had not complained of any pain in this area – you will not, as we have said before, find a 'lesion' as such. What you will find is an area of great significance, as far as your remedial efforts are concerned.

You are no doubt familiar with 'Martindale's postulation.' In my Clinic we have adapted and developed a chart of such for quick reference (see Plate 67). You will see that he is really talking about a minimal lesion. He cites the 'neutral' vertebra as the silent offender. Check the chart and you will be able to identify our patients' symptomology, remembering that if the lesion is in flexion (descending) we correct the 1st of the group (on the neutral) even when we think we should be correcting the second on the third. Always correct the first; but if the lesion is in extension, then treat the 3rd of the group on the neutral. Therefore treat C1 *ON* C2 in flexion, and C3 *ON* C2 in extension (ascending).

Most of us have been taught to think of the spinal vertebrae from above downwards, and so we tend to be fixed in our thinking; but why should we be? It is essential to understand how to treat from below upwards; C3/2, C6/5, D2/1, etc. Versatility is important.

Let us again consider Mrs Collier. Minute facet placement analysis revealed that in addition to the L2/1 (as we will now call it) there was a minimal lesion around D2/1.

There had been no pain at all, not even mild discomfort, in this area until we palpated. Nevertheless, as we are already aware through our study of physiology, any immobility in the spinal column must have an adverse effect, and especially so at D2. Through the innervation at this level there is great influence on heart function and circulation. Restriction at D2 lessens visceromotor activity. Consequently there is a diminution in tone of the superficial spinous muscles and heart activity.

This is the area (between D1–D4) where you can either inhibit or excite the behaviour of the heart, etc. by imposing pressure of varying degrees on the vertebrae. You can induce not only drowsiness, but sleeplessness; as well as that, you can lower the blood pressure. In cases where such pressure is already defective it can be dangerous to experiment. Caution is imperative. In our experience, however, when an otherwise apparently relatively healthy patient such as Mrs Collier complains of persistent tiredness – despite any other complaints, this area should be thoroughly investigated.

Once we mobilized the spine at this level for Mrs Collier within a few days her backache and radiating pain in the leg, sore throat, and tiredness completely disappeared.

Having checked the chart and discovered how you would have treated this patient you may be tempted to think that that is all there is to it. But, of course, nothing is 'ever,' and nothing is 'never.'

In common with all 'rules' on whatever subject, this postulation will not apply to everyone you treat. The exception 'proves' the rule. You will find the occasion when you feel you have a definite restriction at D2 *ON* D3 – if so, follow your findings, despite all 'rules' to the contrary.

LIN YUTANG

'A doctor who prescribes an identical treatment for an identical illness in two individuals and expects an identical development, may be properly classified as a social menace.'

'Any good practical philosophy must start out with the recognition of having a body.'

'The old proverb that "to understand is to forgive" is applicable to our own bodily and mental processes.'

'Science, if anything, has taught us an increased respect for our body by deepening a sense of the wonder and mystery of its workings.'

'The more a physiologist tries to analyse and study the biophysical and biochemical processes of human physiology, the more his wonder increases.'

CHAPTER SIXTEEN

Some More Case Histories

*Mrs Crawford, who was 52 years old, came to us exhibiting symptoms, some of which were reminiscent of Parkinson's disease. She had a low backache; her head, arms, and neck were painful, and she had particular difficulty with walking due to a pain in her left hip. These complaints were accompanied by twitches and tremors in different parts of her body.

She had been treated with traction, physiotherapy, and drugs (some of which had caused severe withdrawal symptoms) and none of these had given any appreciable measure of relief. An under active thyroid had been suspected and so she was taking supplements.

On examination it was obvious that this lady was tired, chronically tired, due to an inability to fall asleep. This was mostly because of a paroxysmal flexing of the left knee which occurred whenever she laid down. Hence she complained of only being able to 'cat-nap' and of never feeling refreshed and able to cope during the day. Needless to say her husband was also losing sleep, and life at home was becoming rather strained.

As well as the jerking of her left knee she exhibited a disturbing tremor, mainly on the right side of the body. A cranio-sacral evaluation revealed a pervasive dysrhythmia – an incoordination within the C.N.S. and P.R.M. It was necessary therefore to restore body fluid balance primarily, and musculo-skeletal integrity.

Beginning with 4VC at the first treatment it was significant that the tremors and jerking intensified. This was to be expected, and the hold was maintained until there was an obvious quietening of the limbs – a matter of 2–3 minutes. At each subsequent visit where cranial techniques were employed a similar pattern ensued. These paroxysms sometimes lasted for ten minutes becoming violent enough to lift Mrs Crawford's limbs from the couch, but these were always followed by a definite 'resignation' with all symptoms abating.

Mrs Crawford began to sleep well, and so to regain the energy, confidence and happy personality that had been the hallmark of her character. Within two

* All names have been changed

months it was a joy to see this vivacious, contented lady coming into the Clinic. Family harmony was restored and this improvement has been sustained over the last four years.

Incidentally, with all cranial techniques, wait a few moments before asking the patient to sit up – and whilst he is still sitting, get him to stretch his arms, and fingers, above his head for a few seconds. (If you keep your hands in contact with the patient's arms or shoulders you will notice the moment of fascial slackation when they can bring their arms down). This will re-orientate the system and minimize any tendency to dizziness/vertigo.

* * *

Jonathan was nine years old, of advanced intelligence, but impatient, destructive – hyperactive.

He walked on the tips of his toes everywhere he went as if he could not wait to be somewhere else. He was big, solid and boisterous – almost uncontrollable, and attended a special school that could harness his active mind into less violent channels.

He could be very withdrawn with adults, and very bullying to his peers. He would 'stuff' food one day, and go without a meal on others. He slept a mere three or four hours a night and was a constant upset to his parents and family.

As with all hyperactive children sacral flexion is the most important aspect of the treatment. The fractious child becomes contented; the unmanageable child cooperative; often within a few minutes of holding the sacrum in flexion. It is often noticeable that the child will begin to yawn and rub his eyes – showing evidence of feeling sleepy – during this procedure. That is a good sign, it proves the treatment is being effective. Gradually with treatment once a week you will notice a change in the child's behaviour, as we did with Jonathan.

He would now sit quietly in Reception waiting for his turn to be treated; his eating and sleeping habits became regularized, and he gained friends at school as his behaviour became more acceptable.

* * *

A young man of about twenty five years, Mr Stacey presented with chronic sinusitis, persistent headaches, a nasal intonation and constant sore throats. He also had various eye complaints.

These symptoms had troubled him for several years, and despite sprays, inhalers, pills, etc. he never really improved.

On examination it was found that he had very crowded central facial fields. The maxillae were internally rotated, the bridge of the nose depressed; there was an obvious torus palatinus, and the right temporal was externally rotated. There was no history of accident and it became apparent that these conditions were almost certainly due to birth trauma. We understood that the birth had been prolonged.

In this particular case it was possible to begin treatment with 4VC, then to start mobilizing the facial structures, with maxillary flare, nasal distraint, and orbital widening. At a later stage it was necessary to adjust the temporal outflare – with resulting balance of the occiput.

So we can see that in some instances it is necessary to use several techniques together. In cases such as we have just described it is possible that you might begin with 4VC to 'start up the pump;' then progress, perhaps, to maxillary and mandibular flare, frontal lift, distraint of the nasals . . . paying attention to any dysfunction at the temporomandibular joint, and any imbalance in the superior and inferior hyoidal muscles and ligaments. Then it might be that you would use a vault hold, E.T.T. or sacral flexion to 'stabilize' all you have done.

* * *

Recently I was treating a young woman who has been attending our Clinic over some months. She was good-looking, basically intelligent, witty, and well proportioned; the type of person most of us would look at more than once. The only problem was that that would-be nice woman Mrs Rushton, was melancholy, cynical, and suicidal. At least, that was her case history, and her marriage was practically at an end.

At this particular visit as she lay on the couch, I was most surprised when she suddenly exclaimed 'You know something? My husband is wonderful! I really love him, he's so romantic. And talk about generous – he's kindness itself. I can hardly believe that he's really mine!'

Now this might not seem so extraordinary. But, if I were to tell you just how much Mrs Rushton had been despising her husband at previous visits to the Clinic, you would understand my surprise. The relationship between them was so bad – even to the extent of her having the occasional day or two away from home in a clandestine affair.

But now, happily, and apparently so suddenly, everything was different. Here she was appreciating her husband as much as ever she had done when they first started courting. I remember during my earlier years of studying cranial osteopathy my tutor saying 'more marriages are mended on our couches than anywhere else.'

How could you clinically identify or classify Mrs Rushton? Remember what was said earlier about fluid stasis – and build up of back-pressure; and you will have the answer. This lady came to us complaining of depression and diabetes mellitus. In her case the memory release, as it turned out, was a blessing, as I undid that kink in the straight sinus; but it might have been otherwise – especially if I had ventured to use any force. We really cannot say this too many times. It is all important. You have to be careful.

SOME MORE CASE HISTORIES

* * *

Mr David Picks had suffered from severe asthma for most of his life. In his middle fifties he had lost all hope of ever being normal in health.

His wife and two grown-up daughters were well used to seeing him in extreme bouts of depression. The asthma attacks left him prostrate and exhausted for days, thus heightening his depression. Being an architect, he explained, is a very demanding profession, and often he was unable to do his work – to cope with precision. He was often on the verge of quitting his job. He was also extremely 'body conscious' noting every little asymmetric inconsistency.

Hence, like many asthmatics that we see in our clinics, he had become a very anxious 'fussy' man, constantly trying one medicine after another, and always carrying a pocketful of remedies around with him 'just in case.'

Mr Picks also complained of pain in head, neck, shoulders, and low back – as you would probably expect.

Mobilization of fluid systems and fascia was induced with sacral balance. (You will recall that we never use 4VC where there is respiratory distress). The musculo-skeletal anomalies were also treated by soft-tissue and neuromuscular manipulation.

Over the next few months Mr Picks steadily improved – learning to live without recourse to inhalers, tablets, exercise, and so on. His anxiety and body awareness abated. He began to cope much better with his work and family circumstances.

It is as well in all cases of respiratory incompetence to check the temporal bones. There may well be an unilateral or bilateral internal rotation. The coccyx should always be examined as well. It is often the key to a delay in the expected recovery time.

This particular patient had a flexion lesion of the coccyx, and an internally rotated temporal on the right.

* * *

Mrs Jessop arrived at the Clinic walking with the aid of two sticks, and convinced that life was no more than a burden.

She said that she was supposed to use a wheel chair but that her elderly husband (they were both in their sixties) had had a major operation for aortic haemorrhage and was too frail to help push the chair.

So here was this lady struggling along on her sticks, having had much conventional treatment and having been told that she would never be out of pain, or walk unaided again. For four and a half years she had been the victim of severe back pain, which caused her to stoop badly. Her left knee was constantly swollen, and 'gave out,' as she put it. This rather timid lady felt

ESSENTIALS OF CRANIO-SACRAL OSTEOPATHY
67 & 68 MRS BRAY'S SKETCHES
(See Page 211)

67 page

BUILD UP OVER TWO WEEKS
(Since accident)

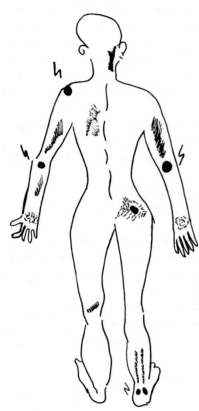

⚡ Intense, sharp pain – in shoulder in repose, others when walking, lifting or pushing.

● Diffuse ache or throb – intermittent

▨ Bruised, aching, feeling when lifting, driving, cleaning blackboard, etc. throbs intermittently

68 ONE WEEK LATER

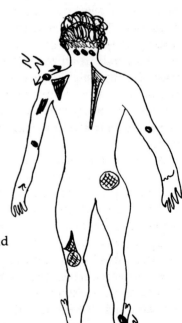

▨ Intermittent aches and twinges

⚡ Bad pain

● Sharp twinges

cheated by circumstances and was now a registered cripple. This was attested to by a recent letter from a specialist at the local hospital.

Examining Mrs Jessop it was not surprising that she exhibited a multiplicity of cranial and sacral lesions, including overlapped maxillae, sacro-iliac strain, and psoitis – consistent with the history as given.

This patient was treated initially with E.T.T. and at the end of this first session rose from the couch and was encouraged to walk across the room without her sticks. Gaining confidence, and now upright, she dressed and went out of the room to where her husband was waiting. 'Look at this' she exclaimed, 'Isn't it lovely, I can throw away my sticks!' Of course, he was thrilled and so were their sons and daughters when they visited her later that week.

On each subsequent visit to the Clinic she showed a marked heightening of confidence and strength, and she spoke of being able to stand at the sink to wash-up, and being able to stand to prepare meals, etc. as she had not been able to do for five to six years.

* * *

A little while ago a struggling Mr Brook was brought into our Clinic. A virtual cripple he could only stand half upright and needed the aid of a stick to balance. In 1968 he had fallen 170 feet down a lift shaft and suffered severe multiple injuries, including seventeen hair-line fractures of the spine. These injuries had rendered him impotent, incontinent of both urine and faeces, in constant pain, and restricted movement for all these years. Lately he had had pain in his right shoulder and hip, and was suffering from nausea, sleeplessness, and an inability to focus.

Can you imagine the embarrassment, not to mention inconvenience this 53 years old married man had to bear? For years he had had to keep to a separate bed.

As an osteopath where does one start with any hope of helping this unfortunate person? On examination his pulse, respiration, and blood pressure seemed reasonably normal; knee jerks were diminished on the right, and his hair was lustreless. I asked him about his diet, only to hear him say that he had great problems. 'Most foods run straight through me, and I have a pain all up my back', he said.

I was not able to elicit any causative disturbances relating to the digestive tract. Nevertheless, checking through the system for obstruction to normal fluid flow, I stopped at the occiput where some measure of distortion was evident, inhibiting the C.S.F. flow, and occasioning an imbalance in the sacrum. I decided that the spinal condition was merely compensatory through the aid of the fascial connective tissue.

With the help of my assistant, I set about rebalancing both the occiput and sacrum. Within a few minutes of my starting the treatment my recumbent patient started to shake from head to foot, and for a few seconds was almost like jelly in my hands. Significantly, during the shaking and the 'jelly' state, all Mr Brook's obvious anatomical distortions appeared to rectify. I immediately stopped the treatment and after a moment asked him to get up from the couch and stand on the floor. This he did quite normally, but with utter amazement, commenting as he took a few steps 'I don't believe it, the pain is gone – I'm walking!'

A more than satisfied Mr Brook left the Clinic assured of a new lease of life. It so happened that it was that weekend that he was due to go to Belgium for an annual Army reunion, and he had previously needed either a stretcher or a wheel chair to accomplish the journey. It appears that this time he went as a normal able-bodied passenger. The next week he returned to the Clinic to keep the first of a planned series of appointments. 'I still don't understand what you did to me, but I'm feeling marvellous! I haven't had any pain in my back, and I've had a dry bed all week. Of course, you don't really expect this to last, do you? My wife is a nursing Sister, and she says it won't. It's most embarrassing. When people ask me what's happened to me, I just tell them that I've been to Lourdes.'

So much for all the good work!

Examining Mr Brook this time I was gratified to see the changes that had taken place. In my mind's eye I could see the man's entire musculo-skeletal system with its multiplicity of pathological changes, as a beseiged city. Due to enemy activity for some time the internal water supply had been severely restricted. But a friendly ally (the cranial osteopath) intervened, breaking the boom, removing the restrictions, and restoring the water supply (the normal fluid flow), whereupon everyone in the city (the viscera, muscles, spinal column . . .) rushed to the taps and other sources (lymph vessels, veins, arteries . . .) for instant refreshing.

As they were revitalized their normal strength returned. Thus we can see that even a semblance of stasis can produce disastrous effects. Fluid flow restriction – which is the enemy – is put to flight, and industry, in the shape of normal health, begins to re-establish itself.

* * *

Typical of the conditions to which we have been alluding was that of a thirty year old woman who came into this Clinic recently. Complaining of low back pain and head aches, she told us how much she had suffered intermittently over the years. There was facial disfigurement, and her gait was quite unattractive. Examination revealed right sphenobasilar symphysis side-bending, impacted right frontal, and fixation of the sacrum in its involuntary axis.

The treatment was relatively simple, when one recalls the magnitude of the result. It was principally a matter of exaggerating the sidebending of the sphenobasilar symphysis, with the respiratory cooperation of the patient, while the sacrum was held in slight flexion.

Who can estimate the value the patient placed upon the change that began taking place in her life – her facial asymmetry for one thing. A delighted Mrs Bunce returned home walking well, pain free, and with a heightened impression of osteopathy.

* * *

Zoe was a beautiful little three year old – a real charmer. With her blond hair and big blue eyes, when she came into the Clinic all eyes were upon her. She had delightful manners and was highly intelligent.

Her mother had brought her to us because she could not walk evenly. Her gait was like the pendulum of a grandfather clock, she rocked from one side to the other in order to progress and it was obvious that her pelvis was not moving as it should and the legs were doing all the work.

Her parents had visited hospitals in various places only to be told that 'nothing could be done' or, even more disastrously, that 'it was normal for some children to walk this way.'

On examination (with the child supine) her right leg was grossly inverted – a dysplasia, in fact. Consequently the pelvis was anteriorly tilted on the right and its movements reduced. This was already causing musculo-skeletal anomalies in the rest of the spine, and these would, of course, become a severe problem if left untreated.

Sacral flexion was instituted accompanied by local moulding techniques to the right leg and foot. Zoe was found to have an occipito-condylar impaction on the left – an anteromedial displacement of the left occipital condyle. This was also dealt with.

Over the next three-four months the exaggeration of gait lessened – the pendular swing getting smaller on each visit and mother reported with great delight after the first month that Zoe had climbed six stairs on her own for the first time. The child was gaining confidence to run around normally – her attempts at this previously had always ended in a fall. How good to know that Zoe can look forward to a normal, healthy, adolescence and adulthood.

* * *

Mrs Bray is a language teacher at the local Polytechnic College. She is in her forties, short, slim, and dark haired, and has regular maintenance visits at the Clinic two to four times a year.

Most often she will bring a sketch of any 'aches or pains' she may have; as on this occasion (Plate 67, 68; p. 208) when she had had a fall two weeks previously. (There were no visible wounds or injuries). These very graphic sketches prove helpful in cranio-sacral evaluation. This lady has happily given her permission for these to be reproduced here for the same purpose. Perhaps you would like to make your own cranial assessment, and suggest a treatment programme for Mrs Bray.

69 CRANIAL HYPOTHESIS

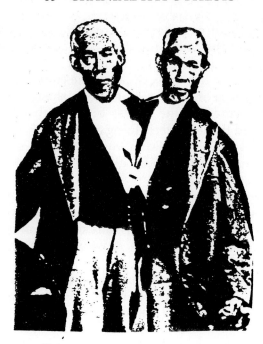

We have spoken of the individual characteristics that pertain even within a family, and it is interesting to find that this was so even in the conjoined twins, Chang and Eng (shown above) who exhibited remarkable differences.

They were opposite in character, temperament, likes and dislikes. They had totally different ideas on hobbies, clothes and food, and it is reported that when one was ill, it did not affect the other; if one drank too much it had no effect on his brother; this, despite the fact that a post-mortem examination revealed the liver and circulatory system to be common.

Born around 1811 of Chinese parentage (arguably in Meklong, Siam) they were connected at the lower chest – at the sternum – by a thick ligamentous band, which had enough 'elasticity' to allow them to almost 'face front' and stand upright. They were taken, via England, to America where they became citizens, and married farmer's daughters, and raised twenty-one children of their own. They lived sixty-three years both dying after Chang had had a short illness. It would seem that Eng died primarily from the shock of his brother's death, rather than from any personal illness.

It is noteworthy to reflect on the factors that can be responsible for such phenomena; and even more interesting to speculate on the possible effects of cranial treatment on one or other of these twins. It would appear that, despite common organs and vessels, the C.R.I., P.R.M., and C.S.F. were separately maintained, enhancing their unique individuality.

I wonder what we would do if we were called upon to treat people such as these. One was irascible and the other equable in temperament. If, as we have seen elsewhere in this book, the very character can change (or be released) during cranial treatments (see p. 206) perhaps we could have created a more harmonious life-style for these two men.

A.E.CLARK-KENNEDY

'The application of science (knowledge derived from exact observation and experiment) to practical medicine (getting people well by any conceivable method!) is gaining so much power and such a hold on us that our real object, the relief of suffering, is sometimes in danger of being forgotten.'

'Diseases could be presented through the minds and bodies of patients in order to correct the bad habit of thinking of them as if they had a real existence apart from the men, women and children who suffer from them.'

'The human body is . . . self-maintaining, self-regulating, self-adapting, self-protecting, and to a large extent self-repairing.'

PART II

70 CRANIAL LANDMARKS

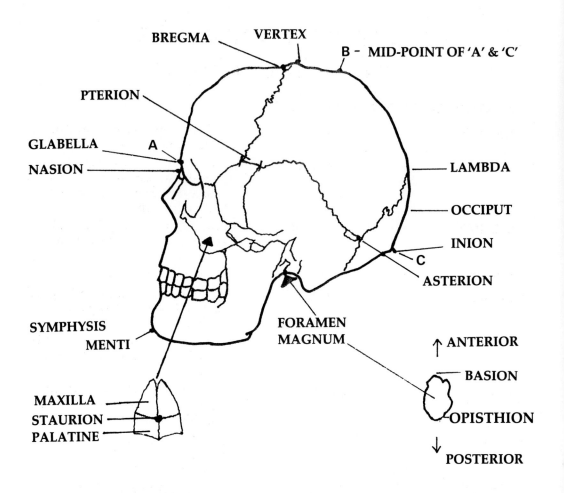

CHAPTER SEVENTEEN

Cranial Landmarks and Other Charts

ANATOMICAL POINTS OF REFERENCE

NASION	(L. nose)	Articular junction with frontal, forms bridge of nose
GLABELLA	(L. bald spot)	Mid-frontal point – being the smooth area between the superciliary arches (eyebrows) on the sagittal plane
BREGMA	(L.Gr.-junction)	Junction of coronal and sagittal sutures. Foetal anterior fontanelle position
VERTEX	(L.top)	Highest point of skull
LAMBDA	(L.letter 'L')	Junction of lambdoidal and sagittal sutures. Posterior fontanelle position
OCCIPUT	(L.back)	Most posterior point of skull. Mid-line of occipital bone and 2–4cm above inion
INION	(Gr. nape of neck)	External occipital protuberance the most prominent part but note:- NOT the most posterior
ASTERION	(Gr.star-like)	Junction of occipital, parietal and temporal sutures. Mastoid fontanelle position
PTERION	(Gr. wing)	Junction of frontal, parietal, temporal and sphenoid bones. An 'H' shaped area of great importance. The anterior portion of the middle meningeal artery is directly underneath. It lies c 3cm posterior to external angular process of orbit

SYMPHYSIS MENTI	(L. growing together/chin)	the line at which the foetal mandible unites
FORAMEN MAGNUM	(L. large hole)	Foramen which allows passage of contents from cranial cavity to spinal cavity. Located at base of occipital bone
BASION	(Gr. base)	Mid-line point anteriorly of foramen magnum
OPISTHION	(Gr. rear)	Mid-line point posteriorly of foramen magnum
STAURION	(Gk. cross)	Central crossing point between median and transverse sutures at the maxillary/palatine borders.

TABLE H   MAIN OSSEOUS COMPONENTS OF THE CRANIO-SACRAL CONCEPT

	SINGLE	PAIRED
VAULT	Frontal (Cranially- count as two)	Parietal
BASE	Occiput Sphenoid	Temporal
FACE	Mandible Ethmoid Vomer	Zygoma (Malar) Maxilla Nasal Lacrimals Palatine Inferior Nasal Concha (Turbinates)
ANCILLARY	Hyoid	Ossicles (Stapes, Malleus, Incus)
PELVIC	Sacrum	Ilia

22 (23) Main Skull
29 (30) including ancillary
32 (33) including pelvic
(Brackets indicate second frontal)

TABLE I ARTICULATIONS

There are many types of joints in the body, but only two kinds are found in the skull – Synarthrosis which has a binding substance such as cartilage, fibrous tissue, etc. and Diarthroses, a freely movable synovial joint with a cavity – e.g. temporomandibular joint.

Synarthrosis
can be sub-divided into
a) *Synchondrosis* – a cartilaginous union with intervening cartilage e.g. sphenobasilar symphysis
b) *Syndemosis* – a ligamentous union e.g. petrosphenoid
c) *Suture* – Sutures/bevels and their movements vary from person to person – an irregular corrugation in one skull may be found as an internal bevel in another, especially at the O.M. suture. Therefore any attempt to 'regularize' a suture to what might be expected (even from this list) could be disastrous. Sutural motion appears to be activated by C.S.F. flow and P.R.M. Elastic, nerve and vascular tissues have been found between sutures. Each suture would appear to be 'bridged' by a continuation of periosteum consisting of cells which are peculiar to growth and repair of bone, and by connective tissue.

Sutures can be divided into:–
Harmonic – (Plana-flat) Edge to edge or apposition of roughened surfaces.
  e.g. ethmoidalmaxillary or vomeroseptal
Gomphosis (schyndylisis) 'Peg and socket' or 'plate receiving' juncture.
  e.g. Sphenoidal rostrum with vomeric ala or sphenoethmoid
Serrate (dentata) Saw-toothed, interdigitated (Sometimes divided into two types)
  e.g. Sagittal or frontonasal
Squamous (Limbosa) Overlapping scale-like e.g. parietosquamous, or a combination – *squamoserrate* – e.g. lambdoid or coronal sutures (saw-toothed and overlapping)

TABLE I ARTICULATIONS (CONTINUED)

SUTURE/JOINT		TYPE	BEVEL Internal	BEVEL External	NOTES
SPHENOBASILAR		Synchondrosis	—	—	via disc (post. 25 years cancellous)
SPHENOPETROSAL	(both parts)	Synchondrosis	—	—	with petrous apex – connected by petrosphenoid ligament of tentorium cerebelli via a disc.
SPHENOSQUAMOUS	(both parts)	Squamoserrate	inf.	sup.	includes S.S. pivot. N.B. POINT OF CHANGE IN BEVELS PREVENTS TRAUMATIC OVERRIDING
SPHENOPARIETAL		Squamous-gliding	⟋		at A.I.A. (anterior inferior angle) Pterion
SPHENOFRONTALIS	at triangular great wing tip at lesser wing in orbit	Squamoserrate Squamoserrate	⟋		limbosa (interlocking) fulcrum
SPHENOZYGOMATIC		Serrate			
SPHENOETHMOID	spine with posterior border of cribriform plate crest with perpendicular plate lateroanterior body with posterior lateral masses	Gomphosis Harmonic Harmonic			
SPHENOPALATINE (Sphenoorbital)	(all four sutures)	Harmonic			the pterygoid fissure with vertical process is described as tongue and grooved
SPHENOVOMERIC	vaginal process with lateral edge of ala rostrum with central ala	Schindylesis Schindylesis	medial	lateral	universal joint, limbosa bevel
OCCIPITOPARIETAL	Lambdoid. (both parts)	Squamoserrate	inf.	sup.	
OCCIPITOMASTOID (Mamillary suture)	O.M. suture.	Notha (corrugated, irregular)			This joint varies in construction / sometimes is a type of harmonic. Notha are for rocking movement. Point of bevel is known as C.S.M. or H.M. pivot

CRANIAL LANDMARKS

Suture		Type		Notes
PETROBASILAR (Petrooccipital)		Synchondrosis		via a disc
PETROJUGULAR (Jugulojugular)	site of Jugular foramen	Synchondrosis		Transverse suture between O.M. and petrobasilar suture. Is a fulcrum-pivot
OCCIPITOCONDYLAR (Atlantooccipitalis)	Cruveilhier's joint	Diarthroses		
FRONTOPARIETAL	Coronal	Squamoserrate medial	lateral	Not always present anatomically, but always accepted functionally
FRONTALIS (Frontofrontalis)	Metopic	Serrate		Interdigital
FRONTOZYGOMATIC (Zygomaticofrontalis)		Harmonic		
FRONTOETHMOIDAL	(All three sutures)	Serrate		
FRONTOMAXILLARY		Serrate Harmonic		
FRONTONASAL	medial border with superior nasal border spine with nasal crest	Squamous Serrate		
FRONTOLACRIMAL		Squamous		Very deep sloping bevel
INTRAPARIETAL (Parietoparietal)	Saggital	Notha		
PARIETOSQUAMOUS (Squamoparietal)		Squamous		
PARIETOMASTOID (Bregmatomastoid)		Notha		Roughened, corrugated at P.I.A.
TEMPOROZYGOMATICA (Temporomalar)		Serrate		
TEMPOROMANDIBULAR		Compound Diarthrosis		A bicondylaris via discs
VOMEROETHMOID		Harmonic		
VOMEROPALATINE		Harmonic		
VOMEROMAXILLARY		Harmonic		
VOMEROSEPTAL		Harmonic		with septal cartilage
ZYGOMATICOMAXILLARY (Malomaxillary)		Irregular		interdigitated

TABLE I ARTICULATIONS (CONTINUED)

SUTURE/JOINT	TYPE	BEVEL Internal	External	NOTES
NASOMAXILLARY	Squamous			
NASOSEPTAL	Harmonic			
INTERNASALIS (Nasonasal)	Serrate			
INTERMAXILLARY (Maxillamaxillary)	Serrate			
LACRIMOETHMOIDAL	Harmonic			
LACRIMOMAXILLARY (both sutures)	Harmonic			
LACRIMOCONCHAL (Lacrimoturbinal)	Harmonic			
CONCHOMAXILLARY (both sutures)	Harmonic			
ETHMOIDOMAXILLARY (both sutures)	Harmonic			
ETHMOIDONASAL	Harmonic			
ETHMOIDOSEPTAL	Harmonic			
ETHMOIDOCONCHAL	Harmonic			
PALATOETHMOIDAL (both sutures)	Harmonic			
PALATOMAXILLARY anterior orbital process with medial orbital surface	Harmonic			
maxillary process with base of hiatus	Harmonic			
lateral edge of perpendicular plate with tuberosity	Irregular			
(Palatina Transversa) anterior edge horizontal plate with posterior palatine process	Serrate			
PALATOCONCHAL	Harmonic			
PALATINA MEDIANA (Interendognathic palatine mediana)	Serrate			
OSSICULAR JOINTS Incudo mallearis	Diarthroses			
Incudo stapedia	Diarthroses			
tympanostapedia syndemosis	—			

CRANIAL LANDMARKS

TABLE J   KEY VERTEBRAE

The following list gives an indication of structures served from the level of each vertebra, as well as those that should be examined/suspected as lesioned (or the site of a minimal lesion) in pathological conditions.

Occiput	Lesions here can cause calcarine fissure; muscular stress induces sphenobasilar lesions		
C.1.	Circulation to scalp, brain, face, pituitary, sympathetic nervous system, special senses	Occipito-Atlantal-Nuchal junction Tiredness, vertigo, migraine, headaches, hypertension, amnesia, insomnia, epilepsy	
C.2	Facial fields – frontal, optic and auditory, mastoid, tongue and sinuses. eye and ear problems, allergies		
C.3.	Cardiac control (with D3) Thyroid (indirectly via clavicular strain from sternocleidomastoid) Facial osseous structures and teeth, cheeks	C.2./C.3 Neuralgia, neuritis, acne, eczema	C.2./C.3./C.4. Vasomotor control, sinuses & nasopharynx
C.4.	Diaphragm. central facial fields – nose, mouth, eustachian tube Hay fever, cattarh, hearing difficulties		
C.5.	Controls rhythm of cardia, vocal cords, pharynx and neck. sore throat, laryngitis, dysrhythmia	C.5./C.6./C.7. Neck, Pharynx & Larynx	
C.6.	Tonsilitis, whooping cough, shoulders		
C.7.	Thyroid gland, goitre, bursitis, shoulders, colds. Controls all ilial lesions.	C.6./C.7. Thyroid & parathyroids	C.6./C.7./D.1./D.2. Thyroid, thoracic duct (and inlet above) drains upper & lower lymphatic fields.

TABLE J KEY VERTEBRAE (CONTINUED)

C.7. (cont'd) *Left side:* diarrhoea, miscarriages, abortions, heavy periods, impotency, irritable bowel, prostate, heart, breast, respiration, asthma, tinnitus. Lesions at upper curvature of stomach

N.B. C.7. is for functional stress of thyroid. If there is no lesion, the primary cause is elsewhere. Haemorrhoids are from blockage of superior lymphatic branch – from below, impeding flow

Right side: constipation, bladder, appendicitis, haemorrhoids, non-malignant uterine tumours, uterine displacements, hiatus hernia. Control for coccygeal and rectal problems. Vertigo, blood pressure (if not temporal lesion)

C.7./D.1–Cervical Prominence thyroid. Sphenobasilar thyroid. sphenobasilar lesions via 3rd cervical plexus. Cardiac mechanisms. Fatigue, halitosis, cough reflex (see C.1.)

D.1. Controls all 5L lesions, acute lumbago, asthma, forearm and hands.
Right side: bladder disturbances, cystitis

D.2. Heart and chest conditions.

D.3. Chest complaints, influenza.
D2/3 Left
Car sickness, rib conditions
D2/3 Right
Diabetes – N.B. always have sugar/insulin to hand when treating diabetics at this level for hypo/hyper reaction

D.2./D.3
Cough reflex (see C1/C7/D1) Upper fascia control (see L.5). sphenobasilar control inhibits drainage of posterior cranial base. Cardiac problems (see C3). Idiopathic epilepsy. Glaucoma, myopia (due to thoracic ciliary – secondary – reflex)
N.B. Not muscular eye problems. Lungs, stomach.

D.4. Gall bladder, jaundice, shingles.

D3/D4 Left
Stomach instability – car sickness, vomiting, nausea.

CRANIAL LANDMARKS

TABLE J   KEY VERTEBRAE (CONTINUED)

	D3/D4 Central Kidney control	*D.3./D.4.* A.T. Still calls D3/4 the key to all recurrent problems (including 3rd rib). Colds, hayfever, catarrh, circulatory problems, due to cardiac pulmonary plexuses anterior to D4	
	D3/D4 Right Intestinal and liver stasis		
D.5.	Liver conditions, fever, hypotension, arthritis. Pancreatic, apoplexy	*D.4./D.5.* Biliary conditions	
D.6.	Indigestion, heartburn.	*D.6./D.7* Stomach & cardiac orifice	*D.5./D.6./D.7./D.8.* Oesophagus and duodenum
D.7.	Pancreas, ulcers, gastritis sympathetic direct plexus with C3	*D.7./D.8./D.9.* Spleen & pancreas	
D.8.	Hiccoughs, spleen, diaphragm		
D.9.	Genito-urinary reflex. Adrenals, some allergies.	*D.9./D.10* Adrenal conditions	
D.10.	Arteriosclerosis, pyelitis		
D.11	Kidneys, acne, boils	*D.10./D.11* Controls spinal extension (above ribs restrain, below psoas restrains)	*D.10./D.11./D.12* Kidneys, jejunum, ilium
D.12.	Haemorrhoidal plexus (see C7) Psoas and Piriformis key. Respiratory excursion inhibitor. Ilium rheumatism		*D.11./D.12./L.1./L.2.* drains lower lymphatic field (but treat at C6/D2.)
L.1.	Colitis, colon, inguinal area.	*L.1./L.2.* appendicitis, ileo-caecal valve	
L.2.	cramp, varicosity, abdominal and thigh pain.		
L.3.	Knee, bladder, key to spinal mechanism, controls upright posture.	*L.2./L.3.* Ovaries, uterus	
L.4.	Sciatic nerve problems, urinary insufficiency, prostate	*L.3./L.4./L.5.* Gonads, colon, rectum	

TABLE J KEY VERTEBRAE (CONTINUED)

L.5.	Fascia control, bed-wetting (Primary). Controls all sacral/innominate problems. (N.B. treat C7/D1 as well), cramp. Lower extremities	*L.4./L.5*	Urinary, bladder, prostate.
Sacrum	Sacroiliac and hip	*Sacrum & Coccyx*	Anal and vesicle sphincters
Coccyx	Respiratory inhibitor (key D12) Rectum, anus		

TABLE K KEY VERTEBRAE: KEY PAIRS

Sphenoid	Ilia
Sphenobasilar symphysis	C7
Sphenobasilar symphysis	Sacrum (& Coccyx) (Ganglion of Impar)
Occiput	Sacrum
C1	C7/D1
C1/C7/D1	D2/D3
C3	C7
C3	D3
C3	D7
C6–D1	D11–L2
C7	D3
C7	D12
C7	L5
D1	L5
D2	L4
D3	L3
D2/D3	L5
D4	L2
D5	L1
D12	Coccyx

CRANIAL LANDMARKS

TABLE L   PHYSIOLOGICAL MOVEMENT

OSSEOUS

BONE	AXIS	MOVEMENTS ON INHALATION (Sphenobasilar Flexion)	NOTES
SPHENOID	Transverse (immediately anterior to sella turcica)	A.P. (anteroposterior) with some lateral expansion inferiorly at pterygoid plates. Sella turcica moves superoanteriorly. Pterygoid plates posterolaterally	N.B. On exhalation all bones return to neutral position
OCCIPUT	Transverse	Base moves superoanteriorly, squama posteroinferiorly	
FRONTAL	Vertical (Through ossification point)	Effectively – moves anterolaterally. The glabella recedes (metopic suture depresses) as falx cerebri pulls on crest. The orbital plates move with glabella medially, & with the sphenoid posteriorly widening ethmoid notch.	Moves with Temporal
PARIETAL	Posterolaterally (Bregma through ossification point)	Anterolaterally, opening the saggital suture – especially posteriorly	Moves with temporals, sphenoid, occiput and frontal.
TEMPORAL	Oblique (along petrous ridge)	Squama externally rotates (petrous ridge moves superolaterally) as sphenobasilar moves upwards. The mastoid process moves posterolaterally.	The rising basiocciput and jugular processes 'spin' the temporals outward as the tentorium cerebelli flattens.

TABLE L PHYSIOLOGICAL MOVEMENT (CONTINUED)

Bone	Axis	Movement	Relation
VOMER	Transverse	Superior border moves posteroinferiorly (with rostrum). Inferior border moves anterosuperiorly (with nasal crest)	Moves with sphenoid, maxilla, etc.
ZYGOMA	Vertical (through frontal process)	moves anterolaterally – widening the oblique diameter of the orbit	Moves with sphenoidal great wings and maxilla
MAXILLA	Oblique (Glabella through first molar)	effectively moves anterolaterally, allowing palatine process to descend posteriorly. The alveolar arch widens, flaring teeth. Posterior edge of frontal process moves laterally, opening nasal cavity	Moved by sphenoid via palatines
NASAL	Vertical	Posterolateral movement	With maxilla and frontal
LACRIMALS	Transverse	Inferior border moves laterally opening naso-lacrimal canal	Moves with ethmoid, maxilla and frontal
INFERIOR NASAL CONCHA	A.P.	Unfolds to allow expansion of meatal air cavity	
ETHMOID	Transverse (through superior end of perpendicular plate)	Clockwise rotation with some external rotation of lateral masses enlarging the nasal fossae. Superior crista galli moves superoposteriorly, (with falx cerebri) inferior perpendicular plate anteroinferiorly	Moves with falx cerebri and sphenoid
PALATE	Oblique (Orbital process through middle of horizontal plate)	In effect, the lower part turns mediopsoteriorly, lateralizing the posterior pyramidal surface, and the upper part moves inferiorly.	Moves with vomer, maxilla, and sphenoid
MANDIBLE	—	Symphysis recedes (to co-ordinate with maxilla) The superior ramus moves posteriorly with the externally rotating temporal. This action widens the alveolar arch.	Moves with temporal bone and in harmony with maxilla

CRANIAL LANDMARKS

ORBIT	Oblique (superomedial to inferolateral angles)	As the sphenoidal great wings move anteriorly so do the eyes. The zygoma and inferior orbital part of the maxilla move laterally and anterolaterally respectively and (although the bones of the medial wall move laterally as well) the oblique diameter of the eye increases	This conical pocket has to have unrestricted oblique movement in order that the eye, muscles, vessels, etc shall function effectively. Dura invades the orbit as periosteum making a direct link with C.S.F. which surrounds the optic nerve.
NASAL FOSSA		The recession of the bones in the mid-line (together with R.T.M.) and external rotation of the lateral ones increases the transverse diameter (decreasing the vertical). This heightens the circulation of blood, lymph and air. This movement creates a pumping action on sinus walls, at the vomer (sphenoidal sinuses) on the frontals and sphenoid (ethmoid sinuses) on zygoma (maxillary sinuses).	Near the olfactory area at the posterosuperior part of the nasal fossa inhaled air is cleaned, humidified, and warmed to be fit for use in the lungs. Returning (exhaled) air avoids this area and follows the floor of the nasal cavity.
SACRUM	Transverse	Superior part moves superoposteriorly. The inferior part moves anteroinferiorly	Dural pull on firm attachments pulls spinal dura superiorly (as F.M. rises). This rotates the sacrum into respiratory flexion
RECIPROCAL TENSION MEMBRANE	Transverse	Falx Cerebri moves anteromedially (with crista galli). This 'pulls up' or flattens the *Tentorium Cerebelli* to move forward *Falx Cerebelli* moves anterosuperiorly *Spinal Dura* rises and shortens, lifting the rest of the R.T.M.	

ESSENTIALS OF CRANIO-SACRAL OSTEOPATHY

TABLE L PHYSIOLOGICAL MOVEMENT (CONTINUED)

R.T.M. cont'd	Poles of attachment	
	Anterior Superior move anteroinferiorly	Mechanical (structural) movements such as exaggerated pulmonary excursion (very deep breathing or holding the breath) can alter or interrupt this P.R.M. but normally it continues throughout life, and even for some time after death – when all other respiration has ceased.
	Anterior Inferior move posterosuperiorly	
	Lateral move superiorly and anterolaterally	
	Posterior move anteriorly, bring occiput forward.	

SUMMARY The cerebellum, choroid plexus, first, second and third ventricles expand laterally and superiorly to increase production and fluctuation of C.S.F. and this altered volume affects metabolism (especially at the hypothalamus and pituitary which move superiorly with the sphenoid). This shortens the A.P. diameter, curling the ram's horn tighter. The venous sinuses alter in shape and increase in drainage capacity. Other veins drain at an increased rate (no change in size).

In homeostasis, due to the guidance, control and limiting effect of the dura (and poles of attachment) the 'pumping mechanism' of the R.T.M. is equal in pressure

a) either side of each suture
b) at poles of attachment
c) all other joints of the body
d) on components of fluid systems
e) between cranial and sacral action

In non-homeostatic conditions (such as in traumatic or pathological disturbance) there is a shift of fulcrum and articular motion creating restriction to some or all of a) to e)

Inspiration (sphenobasilar flexion)
Mid-line bones move into flexion on transverse axes (Sphenoid, Ethmoid, Vomer, Occiput)
Lateral bones (either side of mid-line) rotate externally (Frontals, Zygomae, Maxillae, Palatines, Temporals, Parietals)
This a) lessens A.P. diameter
b) lowers the vault
c) flattens the Tentorium Cerebelli
d) increases transverse diameter
e) changes osseous shape (not cranial volume)

FRED L. MITCHELL

'Treat what you find, not what you are looking for.'

CHAPTER EIGHTEEN

Anatomy of the Vault

FRONTAL
PARIETAL
OCCIPITAL

ANATOMY OF THE VAULT

71 VAULT SUTURAL BEVELS

Diagrammatic representation of overlapping bevels at vault (not to scale).

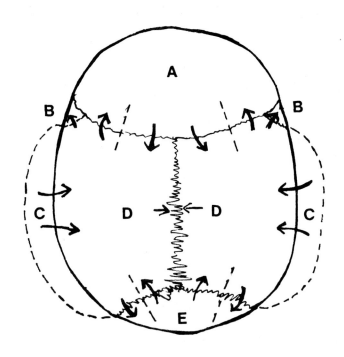

- **A** Frontal
- **B** Sphenoid
- **C** Temporal
- **D** Parietal
- **E** Occipital

↻ Denotes overlap

↘ Denotes changeover point of bevel (mobility point)

FRONTAL BONE

Lt. Frontalis: forehead.

The frontal forms the anterior of the vault and the roof of the orbit, and resembles a cockle shell. It tends to be larger in the male than the female, partly due to the size of the frontal sinuses. As it overlies the behavioural centres of the cerebrum, lesions to the frontal can be the 'governor' of mental/social instabilities, hence many mental states respond significantly to restoration of frontal harmony.

Cranially speaking perhaps the most important point to bear in mind is that the frontal is formed as two bones pre-natally and continues to move as two bones throughout life; one may be in external rotation, while the other is in internal rotation. (This is so despite the fact that only 1:10 people retain a patent metopic suture – from glabella to bregma – into old age). It is always to be treated as two by the practitioner.

It is also important to note – from the cranio-sacral standpoint – that the 'L' shaped area between the frontal and the great wing of the sphenoid (pterion) mirrors the 'L' shaped area at the sacro-iliac joint. The latter acts as a fulcrum with gliding mobility.

The shape of the forehead can be a clue to diagnosis. Anterior flexion – external rotation of the frontal – is often denoted by the sloping forehead, whilst the opposite is suspected with the jutting brow. Frontal lesions are dependant to a large degree on the state of the spheno-basilar symphysis. The other main cause is direct trauma – this is especially so in children.

The frontal, being part of the vault, is formed in membrane and has two main ossification points at the frontal eminences – though secondary points are not uncommon. The anterior 'corner' of the anterior fontanelle is formed by the superomedial edges of the bones and this normally closes between eighteen months and two years of age. The squama consists of two compact laminae with a 'spongy' layer between; and the orbits tend to be thin, smooth and transluscent.

Basically it is possible to divide the frontal into three parts.

The squama

is convex anteriorly and curves upwards and backwards above the orbits. The supraorbital arch (which carries the eyebrows) forms the inferior margin, and the frontoparietal suture the superior and lateral margins.

The most prominent parts of the squama are the zygomatic process which form the laterionferior angles of the frontal and the outer edge of the orbit; the superciliary arch that joins at the glabella and the frontal eminences (ossification points).

Internally the frontal crest behind the glabella forms attachment for the falx cerebri, and ends in a small notch which houses the foramen caecum. At the side of the continuation of the crest – the sagittal sulcus – in a concave groove,

ANATOMY OF THE VAULT
72 FRONTAL BONE

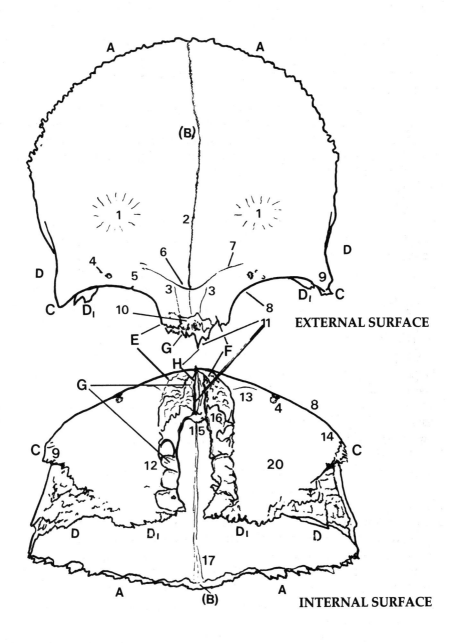

72 FRONTAL BONE

A Coronal suture margin – for articulation with Parietal
B Metopic suture margin – for articulation with opposite Frontal
C Zygomatic process – for articulation with Zygoma
D Pterion – for articulation with great wing of Sphenoid
D_1 Orbital margin – for articulation with lesser wing of Sphenoid
E Internal orbital process – for articulation with Lacrimal
F Nasal notch – for articulation with Maxilla
G Postnasal notch and Ethmoidal air cells – for articulation with Ethmoid
H Anterior nasal notch and spine – for articulation with Nasal.

1. Eminence (ossification point)
2. Metopic suture
3. Site of supranasal folds
4. Supraorbital foramen
5. Supraorbital notch
6. Glabella
7. Superciliary arch
8. Supraorbital margin
9. Zygomatic process
10. Nasal section
11. Nasal spine
12. Roof of ethmoidal air cells
13. Trochlear fossa
14. Lacrimal glandular fossa
15. Ethmoidal notch
16. Ethmoidal foramen
17. Sagittal sulcus
18. Frontal crest
19. Foramen caecum (for emissary vein)
20. Orbital surface

ANATOMY OF THE VAULT
73 FRONTAL BONE

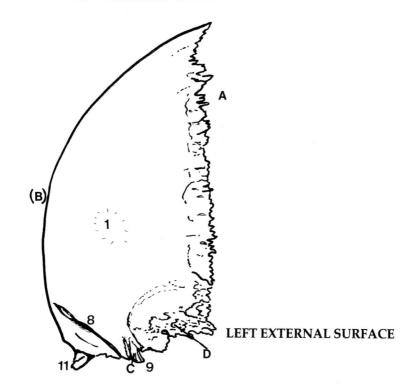

LEFT EXTERNAL SURFACE

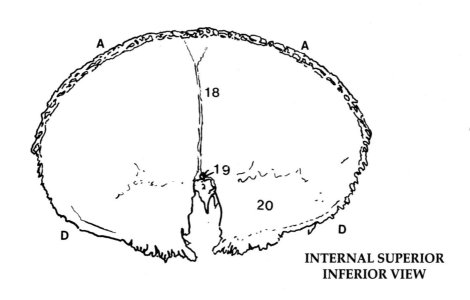

INTERNAL SUPERIOR INFERIOR VIEW

lies the anterior superior sagittal sinus. Pacchionian pits may also be seen, these are for arachnoid granulations which allow C.S.F. to be drained into the sagittal sinus.

The squama also houses the frontal sinuses – between the bony plates – either side of the nasal spine and in front of the ethmoid notch. These vary in size in individuals but one is usually somewhat larger than the other and they normally attain their full size at puberty. Along with the other air sinuses of the skull they lighten the bony mass and contribute to the tone of the voice. It is, of course, vital to the well-being of the patient that these should be drained in cases of catarrh, sinusitis, coryza, etc.

Orbits

A smooth concave surface externally and thickened corrugated internally this part forms the medial roof of the orbit and the ethmoid notch anteromedially. The postmedial part is not usually joined but occasionally fusion takes place. The ethmoidal foramen form the roof of the ethmoidal air cells. Across the margin of the notch run two grooves which form the anterior and posterior ethmoid canals (with part of the ethmoid). There are grooves on the cerebral surface of the orbit that accommodate the cerebral gyri.

Nasal

This anteromedial portion of the frontal forms part of the nasal cavity laterally and part of the nasal septum via a grooved surface on the frontal spine.

The frontal articulates with eight other bones (including its counterpart at the metopic suture). With the sphenoid's great wing at the pterion, and the small wing in the orbit; with the parietal at the coronal suture where, it should be noted, it overlaps the parietal medially and is overlapped by it laterally; with the ethmoid at the posterior of the notch; the nasal anteromedially; the superior portion of the maxilla at the posterolateral nasal part; the lacrimal at the margins of the notch anteriorly; and the zygoma via the zygomatic process.

PARIETAL BONE

Lt. Parietalis: (paries – a wall).

These two rectangular, externally concave, bones which form the posterior roof and sides of the vault are often overlooked in the cranial consideration, being dismissed as of little significance. However, as they immediately overlie the superior sagittal sinus they tend to monitor the distribution of C.S.F. and the cranial venous (sinus) system into which it drains. They also cover and protect the parietal lobe of the cerebrum which is the somasthetic area – responsible for temperature sensations (though not extremes of temperature) and muscular movement. Hence it is possible that the secret of control of such conditions as ataxia and involuntary muscular activity may be found here. When there is injury, information appears to be interfered with and therefore control of muscular activity is impaired. Nevertheless, no pain sensations appear to emanate from this part of the cortex.

Lesion possibilities vary – from direct trauma from many angles; to impaction at the coronal border from referred blows to the frontal. At the temporoparietal junction 'shearing' action trauma can cause local and referred conditions – T.M.J. dysfunctions, for instance can arise here – partly due to the retardation of the temporalis muscle. If there is high convexity at the parietal eminences this may well indicate undue dural tension. This may still be present or might be the pointer to the bones being unable to expand in early life and therefore pushing upwards to compensate.

Formed in membrane the parietals carry some of the deepest serrations to be found in the skull. Ossification takes place from one central point (the eminence) on each bone. As with all vault bones these ossify concentrically the 'corners' being the last to become bone. Hence at the angles of all four borders are found the six fontanelles – anterior, posterior, anterolateral (2), posterolateral (2). It has been known (rarely) for the parietals to be divided into two by a suture at the level of the superior temporal line. A groove indicating this is more apparent on some skulls (at dissection) than others. Note that at the Bregma and Lambda the borders describe almost perfect right angles (90 degrees) in the adult.

Externally a smooth surface superiorly gives way to a roughened area below the two temporal lines for the attachment of temporal fascia (superior line) and the temporalis muscle (inferior line). The temporal lines are lower natally but move upward as the molar teeth erupt. If parietal foramen are present they are usually in the posterior third of the sagittal border and mostly bilateral and visible externally and internally. They transmit an emissary vein from the superior sagittal sinus and sometimes a branch of the occipital artery.

Internally the most prominent features are the fan-like grooves for meningeal vessels and the grooves for sigmoid and sagittal sinuses. The latter at the juncture of the two Parietal bones. Either side of this superior border the falx cerebri attaches. The tentorium cerebelli being attached at the posterior-inferior angles of the parietals. Depressions for arachnoid granulations (pacchionian bodies) are mostly apparent in the skulls of elderly subjects.

The parietals generally articulate with four other bones. (Occasionally the temporal squama articulates with the frontal – in these cases the parietal has no articulation with the great wing of the sphenoid). Normally however, the parietal articulates with the frontal at the coronal suture, the occiput at the lambdoidal suture; the squama of the temporal at the squamosal suture, and the P.L.A. (Posterior Lateral Angle) with the superior border of the mastoid;

74 PARIETAL BONE

A Saggital suture margin – for articulation with opposite Parietal
B Lambdoid suture margin – for articulation with Occiput
C Coronal suture margin – for articulation with Frontal
D Squamosal suture margin and P.L.A. – for articulation with the Temporal
E Sphenosquamosal suture margin – for articulation with Sphenoid

1 Parietal foramen (if present carries emissary vein)
2 Parietal eminence (or tuberosity)
3 Superior Temporal line
4 Inferior Temporal line
5 Grooves for Middle Meningeal vessels (anterior branches)
6 Grooves for Middle Meningeal vessels (posterior branches)
7 Groove for Sigmoid Sinus
8 Groove for portion of superior Sagittal Sinus

ANATOMY OF THE VAULT

74   PARIETAL BONE

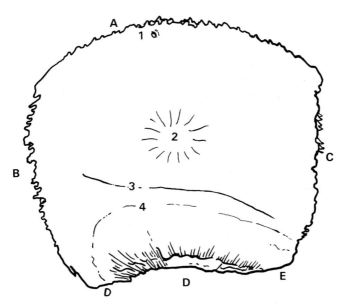

RIGHT EXTERNAL SURFACE

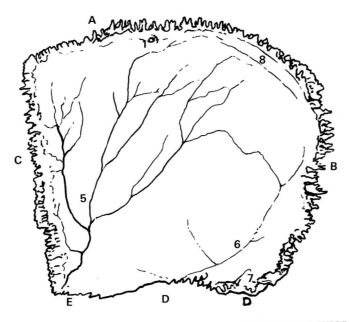

RIGHT INTERNAL SURFACE

and the great wing of the sphenoid at the pterion. (The pterion directly overlies the motor speech centre of Broca on the left hand side – in right handed people). The parietal also articulates with its counterpart at the sagittal suture.

The bevels of the vault should be studied carefully – particularly at the point where the bevels change. As will be seen in the accompanying Plate 71 the parietals are 'held' in such a way that they can be said to be almost springing apart if they were not 'tucked under' and held at the medial part of all four borders.

OCCIPITAL BONE

Lt. Occipitalis: Back of head-neck

Roughly diamond shaped and deeply convex externally the occiput is the posterior portion of the vault and the cranial base and is situated in the posterior cranial fossa. It consists of a central diploe which is sandwiched between two layers of compact tissue. The shape it assumes in ossification influences the shape of the whole cranium. It covers and protects the posterior (occipital) lobe of the cerebrum and the cerebellum and receives attachment of the posterior and lateral poles of the Falx cerebri and the Tentorium cerebelli.

Above the highest nuchal line the occiput is developed in membrane, below this (being part of the base) it develops in cartilage. The lateral condyles develop partly with the squama (about two thirds) and partly with the base (approximately one third). There are two centres of ossification at base and four at the squama.

The medial border at the lambda is the site of the posterior fontanelle, and the lateral border at the asterion is the site of the posterior lateral fontanelles. Because the ossification of the occipital is a lengthy process – the squama ossifying by about 5 years of age and the basi-occiput not until around 8 years old – direct methods of cranial osteopathy are not used until after this is complete. If there is undue distortion at the base during these early years there will be deformity of the whole sphenobasilar symphysis, and therefore the cranio-sacral system, later.

Many lesions occur at the occipital mastoid articulation. These disturb the sinus (venous) and C.S.F. circulation, and inhibit dural tension. Medially, lesions at the occipito-atlantal junction are also numerous, but are not to be confused with dural aggravation at the upper cervicals.

The occiput can be thought of under four headings.

Squama

This curves superoposteriorly and forms the back of the head inferiorly. Externally it is smooth above the nuchal lines, of which there are three (supreme, superior and inferior), and below the surface is irregular to form attachment for several muscles and ligaments such as the trapezius sternomastoid, splenius capitus, and ligamentum nuchae. The most prominent part of the squama is the external protuberance (inion).

The internal surface is divided roughly into four depressions, or fossae, by grooves running transversely and superoinferiorly. The upper sulcus carries the sagittal sinus centrally and gives attachment to the occipital sinus laterally (sometimes there are two present). The falx cerebri and tentorium cerebelli also attach along the length of the sulcus. The right hand transverse sulcus is usually larger than the left as the transverse sinus most often deviates to the right.

Inferiorly the internal occipital crest ends in the vermiform fossa, and a small 'dished' area gives attachment to the falx cerebelli. The eminetia cruciate (internal protuberance) forms the crossover point of the sulcii and is the level of the confluence of sinuses.

Base

This is anterior to the foramen magnum and forms its anterior arc. It is a short 'stump' of bone and where it articulates with the sphenoid is known as the basiocciput. This is a synchondrosis which is said to ossify at around 25 years of age, but actually exhibits movement – therefore flexion, extension, sidebending, and torsion lesions (or combinations of these) are all possible here and form the king-pivot of the cranial osteopath's art.

The pharyngeal tubercle is found on the internal surface of the base about 1cm. from the foramen magnum. To this attach fibres of the raphe of the pharynx. This is the cranial part of the posterior longtitudinul ligament that is found on the dorsal surface of C2/3.

Foramen magnum

Though not an area of bone the foramen magnum is a most important consideration in the occipital structure. An oval hole through which the contents of the cerebral cavity connect with the vertebral canal and thereby the rest of the body, the posterior of the foramen magnum is wider than the anterior and contains the medulla oblongata and at its rim attaches dura mater. This foramen also contains the apical ligament of the odontoid process, branches of accessory and upper cervical nerves, spinal and vertebral arteries.

Condylar/Lateral

Either side of the magnum posteriorly lie the smooth oval surfaces of the condyles and between condyles and magnum is the hypoglossal canal. As already stated this is the most lesion prone area of the occiput. The eventual 'siting' of the condyles determines the functional capacity of the whole basal and vault area from birth onwards.

75 OCCIPITAL BONE

A Lambdoidal suture margin – for articulation with Parietal
B Mastoid margin – for articulation with Temporal B Lateral basal margin – petrobasilar suture – articulation with Temporal
C Occipital condyle – for articulation with Atlas
D Basilar suture margin – for articulation with Sphenoid

1 Occipital protuberance
2 Highest (or Supreme) nuchal line
3 Superior nuchal line
4 Occipital crest
5 Inferior nuchal line
6 Foramen magnum
7 Posterior condylar canal
8 Condyles
9 Jugular process
10 Anterior condylar canal
11 Pharyngeal tubercle
12 Superior (Cerebral) fossa
13 Sagittal sulcus (for sagittal sinus)
14 Transverse sulcus (for transverse sinus)
   (N.B: these sulci are usually of unequal size.)
15 Inferior (Cerebellar) fossa
16 Occipital crest
17 Posterior condylar canal
18 Jugular tubercle
19 Jugular notch
20 Sigmoidal sinus groove
21 Basilar suture
22 Eminentia cruciate. Internal protuberance.
   (also known as Torcular Herophyli)

ANATOMY OF THE VAULT
75 OCCIPITAL BONE

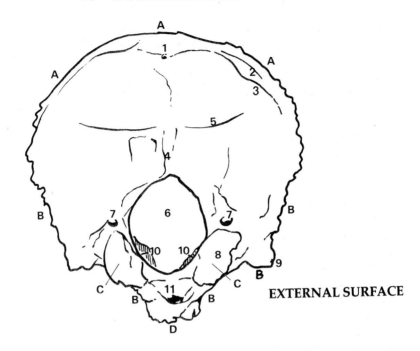

EXTERNAL SURFACE

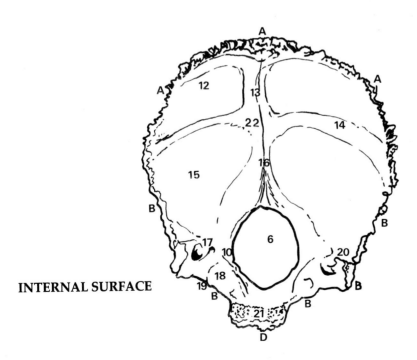

INTERNAL SURFACE

The two jugular processes are the inferior lateral angles of the occiput, roughly level with the condyles. Internally the groove for the sigmoid sinus and jugular foramen will be observed. This latter carries branches of the occipital artery; internal jugular vein; 10th, 11th & 12th cranial nerves; and the inferior petrosal sinus. A groove behind the jugular notch which carries on to the temporal gives the axis-pivot angle of mobility of the base.
temporal gives the axis-pivot angle of mobility of the base.

The occiput articulates with four other bones. The parietals at the lambdoidal suture where, as happens similarly at the coronal suture, the occiput rides over the parietals medially, and is overridden by them laterally: the sphenoid at the basilar process – a synchondrosis – and with the temporal bone where it can be said to articulate on three planes. The OM. (occipitomastoid) suture runs anteroinferiorly, changing bevel at the C.S.M. (or H.M.) pivot. This suture continues anterosuperiorly (as the petrojugular) still in contact with the mastoid. The third plane is at the lateral edge of the base with the petrous portion of the temporal and its apex – the petrobasilar suture.

The fourth articulation of the occipital bone is at the condyles. These receive the superior facets of the atlas.

PARACELSUS

'If a new idea can be fitted into the authoritarian framework we are too apt to accept it uncritically, whereas if it breaks new ground we are too likely to reject it.'

CHAPTER NINETEEN

Anatomy of the Base

SPHENOID
TEMPORAL
BASIOCCIPUT
(See Vault)

ANATOMY OF THE BASE
76 BASAL RELATIONSHIPS

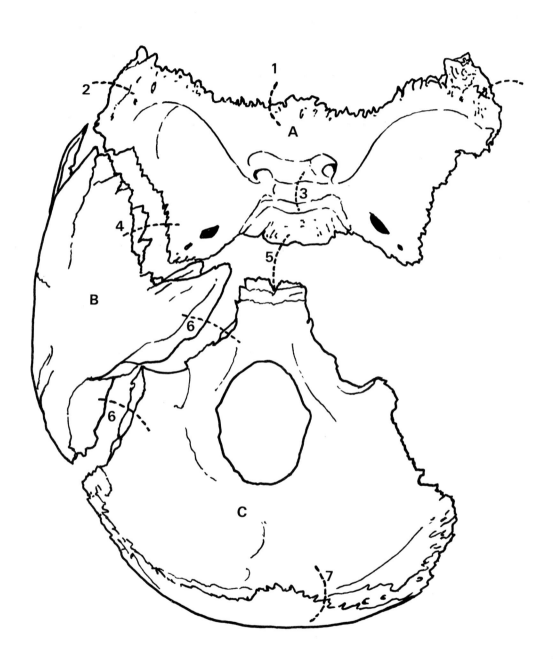

76 BASAL RELATIONSHIPS

A SPHENOID
B TEMPORAL
C OCCIPUT

ARTICULATIONS

1. Frontosphenoid
2. Parietosphenoid
3. Sphenoethmoid
4. Sphenotemporal
5. Sphenobasilar (occiput)
6. Occipitotemporal
7. Occipitoparietal

ANATOMY OF THE BASE
SPHENOID BONE
Gk: spheno = wedge; eidos = form

The sphenoid is an irregular wedge of bone forming part of the base of the skull. It is generally described as being like a bat with outstretched wings – and appears so at each surface (superior, inferior, posterior or anterior), hence its older name of Alar – a wing. The keystone of the cranio-sacral system, it has many muscular and ligamentous attachments, and many foramina, which are described in detail in Table D (p. 67/68). It articulates with all the bones of the vault and base, and the zygoma, palatine and vomer (and occasionally the maxilla) in the face. It forms part of all the cranial fossae, anterior, middle and posterior, and helps form the nose (roof and walls) and orbits (lateral wall and roof).

The sphenoid and sacrum relate and generally mirror movements; the 'L' shaped area at the anterior surface of the sphenoid being matched by a similar area at the anterior sacrum. They are both suspended from other bones in almost the same plane – the sphenoid from the frontal, and between the temporals; the sacrum between the ilia. They both move A.P. with respiratory excursion.

Sutherland maintained that any malfunction/aberration of the sphenoid changes facial and orbital symmetry and expression – and that this is evidenced by disparity in facial fields. The zygoma and palatines act as stabilizers/equalizers between the sphenoid and maxilla.

The central body is hollow and expansile and contains two large sinuses which occasionally invade the basiocciput through the synchondrosis at the sphenobasilar. The superior surface supports the pons varoli, and anteriorly has a depression, the sella turcica (pituitary fossa) which houses the pituitary gland. This fossa rests on air sinuses and is bounded superiorly by the anterior and posterior clinoid processes. The anterior clinoid processes are closer together than the posterior and both are clearly defined on X-rays. The ends differ in shape and are described as pointed, boat-hooked, or rounded. In rare cases the anterior and posterior meet and are described as 'bridged.' Just below the posterior process is the dorsum sellae; the slope behind this sellae is the clivus which is continuous with the basiocciput. Anterior to the sella turcica is an oval eminence, the tuberculum sellae, and the optic groove which ends laterally in optic foramina. This groove is really a short canal between the roots of the lesser wings and carries the optic nerve and opthalmic artery.

Anteriorly the jugum supports the frontal lobe of the brain and olfactory tracts; anteroinferiorly the rostrum projects and receives the ala of the vomer. The crest forms part of the nasal septum, articulating anteriorly with the perpendicular plate of the ethmoid. Laterally the carotid groove which is shaped like an 'f' houses the carotid artery and cavernous sinus; it ends in the lingula.

The posterior border of the body articulates with the occiput at the

77 SPHENOID BONE

A Tip of great wing – for articulation with parietal at Pterion
B Great wing (edge of pterion) – for articulation with Frontal
Lesser wing at posterior orbital plate – for articulation with Frontal
C Anterolateral border of great wing – for articulation with Zygoma
D Ethmoidal spine and crest – for articulation with Ethmoid
Lateral edge of body – for articulation with Ethmoid
E Lateral and inferolateral edges of body – for articulation with Palatine
Pterygoid cleft (fissure) – for articulation with Palatine
F Sphenobasilar symphysis (synchondrosis) – for articulation with Occipital bone
G Dorsum sellae – for articulation with Temporal
Posterior great wing – for articulation with Temporal
Squamous margin (inferiorly and anteriorly) – for articulation with Temporal
H Rostrum and vaginal process – for articulation with Vomer

1	Tip of great wing	21	Pterygoid hamulus
2	Great wing	22	Pterygoid notch
3	Lesser wing	23	Spine
4	Body	24	Dorsum sellae
5	Sphenoidal sinus entrance	25	Posterior clinoid process
6	Optic canal	26	Sella turcica (pituitary fossa)
7	Superior orbital fissure	27	Anterior clinoid process
8	Orbital surface	28	Squamosal border
9	Infratemporal crest	29	Parietal border
10	Maxillary surface	30	Frontal border
11	Pterygoid process	31	Temporal surface
12	Foramen rotundum	32	Zygomatic border
13	Pterygoid canal	33	Ethmoidal spine
14	Concha	34	Jugum
15	Ethmoidal crest	35	Tuberculum sellae
16	Vaginal process	36	Cerebral surface
17	Rostrum	37	Foramen ovale
18	Basi-occiput	38	Foramen spinosum
19	Medial pterygoid plate	39	Middle clinoid process
20	Lateral pterygoid plate	40	Lingula

ANATOMY OF THE BASE
77 SPHENOID BONE

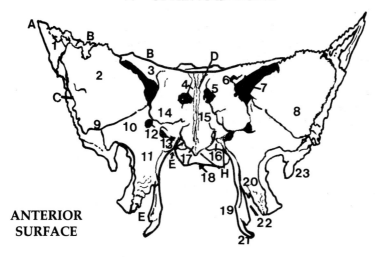

ANTERIOR SURFACE

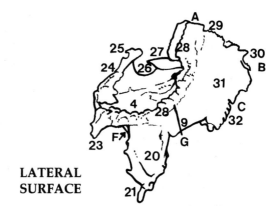

LATERAL SURFACE

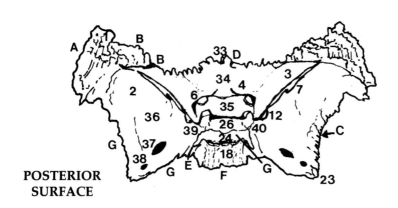

POSTERIOR SURFACE

sphenobasilar symphysis via a disc. Although seen as a synchondrosis, flexion, extension, and rotation are all possible here and X-rays show intraosseous strain, compression lesions, as well as vertical and lateral strains.

The great wings are large strong processes projecting laterally below the lesser wings from the body of the sphenoid. They have great flexibility at their roots; the tips (orbital surfaces) help form the posterolateral wall of the orbit, and the medial margin of the superior orbital fossa. The wings are concave superiorly (posterior surface) and give support to the anterior part of the brain. The inferior surface forms attachment for muscles, including the temporalis. Posteriorly a spine projects from the lateral edge of the wing.

The lesser wings project laterally from the body and move with it. Their roots are at the optic canal, and the posterior border houses the aforementioned anterior clinoid processes and projects into the lateral cerebral fissure. These thin triangular wings help form the posterior orbital roof, and bound the superior orbital fissure which lies between the great and lesser wings. This fissure transmits branches of the 3rd, 4th, 5th, and 6th C.N. as well as blood vessels. A tubercle at the root attaches a tendon for three eye muscles.

The pterygoid processes project inferiorly where the base of the great wing and body unite and are part of the lateral nasal wall. The lateral plate is broader and shorter than the medial plate which is long and thin. The upper parts (roots) are fused but inferiorly the two processes are divided by the pterygoid fissure (cleft). Both plates afford attachment for muscles.

The sphenoid is formed in cartilage except for the anterior part of the great wings which are formed in membrane. At birth the sphenoid is in three parts, the central body and lesser wings, and the two great wings and pterygoid processes. As with other osseous sinuses the sphenoidal cells do not attain their full size until puberty. Where sphenoidal ossification is premature a distinctive depressed nasal bridge is evident.

The sphenoid articulates with seven (sometimes eight) other bones and forms attachment for eleven pairs of muscles. Its anterior articulating surfaces are related to facial flexibility, the rest to basal mobility. Bevels change even along one suture line to take account of movement required at any one part.

The sphenoid articulates with the frontal at the great wing at the triangular edge of the pterion and at the lesser wing with the frontal's posterior orbital plate. The zygoma's orbital process articulates with the great wing's anterolateral border. The ethmoidal spine – which is an extension of the anterior surface of the body, and the sides of the body articulate with the ethmoid's cribriform and perpendicular plates and the labyrinth respectively. The centre and sides of the ala of the vomer articulate with the rostrum and the vaginal processes – found at the root of the medial pterygoid plate. The palatine articulates with the sphenoid at the lateral edge of the body – with the orbital process; at the body's inferolateral border with the sphenoidal process; and at the pterygoid cleft (fissure) with the tubercle (pyramidal process).

The petrous apex of the temporal bone articulates with the dorsum sellae; the posterior edge of the great wing with the anterior border of the petrous (between the petrous and squama); and the squamous margin of the great wing with external bevel of the squama inferiorly, and the internal bevel of the squama anteriorly. The parietal anterior inferior angle articulates with the tip of the great wing (internal bevel) at the pterion, and the occiput articulates by means of a cartilaginous disc at the basiocciput with the basisphenoid at the sphenobasilar symphysis. This joint is said to ossify between 18 and 25 years of age.

Occasionally the sphenoid articulates directly with the maxilla in the orbit, and the ligaments attached to the sphenoid occasionally ossify effectively creating further 'articulations.'

TEMPORAL BONE

Lt. Temporalis = temple/head

The two temporal bones help form the side walls of the skull (squama and mastoid) and part of the cranial base (petrous and mastoid). Complex in both shape and function each bone contains the middle and inner ear (including the ossicles), sinuses, air sacs, and numerous important foramina. Fifteen muscles attach to it as well as several ligaments. With the sphenoid it is, perhaps, the most important osseous element of the cranio-sacral system.

The occiput, especially at the base, is effectively 'slung' between the temporals; hence injury to the back of the head and neck can drive the occiput between them. W.G. Sutherland considered this bone to be one which required much investigation, especially at the inferior mastoid around the jugular notch. At this fulcrum many lesions are possible (including the compaction lesions mentioned) which can inhibit basilar articular mobility.

The temporals follow the movements of the occiput as does the tentorium cerebelli, which attaches to its base at the petrous ridges and the internal surfaces of the mastoid process. This meningeal layer also attaches to the sphenoid's clinoid process – a direct non-osseous 'articulation.'

The temporal bone can be divided into several sections. Basically these are squama, petrous and mastoid portions. Sub-divisions include styloid, jugular, tympanic, and zygomatic parts.

The squamous portion is almost upright and at its upper border fits over the lateral border of the parietal. It is thin, almost translucent and on a skull is seen to be flaring away from the surface. Externally, it is smooth with an elevation running A.P. in the middle of the plate and a groove for the middle temporal artery. The temporalis muscle and fascia attach at the temporal ridge and the superior surface of the zygoma respectively. Internally concave most prominent is the superior bevelled border. Grooves for the middle meningeal vessels and depressions to accommodate the temporal lobe of the brain are also present. The arcuate eminence (petrous ridge) runs from parietal notch to petrous apex, overlies the anterior semicircular canal, and effectively divides the temporal (internally) into the squama (top two-thirds) and petrous portion (bottom one-third). A petrosquamous suture is visible in most skulls.

This portion includes the zygomatic process. This process is a horizontal bridge springing lateroanteriorly from the lower squama to articulate with the zygoma. The length of this bridge is twisted – changing from superior-inferior to anterior-posterior planes. It has three roots, the middle root is most prominent in children, another helps form the mandibular (glenoid) fossa. This fossa is oval-shaped, placed anterior to the external auditory meatus and accommodates the mandibular condyle. It forms a sliding hinge joint which is extremely vulnerable to lesion – a wide yawn can dislocate the jaw. An intervening cartilaginous disc if displaced/injured results in a 'clicking' joint. The plane of the temporal bone determines the positioning of the mandible as do restrictions of the sphenoid and temporal. It was because of this tendency of the mandible to be malpositioned or 'off-set' that Sutherland referred to the wobbling wheel – the mandibular 'axle' restraining the temporal 'wheel.' These fixations put pressure on the membrane which houses the Gasserian ganglion, stretching it, which interferes with the function of the 5th cranial nerve. Dental work is one of the main causes – excess pressure which can warp, twist, or contort the sphenopalatine and Gasserian ganglia, eustachion tube, pterygoid process, spheno-mandibular ligament and, more particularly, the dura, all contribute to facial anomalies such as trigeminal neuralgia (tic doloureux).

The petrous portion is pyramidal, or wedge-shaped, and roughened for attachment of muscles and tentorium cerebelli. It lies in an almost horizontal plane, being directed obliquely medioanteriorly. It forms part of the central cranial base, between occiput and sphenoid and encloses the middle and inner ear (osseous and membraneous labyrinth, eustachian tube, vestibule, semicircular canal, cochlea . . .). Its foramina transmit 5th, 7th (to facial structures) and 8th (to inner ear) cranial nerves. The jugular fossa and foramen – which lie between the petrous portion and the occiput at the petrooccipital suture, give passage to the 9th, 10th and 11th C.N., lateral sinus, and internal jugular vein. This portion has grooves to carry the petrosal sinus, etc. Congestion in this area, therefore, can be responsible for many speech, taste, swallowing and digestive problems as well as headaches, vagueness, confusion, etc.

The styloid process is about one inch long and provides attachment for three muscles and two ligaments. This spike of bone can be said to be a 'continuation' of the hyoid. It lies in front of, and medial to the mastoid process.

The tympanic part of the temporal surrounds the external auditory meatus and is like a thin curved plate that has curled internally to form a canal. In many skulls this leaves a 'gap' between the end of the curl and the posterior wall of the mandibular fossa. The parotid gland is also lodged in this petrous portion.

The mastoid portion is behind the petrous part – between the external auditory meatus and the OM. suture. This portion does not develop until the child's second year. This leaves the facial nerve very near the surface and susceptible to injury. It is rough surfaced, thickened and conical and possesses several foramina – one which, when present, carries an emissary vein to the dura mater. Mucous lined cells investing the mastoid vary greatly in size and distribution – the lower cells tending to contain marrow, the upper ones air. One large air-filled space is the antrum. Its close relation to the inner ear means that inflammation in the ear can be transmitted to the cranial base. Although the mastoid portion itself is not present at birth this antrum is.

The temporal bone is in three pieces at birth (the squama, tympanic ring, and petromastoid) and the rate of ossification varies from person to person. The squama (as part of the vault) forms in membrane. The petrous and mastoid portions (being mostly base) are formed in cartilage. This bone articulates with five others; the mandible anteroinferiorly via a disc at the T.M.J.; the zygoma anteriorly at an oblique line just above the level of the mandibular coronoid process. The sphenoid articulates anteriorly and superiorly at the temporal part of the great wing at the squamosal suture – both with external and internal bevel; at the apex of the petrous portion with the lateral border of the dorsum sellae and the great wings posterolateral border via cartilaginous discs. At the superior squamosal border and posteriorly at the P.I.A. (posterior inferior angle) with the lateral border of the parietals; and with the occiput posteriorly and posteroinferiorly at the 'L'-shaped OM. suture, petrobasilar suture and jugular process.

78 TEMPORAL BONE

A Squamosal suture – for articulation with Parietal
   Superior mastoid margin (P.I.A.) – for articulation with Parietal
B Inferior squamosal suture and Pterion – for articulation with Sphenoidal great wing
   At petrous portion, and apex of petrous portion – with dorsum sellae and great wing
C Zygomatic process – for articulation with temporal process of Zygoma
D Temporomandibular joint – for articulation with Mandible
E Occipitomastoid and petrobasilar sutures – for articulation with Occipital bone Jugular process – for articulation with Occipital bone

1 Squama
2 Groove – middle temporal artery
3 Parietal notch
4 Mastoid portion
5 External auditory meatus
6 Sphenoidal border (squamous and pterion)
7 Occipital margin
8 Mastotympanic fissure
9 Styloid process
10 Tympanic part
11 Tubercle
12 Zygomatic process
13 Grooves – middle meningeal vessels
14 Petrosquamous sinus-groove
15 Sigmoid sinus – groove
16 Mastoid foramen
17 Petrous ridge
18 Petrous portion
19 Apex of petrous
20 Internal acoustic meatus

ANATOMY OF THE BASE
78 TEMPORAL BONE

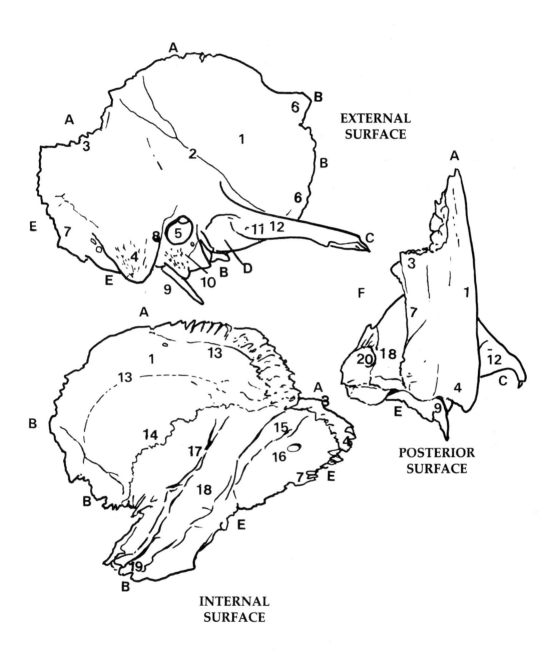

EXTERNAL SURFACE

POSTERIOR SURFACE

INTERNAL SURFACE

JULIEN OFFRAY DE LA METTRIE

'The human body is a watch, a large watch, constructed with . . . skill and ingenuity.'

CHAPTER TWENTY

Anatomy of the Face

MANDIBLE

Anterior (External) Facial Bones
ZYGOMA
MAXILLA
LACRIMAL
NASAL

Posterior (Internal) Facial Bones
ETHMOID
PALATINE
INFERIOR NASAL CONCHA
VOMER

79 FACIAL RELATIONSHIPS

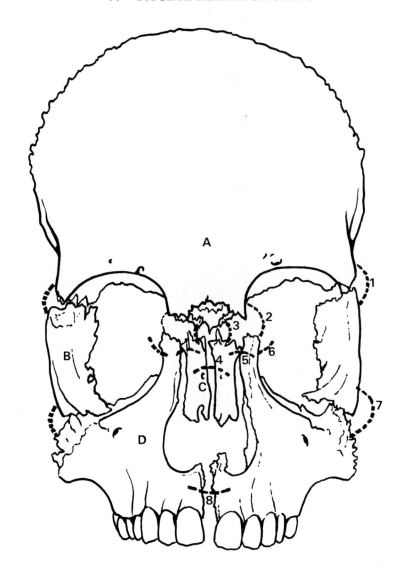

A FRONTAL
B ZYGOMA
C NASION
D MAXILLA

ARTICULATIONS
1. Frontozygomatic
2. Frontomaxillary
3. Frontonasal
4. Nasio-nasal
5. Nasiomaxillary
6. Maxillarylacrimal
7. Zygomaxillary
8. Maxillamaxillary

ANATOMY OF THE BASE

80 FACIAL RELATIONSHIPS
(Diagrammatic – not to scale)

NASAL

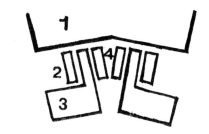

ORBITAL

NASAL

1 Frontal
2 Lacrimal
3 Maxillary
4 Nasal

ORBITAL

A Superior orbital fissure
B Inferior orbital fissure
1 Frontal
2 Ethmoid
3 Small wing of sphenoid
4 Great wing
5 Zygoma
6 Palatine
7 Lacrimal
8 Maxilla

MANDIBLE

Lt: Mandere – to chew/eat
This largest, strongest bone of the skull is also known as the Inferior Maxilla. (Without the mandible the bones of the head are known as the cranium). This bone which forms the chin carries alveolar sockets for the sixteen teeth of the lower jaw. Although formerly considered to be non-weight bearing it is now realized that even pre-natally when the embryo sucks its thumb or fist, this bone is actively bearing weight.

The mandible helps to support and protect various glands and lymph tissue; it is particulary intimately connected with the parotid glands. Its muscular attachments are of special significance to the cranial practitioner as hyper/hypotonicity in any of its many muscles will transmit imbalance – and therefore precipitate cranio-sacral dysfunction – via the petrous portion of the temporal bone to the parietals and then the meninges in one direction; and, again via the petrous portion of the temporal, to the base of the skull and the sphenobasilar symphysis in another. It is advisable then, to investigate and/or treat these muscles (Buccinator, Digastric, Masseter, Mentalis, Mylohyoid, Platysma, medial and lateral Pterygoids, Temporalis, etc.) and the Sterno-cleido-mastoid, before commencing treatment on vault or base.

In embryo this bone is in two halves which come together just before birth. It resembles a horseshoe the ends of which are set almost at a right-angle in adult life. The smooth external surface shows a raised mental protuberance medially at the symphysis menti which becomes roughly triangular inferiorly at the mental point. Either side of this point are small indentations/tubercles which can be palpated externally. One-third of the way along the anterior line of the jaw (under the second pre-molars) are the mental foramen which carry the mental nerves and blood vessels (from the mandibular branch of the 5th – Trigeminal – cranial nerve). An oblique line from the condyloid process to the lateral edge of the body of the mandible is one of its most prominent features. From the convex body the rami rise posteriorly as flattened quadrilaterals of bone, ending in two processes superiorly divided by the deeply concave Sigmoid notch which is crossed by the Masseteric nerves and blood vessels.

The internal surface is also smooth but marked by ridges and depressions. Inferomedially several small projections known as medial spines/genial tubercles occur at the incisive canal: these afford attachments for muscles. Another roughened area at the internal angle carries the medial pterygoid. A large foramen placed centrally in the ramus and bounded by a rounded 'spike' of bone called the lingula, connects with the mental foramen via the mandibular canal.

Apart from carrying the mental nerves and vessels it also carries the dental nerves and vessels which serve the teeth of the lower jaw. The sphenomandibular ligament is attached to the lingula.

Just below the alveolar border on the internal surface of the mandible is an oblique mylohyoid line above which is a depression/fovea for part of the sublingual gland, and below a fovea which houses the sub-maxillary gland.

The anterior, coronoid, process lies anteroposteriorly (the condylar process lying mediolaterally) and fits under the zygomatic arch. It is palpable just under the 'bulge' of the malar when the jaw is moved. Fibres of the Temporalis attach here.

The condylar (capitulum) process at the head of the mandible is divided into a head, neck and pterygoid fovea (the last serves for attachment of the lateral pterygoid). The lateral edge of this can be palpated externally at the auricular tragus when the jaw is moved. The slight depression felt here when the jaw is opened is the neck of the condyle.

In old age the edentulous jaw changes in angulation from about 90 degrees in the adult to an obtuse angle (about 140 degrees) as it was in infancy. Ossification takes place at the symphysis during the first twelve months from membrane formed around the anterior part of Meckel's cartilage, and is from one centre in each half primarily, and several other secondary centres. Cartilaginous deposits are also present at various times and, like the alveolar border in old age, are absorbed into the bone. The superior border becomes thinner, sharper, and harder, as the alveolar is absorbed and the mental foramen comes to lie on top of the jaw.

Mandibular articulations are partly ligamentous and partly osseous. The ligamentous are sphenomandibular and temporomandibular primarily. The only osseous articulation is at the glenoid fossa in the petrous portion of the temporal bone, via a disc, to the conyloid process. This temporomandibular joint is, perhaps, the most weak and unstable joint of the skull, and is subject to imbalance from many factors.

Lesions at the shoulder, neck and collar bone may prove resistant to treatment unless this T.M.J. is considered and treated as well. Dental mis-handling, mal-occlusions, etc. can grossly affect the balance of this joint.

Because of the close proximity to the major Gasserian ganglion of the 5th (Trigeminal) cranial nerve situated in Meckel's cave in the petrous portion of the temporal, pain/pathology at the forehead, scalp, eyelids, temples, nose, teeth, tongue, and hyoid, can all be attributed to a primary T.M.J. dysfunction. Interference with these areas is partly due to a stretched membraneous link involving the sphenoid and temporal bones.

So mandibular lesions can be traumatic or developmental. They can be secondary to grossly internally rotated temporal bones – sometimes from birth, or from a direct blow to the symphysis menti. Other blows can cause unilateral displacements.

81 MANDIBLE

A Articulates with mandibular fossa of temporal

1. Coronoid process
2. Head of condyle
3. Pterygoid fossa
4. Ramus
5. Molars
6. Premolar
7. Canine
8. Incisors
9. Angle of jaw
10. Mental Foramen
11. Tubercle
12. Symphysis menti
13. Protuberance
14. Oblique line
15. Notch
16. Body
17. Lingula
18. Foramen
19. Mylohyoid Groove

ANATOMY OF THE FACE
81 THE MANDIBLE

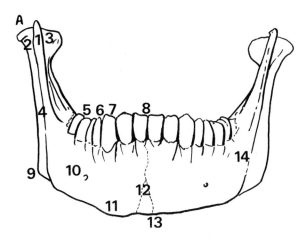

ANTERIOR ASPECT

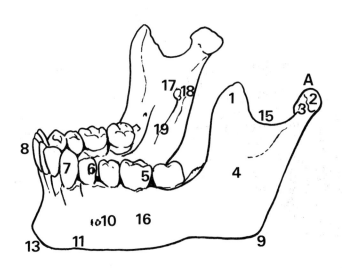

LATERAL ASPECT

ZYGOMA

Lt: jugum-yoke
Mala-jaw, cheek

The zygoma or malar bone has been variously described as quadrilateral or triangular, but it is basically a diamond; or can be seen as resembling a bird in flight – the frontal process representing the wings, and the temporal process the head.

Located either side of the face these two bones help form the temporal and zygomatic fossae, the zygomatic arch, and the inferolateral (side) and lateroinferior (floor) of the orbits – the outer quarter, so to speak. It should be noted that the size of the fossae described have a bearing on any cranial treatment.

Palpably the zygomae are obscured by the orbicularis palpebrarum, the masseter, and temporal muscles and fascia, and the major and minor zygomaticus. If the masseter is hypertonic it may cause a zygomatic lesion, occasioning pain in the cheek and eye.

These bones have an oblique axis in a line from glabella to the head of the mandible and they act as a 'transformer' between temporal and maxilla, and maxilla and sphenoid – slowing down the action of these bones.

The three processes projecting from the main body of each bone vary considerably in size and shape. The lateral (temporal) process is thin and pointed; the superior (frontal) process thicker and blunter with deep serrations which nevertheless possess great flexibility. The medial (maxillary) process is a short thickened wedge with irregular interdigitations allowing the maxilla to be contacted not only externally at the infraorbital border, but also internally in the orbital floor.

The external (lateral) surface of the zygoma is uneven and slightly convex, with a smooth rounded orbital rim, and a concave/convex temporal margin. Approximately one third of the way down the orbital rim is Whitnall's tubercle which is usually palpable and even visible in all but 5% of the population. It serves as an attachment for the lateral palpebral raphe and ligament. Just above the main body of the bone on the orbital rim are found one, or two, zygomatico-facial foramina which carry the orbital branches of the maxillary nerves, and blood vessels. These emerge on the inner rim of the orbit at the zygomaticoorbital foramen. Internally on the concave temporal surface of the zygoma is the zygomaticotemporal foramen.

Formed in membrane from three centres originally this bone can sometimes remain in two parts into adult life. It is a frequently lesioned area; due to its position of prominence it is more susceptible to direct trauma (laterally) than any of its neighbouring structures. It can be unilaterally lesioned by even such a small action as continually resting the cheek on the heel of the hand. It can also be disturbed by referral from maxillary, frontal, temporal and sphenoidal lesions. Any such disturbance to the zygoma must, of course, affect the function of the eye. Conjunctivitis, etc. will often clear if the bone's position is normalized.

The zygoma usually articulates with four other bones. With the zygomatic process of the frontal superiorly, and the zygomatic process of the temporal laterally at an angled or oblique suture – the acuteness of the angle varying greatly in individuals. This construction allows an oblique rocking movement which harmonizes with sphenobasilar mobility. Anteromedially it articulates with the maxilla at the infraorbital process and with the sphenoid's great wing internally where it overlies the maxillary sinus. As the maxilla/zygoma move in respiratory excursion they effectively 'squeeze' air in and out of this cavity.

Where the zygoma meets the sphenoid and the maxilla there is a small non-articulating surface. However, sometimes the sphenoid and maxilla meet directly at this point or there may be a sutural bone between.

MAXILLA

Lt: Maxilla-jaw
These two bones are also known as superior maxillae to distinguish them from the inferior maxilla – the mandible. The maxillae help form three facial cavities – nose, orbit and mouth; or they can be described as helping to form five parts of the facial skull: the sides of the nose; the medial wall and floor of the orbit; the anterior portion of the cheeks; the hard palate, and the upper (dental) jaw. The maxillae articulate with all the facial bones except the mandible (though they could be described as having a non-articular relationship when the teeth come together at the bite). They have a great effect on the cranio-sacral system as a whole via these articulations.

Of complex irregular shape each maxilla can be divided descriptively into five sections. The body is the largest central part and contains the maxillary sinus (Antrum of Highmore); and from this body project four processes; frontal (superomedially), zygomatic (laterally), alveolar (inferiorly) and palatine (anteroposteriorly).

The body of the maxilla is variously described as being pyramidal, quadrilateral, or irregular in shape. Its anterior surface exhibits a deep concavity anteromedially called the nasal notch which ends anteroinferiorly where it joins its counterpart in a nasal crest and spine.

The area below this in the median line is known as the incisive fossa, and laterally there are alternating ridges and depressions – due to the outline of the roots of the teeth – known as canine eminences and fossae. The several foramina in this area carry the dental nerves and blood vessels (from maxillary branch of 5th cranial nerve). At the lateral edge of the body is an articular tubercle. A large infra-orbital foramen situated below the orbital rim carries the infra-orbital nerve (part of the meningeal branch of the trigeminal).

Posteriorly, on the convex surface – parts of which are roughened – is a large jugal ridge. A vertical palatine process is continuous with the vertical process of the palatine bone, and forms an attachment to the other maxilla. Superiorly the smooth orbital surface is pierced by the infra-orbital fissure/groove which is continuous with the infra-orbital foramen externally. The lateral edge of the orbital surface is roughened for articulation with the zygoma (malar) bone.

The maxillary sinus is, arguably, the largest of the facial sinuses. Most of its area is obscured/filled by processes of the ethmoid, lacrimal, palatine and inferior conchae. As with other facial sinuses it does not begin to develop until late childhood.

The nasal surface is continuous with the frontal process of the maxilla which arises superomedially from the body. Both help to form the side wall of the nose, and, where they abut the lacrimal bone, a process/canal is formed for the nasolacrimal duct. The frontal process projects upward to the frontomaxillary suture and is fitted between the nasal bone (medially) and the lacrimal bone (laterally) – this helping to form the medial wall of the orbit. On the medial surface of the body an ethmoidal and a conchal crest are present.

The zygomatic process is triangular and articulates with the zygoma laterally at an oblique suture line. This process is concave on both surfaces.

The alveolar process is the curved anteroinferior border of the maxilla which carries sockets for the 16 teeth of the upper jaw. Each socket (as in the lower jaw) is lined with peridontal membrane (periosteum) – a cushion holding each tooth in place. This process extends posteriorly to the palatine process.

In the roof of the mouth the horizontal plate of the palatine process can be observed. It forms the largest portion (anterior ¾) of the hard palate and the floor of the nostril. As with the palatine bones, to which they are attached posteriorly, mucous membrane is intimately associated with the periosteum. Transverse folds are visible anteriorly – behind the incisive canal. These folds gradually disappear with age. In this area are found the foramina of Stenson and Scarpa that carry the palatine nerves and blood vessels.

Small depressions are also present which house the palatine glands – between the mucous membrane and the bone. A median raphe is noticeable in the mid-line where the maxillae join. When there is a failure to ossify at the lateral edge of the palate, a unilateral or bilateral 'cleft palate' results; often accompanied by a hare lip. A vertical section of the palatine process is continuous with the vertical process of the palatine bone – the posterior part of the nasal crest and spine.

Ossification is in membrane from several centres and begins pre-natally. In the infant the horizontal length of the maxillae is greater than the vertical, and the orbits are proportionately larger than in the adult. By maturity the vertical plane is the largest, due to the development of the alveolar margin and teeth, and the development of the nasal areas and the facial sinuses. In old age much of this vertical height is lost as the alveolar portion is absorbed.

Although direct trauma is not unusual, developmental problems in the maxilla are most common – partly due to the factors noted above of the changes in the horizontal and vertical planes. So lesions here can be unilateral or bilateral. As the infant grows the space between the hard palate and the roof of the nose should increase considerably, encouraging free drainage/flow of air, lymph and blood to facial fields. But a high arched 'gothic window' type palate is often found, denoting an extension head locked in internal rotation – associated with thumb-sucking, mouth-breathing, etc. Conversely a flattened arc – indicating an inferolateral twist – is observed, and is common after early dental extractions, remedial work, has been carried out. These lesions retard drainage in the anteromedial structures and affect facial expression, the function of the eye and other orbital structures (muscles, blood vessels, etc.) and occlusion of the jaws. Several nerves (from the 5th and 7th cranial) are intimately concerned with the maxillary bones. Functionally the maxillae, palatines and vomer act together and follow the sphenoid (though the maxilla does not usually articulate with the sphenoid) so all four should be examined and/or treated in maxillary lesions (e.g. the sphenopalatine ganglion is affected by maxillary crowding).

Lesions can be diagnosed by facial asymmetry protruding tongue, torus palatinus, septal and vomeric depression, observing the facial creases (naso-labial and supranasal) which are usually deeper on the lesioned side. If lesions are noted in infancy judicious moulding of the maxilla can obviate troubles later on.

The many articulations of the maxilla are with nine bones generally, although occasionally the sphenoid's lateral pterygoid plate articulates with the posteroinferior angle of the body of the maxilla at the tuberosity, and sometimes also with the orbital plate of the sphenoid in the orbit.

The maxilla articulates with the nasal part of the frontal in a flexible serrate junction; with the nasal and lacrimal bones either side of the frontal process, and the lacrimal also articulates with the maxilla in the orbit at the medial wall and with the zygoma at the lateral edge of the orbital plate of the maxilla. The zygoma articulates externally with the zygomatic process. It articulates with the palatine bone at the surface of the hard palate and at the vertical plate of the palatine; with the vomer in the median plane at the nasal crest. Inferiorly there are no articulations as this is edged with the teeth. The ethmoid's orbital surface articulates with the orbital surface of the maxilla; and with the inferior nasal conchae at the maxillary hiatus (sinus) and at conchal crest. The articulation with its counterpart is at the palatine process medially.

LACRIMAL

Lt: Lacrimale – tears

The lacrimals are two thin, fragile, roughly oblong plates of bone resembling fingernails – hence their other name os unguis. They are the smallest bones of the cranium and lie in the medial wall of the orbit between the frontal processes of the maxilla and the orbital plates of the ethmoid – in effect dropping into a 'V' space between the two. They also help to form the lateral nasal surface.

These bones ossify in membrane from one centre in each. Trauma to surrounding structures, frontal, maxillae, etc. is the cause of most lacrimal lesions. Therefore treatment of such structures will normalize the lacrimals as well.

The medial (nasal) surface helps form two anterior ethmoidal air cells but has no other distinguishing features.

The lateral (orbital) surface is distinguished by a central vertical crest; behind this the orbital surface is smooth. Anteriorly a groove joins with the posterior border of the frontomaxilla to house the lacrimal sac. This sac overlies the medial palpebral ligament, and is joined by the bifurcated lacrimal duct. It then proceeds inferiorly to become the naso-pharyngeal duct which empties the salty alkaline fluid from the eye into the nose. It is its relationship with the lacrimal apparatus that makes this bone an important consideration cranially.

At the inferior end of the lacrimal crest is a small hook-like process known as the Hamulus. This is sometimes a separate bone and is then referred to as the 'lesser lacrimal.' It helps form the superior part of the nasolacrimal duct.

The lacrimal articulates with four other bones: with the frontals superiorly at the anterior quarter of the notch; and with the ethmoid's orbital plate posterolaterally. Anteromedially it articulates with the frontal portion of the maxilla, and again with its orbital part inferiorly. It also articulates inferomedially with the inferior nasal concha.

NASAL

Lt. Nasus – nose

Two thin, roughly oblong bones lying below the glabella and medial to the orbits, form the bony bridge of the nose. Their size and shape vary considerably in individuals, and help to determine the shape of the cartilaginous section anteroinferiorly to them.

Heavier and serrated superiorly, and thinner and sharper inferiorly, these bones are very liable to direct trauma, causing deviation laterally not only to themselves but also to the nasal septum. They are also liable to impaction – into the nasal part of the frontal. Such injuries hinder nasal mucous flow and fluid drainage from the sinuses, as well as disturbing lacrimal secretion.

Lesions can also result as referrals from maxillary and frontal trauma, and can be unilateral. However, it is usual, partly due to the position of the bones, and partly the difficulty of moving one and not the other, to treat as if both were involved. The position that gives most stability to the practitioner is to engage the nasal portion of the frontal with one hand, whilst moving the nasals anteroinferiorly with the other. It is necessary to check, and usually to treat, the maxillae as well.

Formed in membrane the nasal bones ossify from one centre in each bone. The rotational axis of each is almost vertical.

Each nasal has a lateral (external) and medial (internal) surface. The former is smooth and convex horizontally, concave vertically; (the internal surface being concave across and convex in length). Apart from a foramen carrying a vein, approximately half way down the lateral surface, it carries no distinguishing features. Internally the bone is thick and serrated at the superior border and thinner inferiorly.

It carries an articular crest, and a groove for an anterior ethmoidal vein.

The nasal bone articulates with five units; its counterpart medially – in a triangular manner making them wider apart superiorly than inferiorly; the nasal cartilage at its inferior border; and three other bones. Its articulation with the frontal is twofold – superiorly, with the medial nasal part, and with the frontal spine via the crest. It articulates with the frontal process of the maxilla at the lateral border, and the cribriform plate of the ethmoid via the inferior portion of the crest.

82 ANTERIOR (EXTERNAL) FACIAL BONES

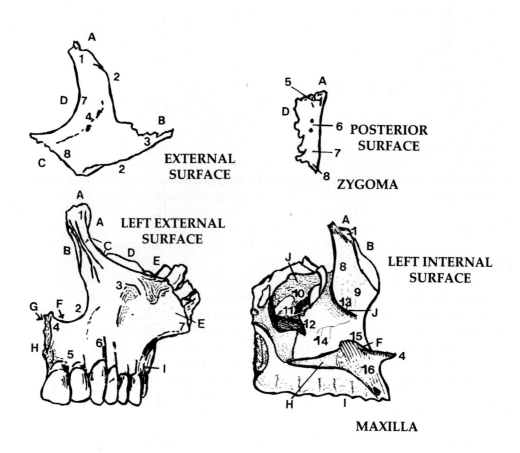

ANATOMY OF THE FACE

82 ANTERIOR (EXTERNAL) FACIAL BONES

ZYGOMA

A Articulates with zygomatic process of Frontal
B Articulates with zygomatic process of Temporal
C Articulates with zygomatic process of Maxilla
D Articulates with Sphenoidal great wing in the orbit

1 Frontal process
2 Free (non-articulating) surface
3 Temporal process
4 Zygomaticofacial foramen
5 Whitnall's tubercle
6 Zygomaticoorbital foramen
7 Orbital margin
8 Maxillary process

MAXILLA

A Articulates with nasal part of Frontal and in the orbit at medial border
B Articulates with Nasal bone
C Articulates with medial edge of Lacrimal
D Articulates with ethmoid's orbital surface
E Articulates with zygoma at maxillary process and in the orbit
F Articulates with inferior border of Vomer
G Articulates with horizontal and vertical plate of Palatine
H Articulates with counterpart at inferior medial border
I Non-articulating (alveolar) border
J Articulates with maxillary process of Inferior Nasal Conchae

1 Frontal process
2 Nasal notch
3 Infraorbital foramen
4 Anterior nasal spine
5 Incisive fossa
6 Canine eminence
7 Zygomatic process
8 Ethmoidal crest
9 Middle meatus
10 Ethmoid
11 Inferior nasal conchae
12 Palate
13 Conchal Crest
14 Inferior meatus
15 Nasal Crest
16 Incisive canal

83 ANTERIOR (EXTERNAL) FACIAL BONES

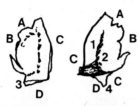

MEDIAL   LATERAL
SURFACES

LACRIMAL BONE

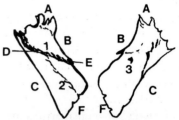

MEDIAL   LATERAL
SURFACES

NASAL BONE

LACRIMAL

A Articulates with medial internal angle of Frontal
B Articulates with orbital plate of Ethmoid
C Articulates with hamulus, nasal process, and orbital plate of Maxilla
D Articulates with lacrimal process of Inferior Nasal Conchae

1 Groove
2 Crest
3 Descending process
4 Hamulus

NASAL

A Articulates with medial nasal and spine of Frontal
B Articulates with counterpart at medial border
C Articulates with frontal process of Maxilla
D Articulates with cribriform plate of Ethmoid
E Articulates with septal cartilage
F Articulates with lateral nasal cartilage

1 Crest
2 Groove for anterior Ethmoid nerve
3 Foramen

276

ETHMOID

Gk: Ethos – sieve, eido – form

The Ethmoid is an irregular cube located at the root of the nose between the orbits, and in front of the sphenoid. It is of light spongy construction, and functionally is part of the cranial base, being formed in cartilage; although the conchal processes can be said to be part of the face – and is usually listed with the fourteen other facial bones – because of its other functions as part of the nose and orbits. In fact, all the bones of the face relate to the ethmoid.

It helps to form the medial wall of the orbit, the superior nasal septum, and the nose: dividing this part of the nose into two cavities. Its lateral aspects are saddle-shaped; the 'pommel' being the ala of the crista galli. From behind it somewhat resembles a moth with a long thick central body, and two heavy 'wings' either side.

The cribriform plate forms the roof of the nose where it is suspended from the frontal at the central ethmoidal notch by the ethmoidal alae. This completes the foramen caecum. The olfactory bulb is found on the grooved superior surface, and is a continuation of the olfactory tract within the skull. The inferior surface of this bulb gives off a bundle of olfactory (1st cranial) nerves which pass through approximately twenty foramina to the mucous membrane of the nose. These are responsible for sense of smell and convey messages to the area of Broca, the anterior commissure, and the uncus.

The superior border of the cribriform plate connects with the anterior superior pole of the dura via the posterior border of a triangular spur called the crista galli (cockscomb). This is a very strong attachment.

The perpendicular plate has more attachments than any other part of the ethmoid. It hangs from the cribriform plate and forms the superior part of the nasal septum.

From the sides of the cribriform plate hangs the laminae of the ethmoidal labyrinths. They have two surfaces, the lamina papyracea forms part of the orbital medial wall. The opposite (medial) surface forms the superior and middle conchae which inferiorly curve evertly. Between these two surfaces the ethmoidal air sinuses are paper thin cells honeycombing the lateral masses. They open into the superior middle meatus (space) of the nose. Under the middle concha is a particular group of air cells which present as a circular mass called a bulla. Alongside this bulla is the hiatus semilunaris containing an opening for the maxillary sinus at the uncinate process.

Septal deviations are referred to the ethmoid; often due to faulty facial development. Lesions here are usually secondary to sphenoidal and frontal, maxillary and zygomatic, dysfunction. So, the ethmoid should always be considered along with these bones. In sinusitis, hay fever, etc. the frontal, ethmoid, and conchae are in expansion. If the maxillae go into internal rotation so will the lateral masses as they follow each other.

84 POSTERIOR (INTERNAL) FACIAL BONES

ETHMOID

A Articulates with ethmoidal notch and nasal spine of the Frontal
B Articulates with crest of the Nasals
C Articulates with septal cartilage
D Articulates with superior anterior border of Vomer
E Articulates with crest of Sphenoid
F Articulates with uncinate process of inferior (and superior) Nasal Conchae
G Articulates with orbital plate of Palatine
H Articulates with frontal process of Maxilla – in orbit
I Articulates with posterior border of Lacrimal

1 Crista Galli
2 Ethmoidal labyrinth
3 Cribriform plate
4 Groove for ethmoidal vessels
5 Ala (of crista galli)
6 Orbital plate
7 Canal for posterior ethmoidal vessels
8 Canal for anterior ethmoidal vessels
9 Uncinate process
10 Middle nasal concha
11 Perpendicular plate

ANATOMY OF THE FACE

84 POSTERIOR (INTERNAL) FACIAL BONES

THE ETHMOID

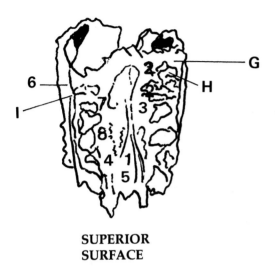

SUPERIOR SURFACE

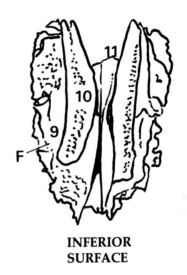

INFERIOR SURFACE

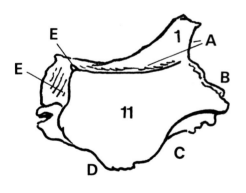

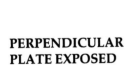

PERPENDICULAR PLATE EXPOSED

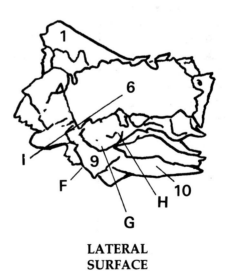

LATERAL SURFACE

279

The motion of the ethmoid can be judged by placing the first finger of one hand on the glabella and the fourth finger on/under the nasion. Freeing the ethmoid can be accomplished by springing the frontals at the anteroinferior border to exaggerate the lesion, then freeing the superoinferior plane by distraining the frontal superiorly and the mastoids anteroinferiorly. Any fixation – and they are common – such as described at the frontoethmoidal articulation limits the falx cerebri and therefore all dural membraneous motion. A frontal lift is sometimes all that is necessary to reduce this occlusion.

Ossification of the ethmoid commences in cartilage and some parts are still cartilaginous at birth. Ossification is not complete until the fourth or fifth year.

The ethmoid articulates with ten other structures two of which are the septal cartilage (at the anteroinferior part of the perpendicular plate) and the anterior superior pole of the falx cerebri, at the posterior part of the crista galli. Articulations with the frontal bone are at the cribriform plate and ala of the crista galli (with the ethmoidal notch and posterior part of the nasal spine) and at the labyrinth with the roof of the ethmoidal air cells. The orbital plate of the frontal articulates with the ethmoid in the orbit.

The nasals and vomer join the perpendicular plate at the anterior border and inferoposterior border respectively. The posterior border of the lacrimal articulates with the ethmoid at the orbital plate. Both the orbital process of the palatine, and the orbital plate and frontal process of the maxilla, articulate with the ethmoid in the orbit – the medial wall of the labyrinth. The superior and inferior conchae articulate with the ethmoid at the uncinate process.

Articulations with the sphenoid are various – with the superior border of the perpendicular plate with the sphenoidal crest; with the lateral mass in the orbit – with the lateral surface of the body and the lesser wing; and by a triangular notch of the cribriform plate with the ethmoidal spine. These give flexible articulation to the cranial base.

PALATINE

Lt: Palatum – division or taste
The two palatine bones form the posterior quarter of the hard palate, the beginnings of the soft palate, and are part of the posterior nasal cavity, and orbital floor. They are therefore concerned with the infra-orbital fissure and pterygopalatine fossa. Like the zygoma they act as a 'transformer' between maxillary and sphenoid – governing the movements of both. The palatines lie between the pterygoid processes and the tuberosities of the maxilla, and lateral to the posterior nares.

Each bone can be descriptively divided into two parts. A horizontal plate articulates with its counterpart at the median raphe and is functionally an extension of the palatine process of the maxilla – forming the palatum durum. When the raphe is forced downwards by depression of the vomer the resulting ridge is known as Torus Palatinus. This medial nasal crest is broad and roughened anteriorly. Buccal mucous membrane adheres closely to this part, and the free posterior portion is curved (forming the anterior soft palate). At the lateral border a branch of the Trigeminal (5th cranial nerve) passes through the greater palatine foramen (carrying greater palatine vessels). The vertical plate has two processes superiorly, one inferiorly.

The palatine is formed in membrane from one centre in the vertical plate. At birth both plates are the same length; in the adult, however, the vertical is twice the length of the horizontal.

Each palatine articulates with six other bones; its counterpart inferomedially – and the vomer – at the horizontal plate; the inferior conchae at the conchal crest of the vertical plate and the middle conchae at the ethmoidal crest. The orbital process also articulates with the ethmoid. The maxilla articulates with various portions of the anterior boder from orbital process to horizontal plate, and the sphenoid similarly with parts of the posterior border (pyramidal, sphenoidal, and orbital process and vertical border).

Palatine lesions are usually secondary to spheno-basilar torsion and rotational side-bending lesions; involving sphenopalatine ganglia and maxilla. (This is except for direct trauma to the roof of the mouth). As the Palatines follow the motion of the maxilla inferiorly and the sphenoidal pterygoids superiorly, it is usual to correct any such lesions to those two bones first, and often the need to treat the palatines themselves disappears. As the palatines also form part of the orbital floor they should not be overlooked as a possible cause of eye troubles. It should also be noted that pain at the temporal fossa may well be referred from a palatine lesion (this is because the innervation – maxillary – is shared). The plate is marked by ridges internally across its width for articulation with the conchae, and these divide the meati. The other surfaces are grooved and uneven for muscle attachments and the passage of vessels. A pyramidal process projects posteroinferiorly and this is also grooved and pitted for passage of the greater palatine vessels and articulation with pterygoids and maxilla.

The orbital and sphenoidal processes are divided by the sphenopalatine notch. This notch becomes a foramen when joined by the sphenoidal conchae which then gives passage to the sphenopalatine and supranasal and nasopalatine nerves and vessels (part of maxillary branch of Trigeminal). The orbital process is the most superior part of the palatine bone and is hollowed internally and occasionally externally, in which case it forms part of an ethmoidal air cell as well as part of the sphenoidal cells which are usually present. Although small this process has three articulating and two non-articulating surfaces – the orbital and zygomatical surfaces are free.

The sphenoidal process is slightly smaller than the orbital and also has articulating surfaces. Occasionally these two processes are joined superiorly and thereby form a foramen; and sometimes there are two foramina thus formed by an extra bony outgrowth between the processes.

INFERIOR NASAL CONCHAE

Lt.Gk: Koncha – a shell
Lt: Turbinate – whirling top
The inferior nasal conchae (or inferior turbinates as they are often known) are situated horizontally in the anterior nares, and form part of the inferior meatus. They are approximately level with the inferior orbital foramen and present as two thin plates of bone curved into scrolls and convex medially. Pointed posteriorly and broader anteriorly each surface is roughened and pierced, pitted, and grooved for the passage of blood vessels. The space created between the inferior and middle conchae forms the opening of the maxillary sinus. There are no muscular attachments but each concha is covered in nasal mucous membrane.

(There are superior and middle nasal conchae but these form part of the ethmoid bone).

Each bone ossifies in cartilage from one centre and is usually only visible via posterior rhinoscopy (an angled mirror at the posterior nasal part of the pharynx) but when in lesion they are visible from the anterior nares. Lesions are mostly unilateral and secondary to sphenobasilar, ethmoidal, maxillary or palatine trauma – hence a deviated septum or unilateral breathing difficulties may well be present and correction of such lesions are, of course, dependant on cause. These bones may be functionally thought of as extensions of the ethmoid.

The concha articulates with four other bones. Taken from behind forward these are the palatine – at posterior/superior border via palatine crest; with the uncinate process of the ethmoid via ethmoidal process of concha; with the lacrimal via superior lacrimal process; and the maxilla at the anterior border and maxillary process via maxillary crest.

VOMER

Lt: Vomis – plowshare
This thin 'V' shaped bone resembles the knife plate of a plough (ploughshare). The two fused laminae closely adhere inferiorly but are evertly flared (curved)

at the upper margins. Roughly trapezoidal in shape the vomer lies in the sagittal plane at the posterior nasal fossa dividing the space into right and left nasal areas. It forms the posterior and inferior parts of the nasal septum, abutting the sphenoidal sinuses at the superior border and the choana posteriorly.

Both surfaces of the vomer are obliquely grooved for the passage of the sphenopalatine nerves and vessels, and furrowed to carry other blood vessels. Mucous membrane is continuous with the periosteum and as this allows for very little sub-mucous membrane, polyps are not usually found in this part of the nose. There are no muscular attachments to this bone.

The vomer should be considered as one unit functionally with the maxillae, palatines, and the perpendicular plate of the ethmoid, as it provides continuity between the sphenoid and the hard palate to which it is firmly attached. Vomeric deviation is often perceived, and is usually secondary to sphenoidal action and is not directly related to septal deviation. Therefore any lesion here is usually developmental, rather than from direct trauma, but, however, distorted, it will retain movement as (in common with most other facial bones) it has a degree of springing, and its pump action helps to drain facial sinuses, especially the sphenoidal sinus. However, distortion will affect the spheno-basilar symphysis.

The vomer may alternatively be pushed down, sometimes actually bisecting the median suture of the maxillary/palatine hard palate and is then seen as a ridge-known as torus palatinus – indicating a shortening of the space between the hard palate and the roof of the nose. Hence it will be readily seen that it is always necessary to examine, and often treat, the vomer in maxillary and sphenoidal lesions. When the sphenoid is in flexion it transmits tension down through the vomer to the maxillae and palatines, and therefore observing the roof of the mouth and noting any concavity/convexity shown there will indicate a similar position at the sphenoid – in the same way as observing the plane of the sacrum tells you what is happening at the occiput. You will, of course, see the same pattern described in the median plane of the facial fields (see Chapter 10).

One finger on the staurion will test vomeric motion and by also tipping the sphenoid as necessary the vomeric action will be therapeutically altered.

The two laminae are formed in membrane and originally have a central cartilaginous plate sandwiched between them. This part is later absorbed but the rest is prolonged anteriorly to complete the nasal septum and superiorly ossifies to become the perpendicular plate of the ethmoid. Ossification of the vomer is usually complete by adulthood.

The vomer has seven articulating surfaces – six osseous and one cartilaginous. Superiorly it articulates with the rostrum of the sphenoid medially at the central groove of the ala; and at the lateral borders of the ala, with the vaginal processes of the medial pterygoid plates. (This union

85 POSTERIOR (INTERNAL) FACIAL BONES

PALATINE

A   Articulates with medial and lateral pterygoid plates and body of Sphenoid
B   Articulates with palatine and orbital process and maxillary sinus of Mastoid
C   Articulates with posterior inferior border of Vomer
D   Articulates with posterior superior border of Inferior Nasal Conchae
E   Articulates with lateral mass of Ethmoid
F   Articulates with counterpart at perpendicular plate

1   Orbital process
2   Conchal crest
3   Maxillary process
4   Pyramidal tubercle
5   Perpendicular plate
6   Sphenoidal process
7   Sphenopalatine notch
8   Nasal crest
9   Horizontal plate

INFERIOR NASAL CONCHA

A   Articulates with conchal crest of Palatine bone
B   Articulates with uncinate process of Ethmoid
C   Articulates with descending process of Lacrimal
D   Articulates with conchal crest and medial surface of Maxilla

1   Lacrimal process
2   Anterior process
3   Medial aspect
4   Posterior process
5   Ethmoidal process

VOMER

A   Articulates with rostrum of Sphenoid
B   Articulates with perpendicular plate of Ethmoid
C   Articulates with septal cartilage
D   Articulates with nasal crest of Maxilla and Palatine

1   Ala
2   Posterior border
3   Nasopalatine groove
4   Anterior border

85 POSTERIOR (INTERNAL) FACIAL BONES

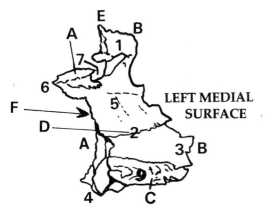
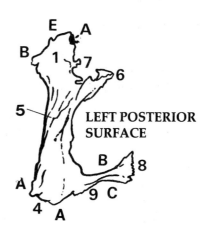

PALATINE

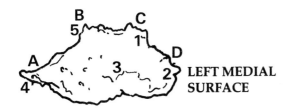
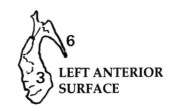

INFERIOR NASAL CONCHAE

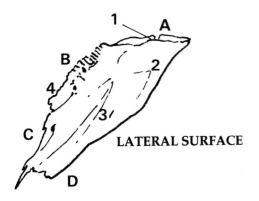
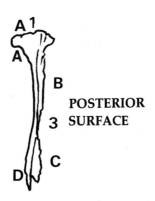

VOMER

occasionally forms a vomerovaginal canal which, if present, carries the pharyngeal branch of the sphenopalatine vessels). This rostrum/vomeric articulation is a modified ball and socket joint, and has been referred to as a type of 'universal joint.'

Inferiorly the vomer articulates with the nasal crests of the maxilla (anterior two-thirds) at the incisive crest, and the palatines (posterior one-third). The anterior border carries the septal cartilage (anterior two thirds) and the perpendicular plate of the ethmoid (posterior one-third). The posterior border forms the posterior edge of the nasal septum, and is smooth and unarticulated.

Two of these articulations are schindelyses – at the sphenoidal rostrum and at the vaginal process, the rest are harmonic (edge to edge).

VILHJALMUR STEFANSSON

'If everything is well managed, if there are no miscalculations or mistakes, then the things that happen are only the things you expected to happen and for which you are ready and with which you can therefore deal.'

CHAPTER TWENTY ONE

Ancillary Bones of the Skull

HYOID
AUDITORY OSSICLES
SUTURAL (WORMIAN)

THE HYOID

Hyoideus Gk (shaped as Upsilon 'U')
This horseshoe, or anchor shaped bone is ancillary to the cranial system but of great significance due to its many attachments of fascia, ligaments, and muscles, which pertain to the function of the neck and skull. It is not the anatomy of the bone itself, therefore, that is important here, but the action of the soft tissue attachments.

Similar in shape to the mandible, albeit much smaller, it is held in suspension in the anterior pharynx at the level of 3C/4C – just above the thyroid cartilage, and beneath the submaxillary gland. The posterior tips of its greater horns can be palpated just under the angles of the mandible, adjacent to the anterior border of the sternocleidomastoid, where it is suspended from the styloid process via the stylohyoid ligaments.

Formed in cartilage, ossification usually commences in utero, although the synovial joints between cornu (horns) and body do not normally ossify until middle age.

The hyoid's posterior surface is concave and directed posteroinferiorly. The lesser horns (cornu) are cone-shaped tubercles on the superior surface at the angle of the greater horn and the base.

This bone is separated from the epiglottis by free areolar tissue, a bursa, and the thyrohyoid membrane. The muscular innervation is from branches of the cranial and cervical nerves.

TABLE M HYOIDAL MUSCLES & LIGAMENTS

NAME	ATTACH-MENT	ORIGIN	INSERTION	NERVE SUPPLY	FUNCTION
PRIMARY GENIOHYOID	↑	posterior surface symphysis menti	anterior Hyoid body	1st Cervical via 12th cranial nerve	moves tongue and Hyoid anteriorly and elevates Hyoid. If hypertonic or contracted can cause tight, taut, throat and forced depression of the lower jaw. Found particularly in depressive, anxiety or general emotional states
STYLOHYOID	←	Styloid process of Temporal	lateral surface of Hyoid	branch of 7th Cranial	moves Hyoid ant/post.
MYLOHYOID	←	Mandibular mylohyoid line	Body of Hyoid	branch of 5th Cranial	raises Hyoid and tongue; aids in mouth action (mastication, blowing, sucking, etc). Watch for referred related dysfunction from Hyoid to c-s system and visa-versa. Lesions found particularly in emotional states, etc.
STERNOHYOID	→	medial end of clavicle, manubrially; sternoclavicular ligament – occasionally from 1st and 2nd rib.	inferior body of Hyoid	1st, 2nd, 3rd Cervical	Depresses Hyoid inferiorly and stabilizes same
THYROHYOID	→	Lamina of Thyroid cartilage	inferior border of Hyoid	1st & 2nd Cervical	elevates Thyroid cartilage. Many significant relationships to c-s system
OMOHYOID	→	Double-bellied muscle with connecting		2nd & 3rd Cranial	moves Hyoid inferiorly; influences c-s system via

TABLE M HYOIDAL MUSCLES & LIGAMENTS (CONTINUED)

OMOHYOID (cont'd)	central tendon (which is bound by cervical fascia) a) suprascapula b) central tendon	central tendon & s.c.m. via clavicle posterior Hyoid		Thoracic inlet
DIGASTRIC	Double-bellied muscle a) anterior: inf. border of mandible – digastric fossa b) posterior: temporal mastoid notch.	via tendon into lateral edge of Hyoid	branch of 5th Cranial branch of 7th Cranial	Both elevate Hyoid and aid jaw opening a) moves Hyoid anteriorly b) moves Hyoid posteriorly. Transmits tension from Hyoid to temporal & mandible causing c-s dysfunction. Associated with aphonia
SECONDARY GENIOGLOSSUS HYPOGLOSSUS MIDDLE CONSTRICTOR CHONDROGLOSSUS	These muscles are also attached to the Hyoid but of secondary importance to the cranio-sacral system		12th Cranial 12th Cranial branch of 10th & 12th Cranial 12th Cranial	Generally control action of tongue constricts pharynx
LIGAMENTS HYOEPIGLOTTIC	Epiglottis	base attached to superior border of Hyoid		triangular band of elastic tissue
STYLOHYOID	styloid process of temporal	lesser horn of Hyoid		forms posterior part of Thyrohyoid membrane
LATERAL THYROHYOID (Berry's ligament)	superior horn of Thyroid cartilage	base of Hyoid		
FASCIA	Basically the investing portion of the deep cervical fascia arises from the 7C and the ligamentum nuchae (arising from the occiput). It invades all the vessels and free spaces of the neck (posterior & anterior traingles) and anteromedially inserts into the symphysis menti and the Hyoid bone			

Most of the muscles which open the mouth and supply the tongue are attached to the hyoid and they are best summarized as the accompanying table shows.

AUDITORY OSSICLES

Lt. Ossicula auditus (small bones of hearing)

These are three bones situated in the irregular middle ear cavity of the petrous portion of the temporal bone. They are part of the mechanism of the reception of sound – the higher tones in particular. The middle ear is lined with respiratory mucosa.

Because of their shape they are called malleus (hammer), incus (anvil), and stapes (stirrup). They act as a bridge between the tympanic membrane and the oval window transmitting sound between them by the handle of the malleus moving with the tympanic membrane anteriorly on the incus, which in turn pushes the base of the stapes forward. The rest of the malleus and the incus rotate around their connecting axis.

Being effectively part of the cranial base the ossicles are formed in cartilage, excepting at the anterior process of the malleus which ossifies separately in membrane. The articulations are synovial joints.

Malleus This has a bulbous handle and tapering tail. The handle is attached to the tympanic membrane laterally and articulates with the incus medially. Some of the fibres of the anterior ligament, and the tensor tympani, attached to the middle third of the bone and the tympanic cavity, reach the spine of the sphenoid.

Incus This bone mainly acts as an articulating surface between the malleus and the stapes. Its angles accommodate to those of the malleus, being a bulbous head at one end, and a tapering tail at the other which attaches to the head of the stapes.

Stapes This is the most accurately named of the three as it does resemble a riding stirrup. Its head articulates with the incus and the footplate is fixed to the oval window by fibres of ligament.

It should be noted that any severe injury to the base of the skull can cause considerable haemorrhage, and leakage of C.S.F., which will be void via the inner and outer ear, due to the invasive mucous membrane around the ossicles which arises from the pharynx and connects via the roof of the middle ear cavity with the dura.

SUTURAL BONES

These **ossa triquestra** (triangular bones) also called Wormian after a Danish anatomist Olas Worm (1588–1654) are often present as small irregularly shaped 'islands' of bone in between sutures and are usually bilateral. They have separate ossification centres from the main bones. Mostly occuring at the lambdoidal suture and at the site of the posterior fontanelle, they are also to be found occasionally in the orbit and other fontanelle sites.

When present at the anterior lateral fontanelles they are given the name Pterion ossicles. As these occur in the vault they are formed in membrane. In size they usually range from tiny 'pin head' excursions into the outer table of bone to finger-nail size and as such have little significance in cranial work – being only two or three in number.

In extreme cases however, more than a hundred have been reported – particularly in cases of hydrocephalus; or, two of these sutural bones have been known to be so large as to almost divide the occipital bone into three parts (see illustration 86). The possible effect of these, cranially speaking, must cause us to pause when attempting occipital techniques.

86 ANCILLARY BONES OF THE SKULL

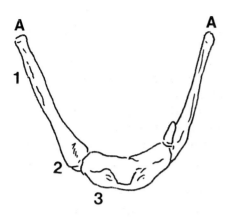

THE HYOID

A Stylohyoid articulation

1. Greater horn (cornu)
2. Lesser horn (cornu)
3. Body

THE OSSICLES

A Malleuoincudo articulation
B Incudostapedial articulation

1. Head
2. Neck
3. Handle
4. Body
5. Short limb
6. Long limb
7. Head
8. Footplate

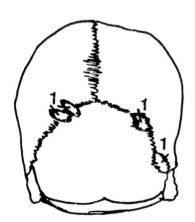
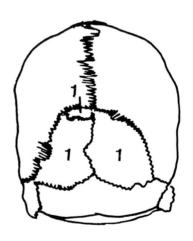

SUTURAL BONES
Note large area of occiput covered by sutural bones in second illustration.

1. Sutural Bones

IZAAK WALTON

'Look to your health; and if you have it, praise God, and value it next to a good conscience, for health is the second blessing that we mortals are capable of, a blessing that money cannot buy.'

CHAPTER TWENTY TWO

The Foetal Skull

87 FULL TERM FOETAL SKULL

FONTANELLES

A Anterior (Frontal)
B Posterior (Occipital)
C Anterolateral (Sphenoidal)
D Posterolateral (Mastoid)

1 Left Frontal (squamous portion)
2 Right Frontal
3 Metopic suture
4 Coronal suture
5 Left Parietal
6 Sagittal Suture
7 Right Parietal
8 Lambdoid suture
9 Occiput
10 Septal cartilage
11 Superciliary arch
12 Zygoma
13 Maxilla
14 Symphysis menti
15 Mandible
16 Sphenoid (Great Wing)
17 Temporal
18 Tympanic ring
19 Parietal tuberosity
20 Frontal tuberosity (ossification points)

ESSENTIALS OF CRANIO-SACRAL OSTEOPATHY

87 FULL TERM FOETAL SKULL

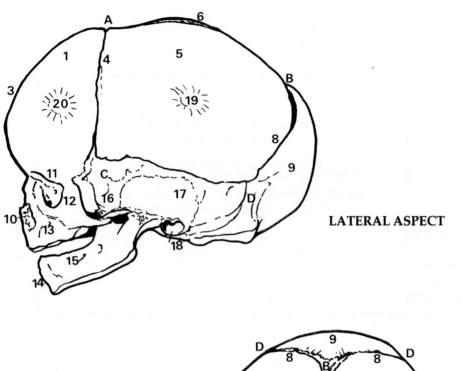

LATERAL ASPECT

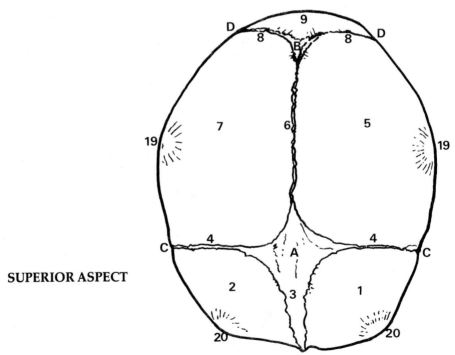

SUPERIOR ASPECT

THE FOETAL SKULL

> ## PLATO
>
> 'This is the great error of our day in the treatment of the human body, that physicians separate the soul from the body.'

CHAPTER TWENTY THREE

The Sacrum & Coccyx

SACRUM

COCCYX

THE SACRUM

Lt. Sacralis – sacred
This large irregular, or wedge-shaped bone, forms the inferior end of the cranio-sacral system, and its movements mirror those of the occipital bone to which it is linked by spinal dura. An 'L' shaped area at the sacro-iliac joint is similar to that of the 'L' shaped area at the sphenoid and frontal at the pterion.

The sacrum is suspended between the ilia by strong ligamentous bands and varies considerably in size, shape, angulation, and volume. It was named for its close associations with the new life that occurs in pregnancy within the pelvic bowl, and indeed it forms the posterior wall of that cavity. The promontary on the anterior surface can be so angled as to reduce the A.P. diameter of the pelvic brim creating difficulties in childbirth. The female sacrum (and pelvis) tends to be shorter and broader than the male, the vestigial articular tubercles are more prominent and larger in men.

The lateral borders of the sacrum can be more convergent at their superior aspect, or at their inferior, or they may lie in parallel planes, the angles of the articulating surfaces altering with each type.

The sacrum consists of five (or sometimes four or six) fused vertebrae, the amount of fusion present being determined mainly by age. (It ossifies from above downward during the first twenty five years of life). The 'sacral base plane' is actually at the superior surface which is transversely horizontal. Magoun stated that the A.P. angle should be 30–35 degrees ideally, but maintained that 15–67 degrees was functionally weight bearing and acceptable, and although many may question this, Fryette agrees with his

THE SACRUM AND COCCYX

findings. The sacrum via the sacro-iliac joints transmits body weight outwards to the hip joints. Like the sphenoid the sacrum has a transverse axis, the upper part moving posterosuperiorly on inspiration, the apex anteroinferiorly.

The anterior (pelvic) surface is concave and triangular (the base uppermost) and exhibits four pairs of foramina which transmit anterior rami of the first sacral nerves. The transverse grooves between the foramina represent the lines of fusion, the intermediate crests, the articular facets.

The convex posterior (dorsal) surface also have foramina which carry posterior rami of sacral nerves. It has central crests which are rudimentary spinous processes, and lateral crests (eminences) which are rudimentary transverse processes.

The lateral surfaces emphasize the angulation which forms the most inferior curve of the spine. The arachnoid and dural membranes close at the level of the second segment. An oval sacral hiatus superomedially is for the sacral canal, and encloses the end of the spinal cord, cauda equina roots, filum terminale, blood vessels, nerve filaments and adipose tissue.

The sacrum can move laterally, superiorly, inferiorly and by rotation. Physiologically flexion, extension, torsion and side-bending rotation are all possible. Eight muscles attach to the sacrum; piriformis and iliacus anteriorly; gluteus maximus, multifidious, sacrospinalis, erector spinae and latissimus dorsi posteriorly – more muscles being necessary to extend the spine against gravitational pull, than to flex it.

Many ligaments criss-cross the sacroiliac spaces etc. the ten major ones are the supraspinous, iliolumbar, short and long posterior sacroiliac, sacrotuberal, sacrococcygeal, lumbosacral, anterior sacroiliac, superficial posterior, and anterior longtitudinal.

The sacrum consists of cancellous tissue, sandwiched in compact tissue. It arises from over thirty centres of ossification. It fuses at approximately the same time as the sphenobasilar symphysis. It usually articulates with four other bones; the base of the fifth lumbar at a central articulating facet having a disc between, and by the superior articular facets which tend to face posteromedially and articulate with the inferior facets of the fifth lumbar. It also articulates with the ilia at large ear-shaped facets laterally. This joint is amphiarthroidal in children, but acquires a synovial cavity and becomes diarthroidal in the adult. Hence in children a definite 'spring' action is observed on palpation. This is replaced by a gliding action in the adult. The fourth articulation is at the cornu with the sacral cornu of the coccyx inferiorly.

It should be noted that both sacralization (fusion with the fifth lumbar to form six sacral segments) and lumbarization (incomplete fusion to effectively form six lumbar) are not unusual and can seriously limit movement, especially flexion and extension. As the anterior ligaments are weaker than the posterior, the anterior portion can easily 'gap' and cause problems; especially where there is lateral body rotation.

88 THE SACRUM

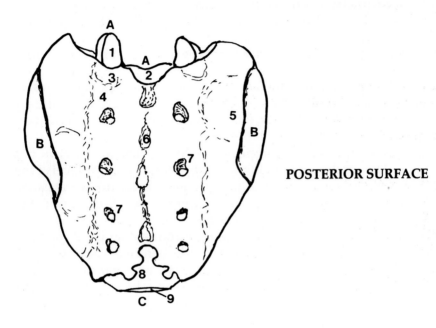

POSTERIOR SURFACE

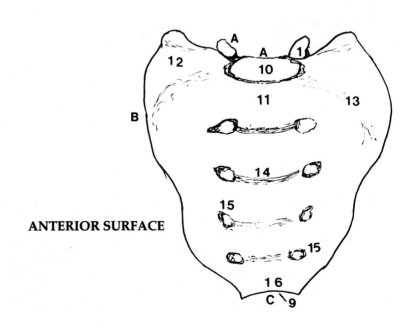

ANTERIOR SURFACE

THE SACRUM AND COCCYX
88   THE SACRUM

A Superior facet – for articulation with fifth Lumbar.
   Superomedial facet – for articulation with fifth Lumbar
B Sacroiliac joint – for articulation with Ilia
C Sacrococcygeous joint – for articulation with Coccyx

1 Superior articulating facet
2 Sacral canal
3 Tuberosity
4 Intermediate sacral crest
5 Lateral sacral crest
6 Median sacral crest
7 Posterior foramina
8 Cornu
9 Hiatus
10 Base
11 Promontary
12 Ala
13 Linea Terminalis
14 Transverse Ridges
15 Anterior foramina
16 Apex

THE COCCYX

The coccyx – as has already been mentioned – is an often disregarded, seemingly unimportant, rudimentary (or modified) group of bones at the inferior part of the vertebral column. It is not weight bearing but retains flexibility and aids in respiratory excursion, as well as serving as an attachment for certain muscles and ligaments.

It is usually found to be in two portions, an upper somewhat oblong part (1st coccygeal vertebra) and a triangular part below (2, 3, 4th coccygeal vertebrae). The exact number of bones present vary from 3 to 5 and the 1st may be fused to the apex of the sacrum, especially in females over 45 years old. Very occasionally the coccyx remains as 4–5 separate units and retains cartilaginous 'discs' between the segments.

Approximately level with the ischial spines inferiorly the coccyx is continuous with the curve of the sacrum (concave anteriorly). Foramina are usually absent, but the filum terminale does extend to the 1st vertebra and bonds with the sacrococcygeal ligament.

The extent of transverse processes, pedicles, spines, etc. varies greatly but are generally absent on all but the 1st and 2nd vertebrae, and then they are vestigial and known as eminences. Where transverse processes are found on the first vertebra they articulate with the inferior lateral angle of the sacrum.

There are two horn like projections rising from the base of the coccyx (superior border of 1st coccygeal vertebra) known as cornu. These articulate with sacral cornu above, and the space that intervenes medially between the 5th sacral body and the intercornual ligament, affords passage for the 5th sacral nerve. Also present anteromedially, in most cases, is a facet for articulation with the anteromedial facet of the apex of the sacrum (5th sacral body).

The coccyx is formed in cartilage from mesoderm and ossifies from one centre in each bone. The first begins to ossify at birth, the rest at various intervals until the fourth is usually complete by late adolescence. Group ossification is from below – the second occasionally fusing with the first at approximately 35 years of age.

The coccyx is generously supplied with ligamentous and muscular attachments to strengthen and give mobility to the inferior triangle of the spinal column. The muscles which move the coccyx anterosuperiorly are the coccygeus and the levator ani, (which is really a group of muscles forming the pelvic diaphragm). The former arises at the Ischial spine and inserts on the lateral surface of the lower sacrum and coccyx. The latter arises post-pubis and from the ischial spine and inserts into the anterior tip of the coccyx. Both form part of the pelvic floor, supporting internal organs and resisting uterine and bladder prolapse. They also help regulate intra-abdominal pressure and micturition.

The gluteus maximus and sphincter ani attach to the posterior surface of the coccyx and counteract the pull of the first two muscles described – their action being posteroinferiorly.

The gluteus maximus arises on the posterior lateral surface of the coccyx (and the sacrum and ilia) and inserts into the iliotibial tract and femoral tuberosity. It extends, abducts and laterally rotates the thigh. The sphincter ani originates at the posterior tip of the coccyx and adjacent fascia and inserts into anal perineum and is the anal constrictor. It is obvious therefore that a distorted coccyx can be involved in a uterine displacement, frequency of urine, pelvic floor collapse, constipation, etc.

The ligamentous attachments are varied. The intercornual ligaments are between the sacral and coccygeal cornu; the anterior sacrococcygeal ligaments are cruciate in form – attaching at the last segment of the sacrum and the last segment (anteriorly and laterally) of the coccyx. The deep and superficial posterior sacrococcygeal ligaments are actually a fan-like continuation of the supraspinous ligament and extend from the sacral hiatus to the posterior surface of the coccyx. The lateral sacro-coccygeal ligaments attach at the tip of the transverse process of the 1st vertebra and insert in the inferior lateral angle of the sacrum. The sacrospinous is attached along the lateral edge of both sacrum and coccyx and inserts into the apex of the ischial spine and with the sacrotuberous ligament (which has similar attachments) divides the sacral space into two foramina (greater and lesser sacrosciatic foramen).

Cranially speaking it is this ligamentous and muscular activity that is most important as it controls the A.P. movement that occurs on inhalation/exhalation, and, together with the sacrum and its attachments, completes the occipital-sacral-dural harmonic excursion.

THE SACRUM AND COCCYX
89 THE COCCYX

ANTERIOR ASPECT   RIGHT LATERAL SURFACE   POSTERIOR ASPECT

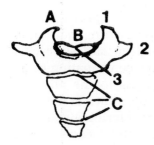 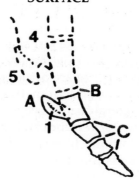 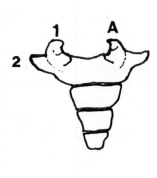

A Cornua-cornual articulation (for articulation with sacral cornu)
B Sacrococcygeal articulation (for articulation with sacral apex)
C Coccygeal-coccygeus articulation (for articulation with other coccygeal vertebrae)

1 Cornu
2 Transverse Processes (Eminences)
3 Articulating facet
4 Sacrum (indicated by dotted line)
5 Sacral Cornu

THÉOPHILE DE BORDEU

'Every organ serves as a workshop for the preparation of a specific substance which enters into the blood: such substances are useful to the body and are needed in order to maintain its integrity.'

Acknowledgements & References

C. BERNARD   Quoted in *Progress in Medicine* I. Gladston, Alfred Knopf, 1940
BEST & TAYLOR   *The Human Body*, Chapman & Hall Ltd, 4th Ed., 1963
BIBLE   Authorized edition
DENIS BROOKES   Unpublished Lecture notes
T. BORDEU   Quoted in *Progress in Medicine*, I. Gladston, Alfred Knopf, 1940
F. CHAPMAN   *Chapman's Reflexes* (Ed. Interpreter), Dr C. Owen, Academy of Applied Osteopathy (Reprint), 1969
A.E. CLARK-KENNEDY   *Medicine in its Human Setting, Patients as People,* Faber & Faber, 1954 & 1962 respectively
DESCARTES   *Medical Meanings*, Harcourt Brace Jovanovich, 1984
DUCHESS OF NEWCASTLE
H.H. FRYETTE   *Principles of Osteopathic Technique*, Academy of Applied Osteopathy, 1966
IAGO GLADSTON   *Progress in Medicine*, Alfred Knopf, 1940
GRAYS ANATOMY, Longmans, Green & Co, 1949, 30th Ed. Bounty Books, New York, 1977, Revised 15th
HIPPOCRATES   *Hippocrates & Galen*, Encyclopedia Brittanic, W. Benton, 1952
JOHN HUNTER   *The Reluctant Surgeon*, John Kobler, Doubleday & Co, 1960
P.E. KIMBERLEY   American Academy of Osteopathy Published Papers of proceedings, Various dates
R.C. LIPPINCOTT   A.A.O. proceedings (see above) & *Manual of Cranial Technic.* (2nd Ed.), 1948, Edward Bros. Inc.
K.E. LITTLE   A.A.O. Papers
J.M. LITTLEJOHN   Reprints of own papers, Maidstone Osteopathic Clinic (J Wernham), 1970's
H.I. MAGOUN   *Osteopathy in the Cranial Field*, A.A.O. papers, 1966
J.O. METTRIE   Readers Digest Quotations, 1978
F.L. MITCHELL   A.A.O. Papers
PARACELSUS   Quoted in *Progress in Medicine*
L.E. PAGE   *Osteopathic Fundamentals*, Tamor, Pierston, 1981
PLATO   Quoted in *Progress in Medicine*
DR. SCHOOLEY
H. SEYLE   *The Stress of Life*, McGraw-Hill Book Co., 1978
V. STEFFANSSON   Reader's Digest Quotations, 1978
A.T. STILL   Autobiography and other sources A.A.O. Reprint, 1981
O.M. STRETCH   Lecture Notes

ACKNOWLEDGEMENTS & REFERENCES

W.G. SUTHERLAND *The Cranial Bowl*, Osteopathic Cranial Association, Post 1947 (reprint)
R.B. TAYLOR
I. WALTON Reader's Digest Quotations, 1978
PERRIN T. WILSON A.A.O. Papers
LIN YUTANG *The Importance of Living*, The New English Library (Four Square), 1962

Other Sources

ANTHONY & KOLTHOFF *Anatomy & Physiology*, C.V. Mosby Co., 1975
APPLETON, HAMILTON, TCHAPEROFF *Surface & Radiological Anatomy*, W. Heffer & Sons Ltd., 2nd Ed.
B.E. ARBUCKLE Selected writings, Reprinted by A.A.O., 198?
DORLAND'S *Illustrated Medical Dictionary*, W.B. Saunders, 25th Ed., 1974
C.H. DOWNING *Principles and Practice of Osteopathy*, Tamor Pierston, 1981
W.F. GANONG *Review of Medical Physiology*, Lange, 7th & 9th Ed. 1977 & 1979
F. WILSON HARLOW *Modern Surgery*, W. Heinemann, 1956
J.M. HOAG, W.I. COLE & S.G. BRADFORD *Osteopathic Medicine*, McGraw-Hill Book Co., 1969
J.F. LOSSOW *Structure & Function in Man* 4th Ed., W.B. Saunders Co., 1978
L.C. FLOYD McKEON *Osteopathic Polemics*, C.W. Daniel, 1938
MINN, HUTCHINGS, LOGAN *Colour Atlas of Head & Neck Anatomy*, Wolfe Med. Pub., 1981
J.E. UPLEDGER & J.D. VREDEVOOGD *Craniosacral Therapy*, Eastland Press, 1983

Glossary

A.A.O.: American Academy of Osteopathy
Aberrant: (L. wandering from normal way) deviation from the norm
Accommodate: (L. put on, adjust) adapt
A.C.T.H.: Adreno-corticotropic hormone (Corticotropin). Pituitary gland secretion acting on adrenal cortex.
Adeno: (G. glandular) Acorn shaped structure
  Adenohypophysis: Anterior pituitary gland
  Adenoma: benign tumour of glandular tissue
  Adenosine: Cyclic A.M.P.
A.D.H.: Anti-diuretic hormone. Vasopressin
Adjustment: Realignment of certain structures, in relationship to others
A.D.P.: Adenosine diphosphate. An hydrolysis of adenosine triphosphate
Adrenergic fibres: Nerve fibres which liberate norepinephrine and epinephrine. Axons where terminals release.
A.I.D.S.: Acquired immune deficiency syndrome
Aldosterone: Adrenal cortex steriod
Allergy: (G. other disease) Hypo/Hypersensitivity to certain substances. Although often considered a modern word it appears to have been coined by an Austrian doctor Clement von Pirquet for an altered ability to react to stimuli. Now used mostly to denote hypersensitivity
Allopathy: (G. other, disease) treating disease by antagonistic means
Amenorrhoea: (G. no monthly flow) Absence of menses. Amenia
A.M.P.: Adenosine M monophosphate
Amphi: (G. on both sides) Amphiarthrosis: Cartilaginous slightly movable joint connected by fibro-cartilage
Amygdala: (G. almond) Amygdaloid nucleus at end of caudate nucleus. A mass of subcorticol grey matter in the tip of the temporal lobe, anterior to the inferior horn of the lateral ventricles.
Anastomosis: (G. through a mouth) Strictly 'to give a mouth to.' A connection, natural (Circle of Willis) or artificial (Surgical). Coined by Galen as a communication of two channels.
Androgen: (G. to produce a man) Any agent that produces male characteristics (in either sex) or effects.
Anomaly: (L.G. inequality) Deviation from norm. Originally used to denote congenital/hereditary defects particularly.
Ant: Anterior, front, ventral.
Anteflexion: (L. bend forward) applied to position of uterus in pelvic cavity, in normal and abnormal conditions.
Anteversion: (L. turn forward) falling forward without bending, tilted forward
A.O.: Atlantooccipital
A.O.A.: American Osteopathic Association

GLOSSARY

A.P.: Anteroposterior
Arachnoid: (G. A spider, or its cobweb)
Arachnoid Mater *(See meninges)*
Armamentarium: (L. – collection of weapons) Medically, the whole of a practitioner's equipment, or remedial treatments.
Ascites: (G. & Fr. sack, wineskin) Hydroperitonia. Serous fluid accumulation (often applied especially to the abdomen).
Asthenia: (G. weakness) without strength
A.T.P.: Adenosine Triphosphate, an energy storing compound present throughout the body.
Atrophy: (G. no nourishment) shrinkage, wasting.
Attitudes (Body); That position assumed by the patient that indicates changes from norm.
Axis: (L. axle, pole) That imaginary line around which a structure moves (revolves), or could revolve. Rotational movement of a bone – in the skull particularly – in sphenobasilar flexion or extension (P.R.M.).
  In this book each bone has been described as having an axis of motion. This is not to say that this movement is always the same in all people, but to give an 'aide memoire' to the practitioner, of the individual bony (minute) movement and its place in the cranial sutural mechanism.
Balance: (L. scales) This is a relative term, as total balance is virtually unknown in any one body, all the time. However, it is used to convey that reaching of the 'still-point' which indicates harmonic tissue integrity in the meninges (brain and spinal cord), and therefore in the whole body. (Membraneous).
Osseous: Structural integrity.
Basicranium: (G. base of skull) That area forming floor of cranial (brain) cavity, consists of basisphenoid, basitemporal, and basiocciput, with part of the ethmoid.
Basilar/Basion: (G. base) Terms referring to cranial base.
Bevel: (Fr. Slanting edge) angle of internal or external edge of cranial bone at suture line. (See Sutural bevel chart). Indicates any angle other than a right angle.
Birth Injury: Birth trauma. Neonatal injury. That occuring during the birth process from induced causes (Induction, forceps, mishandling, etc.) or functional (delayed birth, birth canal too small, nil expansion phase, placenta praevia, etc).
Bowl: 'The Cranial Bowl' William Garner Sutherland's book, published privately 1939.
  Cranial Bowl-calvarium containing brain. The vault; or vault and base.
  Pelvic Bowl: basin formed by ilia, sacrum, and pelvic diaphragm to contain organs etc.
B.P.: Blood Pressure
Brachycephalic: (See head)
B.T.R.: Bi-Temporal Rolling
C: Cervical vertebrae
C: Coccyx
c: (L. about) approximately
C/Ca: (L. crab) Cancer, carcinoma, malignancy.
Calcitonin: Thyrocalcitonin. Thyroid glandular hormone – an antagonist to parathormone.
Calvaria: (L. bald scalp) That part of the skull which encloses the brain, bounded by vault and base.
Chatecholamines: Norepinephrine, epinephrine and dopamine.
Caudal/Caudad: (L. tail) towards the tail, or past the tail i.e. carrying on to the feet.
C.C.K.: C.C.K.–P.Z. Cholecystokinin = Pancreozymin.
Cephalic/Cephalid: (G. head) towards, or beyond the head.
Cephalic Index: (See also Head) The maximum head width x 100 ÷ by maximum head length.
C.I.: Cephalic Index.
Circadian: (L. daily rhythm) 24 hour cycle.
Clinoid: (G. bed-post) Four processes (two anterior, two posterior) at dorsum sellae.
Clivus: (L. slope) Posterior surface of posterior sphenoid. That sloping part behind the dorsum sellae which ends at the foramen magnum of occiput.

C.N.: Cranial nerves. Usually designated by roman numerals I – XII
C.N.S.: Central Nervous System
Coccyalgia, Coccydynia, Coccygodynia: All indicate pain in coccyx or coccygeal area.
Cogs, gears, etc: Terms used to suggest a 'knock-on' effect (from one part to another, or one structure to another). Or the part one bone plays between others to act as a 'transformer'. To transmit motion from one interdigitated surface to another.
Collagen: (G. to make glue). Albumeric protein supporting connective tissue.
Commisure: (L. a seam, joining together). A fibrous or nervous band (usually) uniting tissue. Junction of adjoining anatomical structures.
Compression: (L. squeezing together) The state of an osseous (or other) structure being held in a smaller space than usual – crowded. Also indicates a compression fracture. Bulb compression: alternative name for 4VC
Concavity: (L. hollowed out area). Is indicative of sphenobasilar lesion. Is observable in the face, spine, and in the (supine) body position.
Congenital: (L. born with). Present at birth. (related to pathology) Used to distinguish from 'hereditary' – conceived with.
Contralateral: To the opposite side diagonally.
Convexity: (L. having a rounded, elevated surface) opposite side of object having a concave shape.
Co-operation: Patient: those actions requested of the patient by the practitioner which will enable the capacity of a procedure to be enhanced, e.g. respiratory or pedic assistance.
  Pedic: Using a change in plane of the angles of the feet (with the patient supine) to assist in cranial techniques.
  Practitioner: Either the use of more than one practitioner in a particular cranial technique; or, the practitioner waiting for the body language to reveal what to do next, and then to co-operate with that revelation.
  Respiratory: that assistance that can be harnessed to exaggerate, adjust, etc. cranially. To achieve membraneous/ligamentous equilibrium, together with muscular resistance which restores articular or sutural harmony. This is used in non-clinical conditions to stop hiccups, slow heart-beats, and so on, by holding the breath.
Coronal: (L. a crown) transverse suture of vault of skull.
Corpora Quadrigemina: Four small round eminences on the mesencephalon.
Corpus Callosum: Sickle-shaped white matter in brain connecting cerebral hemispheres.
Corticotropin: Anterior pituitary hormone acting on adrenal cortex. A.C.T.H.
Cortisol: Glucocorticoid of adrenal cortex.
Coxsackie Virus: Virus producing a type of non-paralytic poliomyelitis.
Cranium: (L. skull) skull without the mandible.
C.R.I.: Cranial Rhythmic Impulses.
Crista Galli: (L. cock's comb) A projection of the Ethmoid which forms attachment for the Falx Cerebri.
Cruveilhier's Joint: Atlantooccipital articulation.
C.S.F.: Cerebrospinal Fluid.
C.S.M.: Condylosquamomastoid suture.
Cure: (L. care, attention) does not mean 'to heal completely' as in current use.
Cyclic A.M.P.; cA.M.P.; Cyclic adenosine 3'5' monophosphate; adenosine 3':5' cyclic phosphate.
D: Dorsal Vertebrae.
Decompression: Technique used to combat compression lesions, etc.
Deglutitional Stress: (L.) difficulty in swallowing.
Dentate Ligaments: (L. Ligamentum Dentata – toothed ligaments) a fibrous band. 21 projections of dura mater along the spinal cord, from the level of the first cervical nerve and foramen magnum to D12/L1.

GLOSSARY

Diencephalon: (G. between, through brain) Part of brain between mid-brain and cerebral hemispheres.

Diploe: (G. twofold) The intervening layer between plates of bone.

Dolicephalic: (See head)

Dopamine: A stage in the production of noradrenaline, from dopa.

Dropsy: (L.G. water) older term for ascites.

Dura Mater: (See meninges)

Dysrhythmia: (G. abnormal rhythm) disturbance in rate of rhythms.

E.C.F.: Extra cellular fluid.

e.g.: (L.) for example.

Embryo: (G. Fr. to swell) Growth. Foetus before 8th week i.e. period during which the foetus develops major organs/structures.

Eminence: (L. prominence) jutting out part.

Emissary: (L. drain or outlet)
Emissary vein: occasional veins connecting inside structures to outside of skull.

Empirical: (L.G. by trial, by experience). Knowledge based on constant trial 'in the field', (rather than by proof) A self-trained practitioner.

Endorphin: (Endo[genous mo]rphine) opiate peptides discovered in China in 1970 and developed in West in 1974. So far discovered in C.S.F., brain, spinal cord, digestive and reproductive tracts. Appear to have stimulating or inhibiting properties on metabolism. Over secretion encourages weight gain and hibernation, oblivion to painful stimuli (such as heat, injury, etc) Acupuncture and neuromuscular techniques appear to stimulate production.

Endocrine: (G. to separate within) Secreting into blood, lymph, tissue, substances which act on other structures – organs, etc. Ductless glands.
Endogenous Endocrinology: study of endocrine system.

Epicritic: (G. determination) Fine sensibility. Determining an accurate definition of sensation and touch.

Epinephrine: Vasopressin. Adrenal medulla hormone.

Epithalamus: (L. on inner chamber) part of brain comprising pineal body, habenula, and stria medullaris.

Equilibrium: (L. balanced scales) State in which opposing factors equal each other; a steady state of counteracting balance.

E.T.T.: Energy Transference Technique.

Exaggeration: This technique harnesses the articular mechanism's self-correcting facility. To increase a lesion (e.g. a concavity) to encourage a 'spring-back' effect.

Exocrine: (L. to separate out) Secreting via a duct.

Extension: Opposite primary respiratory phase to flexion. Moving joint surfaces away from each other. External rotation of s-b symphysis.

Falx: (L sickle) plural falces. Falx cerebri, Falx cerebelli: Parts of reciprocal tension membrane. (See meninges).

Fascia: (L. bandage) Fibrous tissue bands enveloping a structure or group of structures, or dividing it from adjacent structures.

Feedback: A back flow of some part of the material that has left the system/organ in order to influence its function.
Negative feedback: a continual re-input of part of a systems/organs outflow, to maintain that outflow's regularity.

Flexion: (L. to bend) Opposite primary respiratory phase to extension. Internal rotation of s-b symphysis.

Fluctuation: A wave-like motion evinced in fluids (C.S.F. in particular) which is not circulatory but tidal.

F.M.: Foramen Magnum.

Foetus: (L. to produce, offspring) used to be used as from the 8th week of uterine life, now used more loosely to include from conception to birth.
Foramen: (L. opening) Hole.
Fossa: (L. ditch, trench) hollow or depression.
Fovea: (L. a small pit) a small depression.
4V.C.: Fourth Ventricle Compression.
Fr.: Derived from French language.
F.S.H.: Follicle stimulating hormone. Secretion of pituitary acting on ovary.
Fulcrum: The 'axis' of the s-b membraneous cranial mechanism around which the articular structures move. It is a shifting fulcrum but centres around the straight sinus – a line known as Sutherland's Fulcrum at meeting of falx cerebri and tentorium cerebelli.
G./Gk.: Derived from Greek language.
Ganglion: (G. knot) 1) tumour beneath the skin. 2) a place where bundles of nerves mass together.
    Gasserian ganglion: Ganglia trigeminale. Named for Gasser, an Austrian surgeon of the 16th century, who described this ganglion of the trigeminal nerve.
Genetic: (G. generation) hereditary factors, origin, birth.
G.H.: Growth hormone, from anterior pituitary.
Glucagon: Pancreatic alpha cell hormone.
Gonadotrophin: (or gonadotropin) Anterior pituitary hormone (also found in urine of pregnant woman) having effect on sex organs.
G.T.H.: Gonadotrophic hormone.
Head: Brachycephalic (G. slow head) Short wide head. 'Melon' head. Breadth 4/5ths of length. C.I. 81.00 to 85.4.
    Dolicephalic: (G. long-headed) Mecocephalic. 'Banana head'. Breadth less than 4/5ths of length. C.I. 75.9 or less.
    Mesocephalic: (G. middle head) Mesaticephalic. Medium head. 'Orange head.' C.I. between 75.00 – 80.9.
    Metriocephalic: (G. middle head). V.I. 72–77
    Nanocephalic: (G. dwarf) Small head.
    Oxycephalic: (tower or pointed head). Steeple head. V.I. over 77.
    Pachycephalic (G. thick skull) Excessively thick cranial bones (particularly in Vault) Seen in acromegaly.
    Plagiocephalic: (G. off-set) non-symmetrial head. Unequal development. Uneven closure of sutures.
    Platycephalic (wide head). Breadth/length Index less than 70.
Hiatus: (L. gap) opening.
Histamine: An amine which can vasodilate, bronchoconstrict, and increase gastric secretions.
H.M. pivot: 'Hinge-mastoid' pivot.
Homoeostasis: (G. constant) A steady state of being. Optimum state of body health. Achieved by negative feedback mechanism (N.F.B.) supplying a perpetual motive force.
5H.T.5 Hydroxytryptamine: Seratonin.
I.C.F.: Intracellular fluid.
I.C.S.H.: Interstitial cell-stimulating hormone. Luteinizing hormone. Secretion of anterior pituitary acting on gonads.
i.e.: (L. that is)
I.F.: Interstitial fluid. E.C.F.
Inf.: Inferior.
Infundibulum: (L. funnel) When used on its own usually refers to Hypothalamic Infundibulum – part of pituitary stalk.
Insulin: (L. in an island) Pancreatic beta cell hormone.
Inter: (L. between) among
    interosseous: between two bones.

GLOSSARY

Intra: (L. within) on the side, inside.
   intraosseous: within the bone.
L/Lt.: Latin derivation.
L: Lumbar vertebrae.
'L' shaped area: Shape observed at frontoparietosphenoid junction. Also mirrored at sacro-iliac joint.
Lesion: (L. to injure) discontinuity of tissue. Any injury due to trauma, pathology or degeneration which causes abnormality in tissue.
Lifts: Cranially – a method of releasing bones (particularly of the vault) from surrounding crowded areas, to restore function.
L.H.: Luteinizing Hormone. (See I.C.S.H.).
Lipid: Fat or fat-like.
Mater: (L. Mother) See meninges.
Membrane: (L. skin) thin layer of tissue lining hollow organs or vessels.
Meninges: (G. membrane)
   Dura Mater: (L. hard – strong protective mother) Outer meningeal layer of brain and spinal cord. Of two layers with venous sinuses and gasserian ganglion between.
   Arachnoid Mater: (webbed layer) middle meningeal layer.
   Pia Mater: (soft, tender mother) Inside meningeal layer; reticular, cartilaginous and elastic fibres.
mm Hg: pressure of millimetres of mercury. Measurement of manometer reading of blood pressure.
Mobile: (L. having movement)
   Cranial articular mobility: movement of cranial bones at sutures.
Motile: (L motion) Innate capability for motion.
Moulding: Method of correcting by hand, bony abnormalities of shape and contour which are causing restriction of function – particularly at cranium and sacrum.
M.S.H.: Melanocyte stimulating hormone. Anterior pituitary peptide.
Nares: (L Nose: naris-singular) external nasal orifices.
Neurohypophysis: Posterior pituitary gland.
O.A.: Occipito-atlantal joint.
Obelion: (G. a spit) crossing point of sagittal suture at place of parietal foramen.
Oblique diameter: The internal or external rotation of the zygoma, together with movement of the frontal, nasal, lacrimal and maxilla at the facial mid-line help change the superomedial, inferolateral diameter of the eye to appear larger (more prominent) or smaller (less prominent). This oblique diameter is the angle of normal eye movement.
Oestrogen: (L. gadfly) female sex hormone.
Oligodenrolgia: Cerebral connective tissue cell.
O.M.: Occipitomastoid suture.
Origin & Insertion: Terminology for muscular attachment.
Oxytoxin: (G. swift childbirth) any agent, natural or chemical, that promotes childbirth.
Palate: Gothic: a high arched palate resembling a gothic window.
Palpation: (L. to touch or feel with the hand) The use of tips of fingers, or whole hand, to diagnose/evaluate pathology by light pressure on skin and underlying organs.
   Cranially – using fingers to sense restriction/yielding of articular mobility.
Pelvis: Frozen: Medically a pathologic condition denoting Ca., infection, etc.
   Cranially see Chapter 13
P.I.A.: Posterior inferior angle.
Pivot: Change-over points of bevel on a single suture line (e.g. a change from external to internal bevel). A pivot is a point of motion.
P.L.A.: Posterior lateral angle.
Poles of Attachment: Points of meningeal attachment to skull (Superior anterior, superior inferior, lateral and posterior). To these can be added points at foramen magnum, cervical (1

& 2), dentate ligaments and sacrum.
P.R.M.: Primary Respiratory Mechanism.
The P.R.M. maintains life and includes the action – motility of the C.N.S., C.S.F., the meninges, cranial bones and sacrum.
It was so named as it is concerned with cell interchange of fluids, gases, etc (as is the pulmonary respiratory mechanism) and involuntarily moves into flexion/extension to maintain the balanced integrity of every bodily part.
Pterion: (G. wing)
Ptosis: (G. falling) drooping or sagging of a structure.
P.W.F.: Pineal weight factor.
Quadrant Analysis: A method of assessing and evaluating cranial movements/lesions, etc. by dividing the cranium (more particularly the vault) into four sections (bisected sagittally and coronally).
Raphe: (G. seam) a uniting line of two similar parts.
R.B.C.: Red blood cells. Erythrocytes.
R.E.M.: Rapid eye movements.
Retro: (L. backward)
   retroflexion: 'bent back' Body of uterus on cervix
   retroversion: 'turn back' Fold back of uterus and cervix.
Rostrum: (L. beak) Part of sphenoid.
Rotation: The movement around an axis described by structures, especially cranial and long bones, in flexion and extension. The movement of each paired bone (peripheral) expanding in flexion and the midline (unpaired) bones rotating on a transverse axis.
R.T.M.: Reciprocal tension membrane: The functional unit of meninges (cranial and spinal) which operate the cranial articular mechanism.
S: Sacral vertebrae.
Sacral rocking: The involuntary palpable motion described by the sacrum (between the ilia) about a transverse axis at S2 level.
s-b: s-b-s: Sphenobasilar (symphysis)
s-b: side-bend
   Hence: s-b,s-b, – sphenobasilar, sidebending lesion.
s.c.m.: Sternocleidomastoid muscle.
Scoliosis: (G. bending) Hippocrates used this term to denote a spinal curvature.
Side-bend: A movement of the vertical or axial plane of a structure or group of structures (e.g. cranial base or spine) inclining laterally. The term is used both to denote a lesion and as a functional test. Cranially, refers to position of sphenobasilar symphysis on superoanterior, inferoposterior axis.
Sickles: (L falx. 'Three sickles') Refers to either the falx cerebri and two halves of tentorium cerebelli or to the Falx cerebri and cerebelli together with the tentorium cerebelli.
Skull: (Scandinavian, bowl) Cranium, face and mandible.
Sphenobasilar: Extension: an exaggeration of the inferior movement exhibited by the s-b (and allied bones) in expiration – which flattens the cranial base.
   Flexion: an exaggeration of the superior movement exhibited by the s-b (and allied bones) in inspiration – which raises the cranial base.
   Symphysis: the synchondrosis at basiocciput and basisphenoid.
S.M. Pivot: Squama (of occiput) and Mastoid portion (of Occiput).
S.S. Pivot: Sphenosquamous sutural pivot.
S.T.H.: Somatotropic hormone. Growth hormone.
Sup: Superior.
Suture: (L. seam) 1) Cranial articulating surface 2) surgical seam.
S.V.: Stroke Volume.
S.W.S.: Slow wave sleep.

GLOSSARY

Symphysis: (Gk growing together) A fibrocartilaginous joint. Found mainly in skull, sacrum and pelvis.

Synchondrosis: (G. growing into one) A joint where the cartilaginous 'disc' is replaced by bone. Therefore refers mainly to bones in foetal state or in infancy.

t.b.: Tuberculosis.

T.H.: Thyrotropic hormone. Thyroid stimulating hormone.

Tinnitus: (L. tinkling) Continual noises of varied pitch in ear.

T.M.J.: Temporomandibular joint.

Tonus: (G. tone) stretching tightening force. Its degree of strength and vigour. Originally meant partial constriction of muscle. Current use is to convey good quality of tone – healthy muscle.

Torsion: A twisting movement of the occiput and sphenoid (particularly) in opposite directions about the s-b axis.

Trophic: About nutrition.

Tropic: Change or a turning about.

N.B.: These terms tend to be used interchangeably as suffixes.

T.S.H.: Thyroid stimulating hormone. Thyrotropin.

Ventricle: (L. small cavity) When used on own usually refers to four ventricles of brain.

V.I.: Vertical Index. Height of Skull x 100 ÷ by length.

V-Spread: A technique for reducing restrictions at a suture or other part of the body. This is a form of E.T.T.

W.B.C.: White blood cells.

DUCHESS OF NEWCASTLE

'Motion is the life of all things.'

INDEX

Acini
  Pancreas 94
  Thyroid 86/7
Accommodation 7, 41, 123, 128, 134/5, 147, 170
Acqueduct 23
  Cerebral 35
  of Sylvius 79
Aqueous Humour 45
A.C.T.H. 46, 84, 98
Addison's Disease see Disease
Adenohypophysis see Pituitary Gland
A.D.H. 78, 85
Adjustment 25, 41, 56, 123, 163
Adrenaline 78, 97
Adrenals 97/8
  Structure & Function 78, **95**
  Hormonal Secretion 84, 97/8
A.I.D.S. 93
Aims xi–xii, 147, 164
Ala see Sphenoid
Aldosterone 97
Allergies 8, 145, 147, 162, 173
Anaemia 49
Anaesthetics 131, 174
Analgesics 174
Anatomy: Osseous see also Individually named bones, etc.
  Ancillary Bones 228–293, **293**
  Base 248–259, **249, 259**
  Face 261–286, **267, 274, 276, 279, 285**
  Gray's 3, 10, 38, 56
  Sacrum & Coccyx 298–304, **300, 304**
  Vault 232–246, **233, 235, 237, 241, 245**
Ancillary Bones see Anatomy
Aneurysms 106, 163
Anti-Bodies 46, 86
Antrum 257
  of Highmore 269
A.O. Assn see O.A.A.
Appendicitis 53, 185
Appetite 84

Loss of 162
Arachnoid: see also Meninges
  Granulations 30, 238/9
  Membranes 38, 299
  Villae 35, 39
Arbuckle Beryl E xiii
Arcuate Emminence see Emminence
Art 243
  Palpatory diagnostic 116
  Surgical 3
Arterosclerosis 163
Arthritis 49, 106, 155
Articulations xiii, **4**, 145, 255
  see also Individual Bones
  Chart of 219–222
  Motion 15, 135
  Sutural 103, 139
Ascites 49, 106
Asthenia 163, 190
Asthma 8, 106, 125, 170, 207
Astigmatism 154, 164
Ataxia 239
Attachments see Articulations & Poles of attachment
Attitudes see Body
Axis 195
  Oblique **150**, 153, 268
  of individual bones 193, 211, 256, 268, 273, 298
  of rotation 25, 246

Backache 61, 133, 181, 191
Banana
  Head 22, see also Head
  Skin slip 170
Banting F.G. (& C.H. Best) 96
Base see Cranial Base
Basicranium see Cranial Base
Bell's Palsy 8
Bernard Claude 157
Best C.H. (& F.G. Banting) 96
Best C.H. (& N.B. Taylor) 75, 89
Bevels 7, **233**, 256
  Chart of 220–222
  Sutural 140, 151, 164, 242, 254
Bible x

Birth **129**, 133, 145, 177, 298
  Induced 133
  pattern 128, 131, 173
  trauma 8, 128, 131–133, 206
Bi-Temporal Rolling see Techniques
Bladder 185, 191
Blood
  circulation 35, **42–43**, 45, 77
  plasma 45, 79
  pressure 57, 58, 78, 83, 85, 97, 137, 202
  sugar 81, 85, 96
Body 3, 5
  attitudes **130**, 132
  systems xi
  weights 45, 48, 298
Bones 3, 5, 7, 131, 145 **see also** Individual names
  ancillary 5, 288–292, **293**
  fractures of 209
  long 19, 25, 30, 41, 190
  malpositioned 19
  pelvic 177, 179, 298–304
  sutural 292, **293**
  Wormian 292
Bordeu Théophile de 305
Bowl
  Pelvic 98, 178, 181, **182**, 298
  'The Cranial Bowl' xi, 3, 7, 131
Bowsher D 35
Brain 23, **32**, 33, **34**, 38, 75, 128, 238, 256
  cerebellum 30, 33, 39, 140, 238, 242
  diencephalon **34**, 79, 84
  epithalamus **34**, 79
  medulla oblongata 243
  weight 35
Broca (Area of) 242, 277
Brookes Denis xii, xiii, 3, 22, 33, 75, 115, 147
Burns Louise xiii

Calcium 46, 86, 91
Calvarium 41

Cancer (Malignancy) 46, 49, 106, 177
Cardia 17, 23, 49, 78, 81, 201/2
Cartilage 7, 41, 64, 128, 134, 242, 254, 265, 280
   Meckel's 265
   Septal 147, 251, 273, 277, 282
Case Histories 164, 199–201, 204, **208**, **212**, 213
Cataract 73
Catarrh 145, 164, 190, 238
C.C.K.-P. 94, 96
Cells 46, 79, 96, 103 **see also** Sinuses
   Alpha & Beta 96
   Air 238, 257, 256, 270, 277
   Bulla 277
   Columnar 91, 100
   Cuboid 100
   Epithelial 84, 91, 92, 98, 153
   Granulamatous 89
   Hassel's (Arthur) 92
   Leydig's 100
   Sertoli (Enrico) 100
Cephalic Index 309
Cervic 179, 181
Cervical **see** Vertebrae
Chapman's **see** Reflexes
Chest, Barrel 51
Children 28, 45, 92, 94, 111, 133, 145/6, 170, 205, 211, 299
   Growth patterns 81, 86
Choroid Plexus 35, 39
Circadian 81
Clark-Kennedy A.E. 214
Clinoid Process **see** Process
C.N.S. 35, 65, 125, 204
Coccyx 169–171, **169**, 302–304, **304**
   Articulations 303
   Lesions 179, 207
   Treatment **169**, 171
Commissure 27, 277
Complexion Changes 107, 114, 154, 162
Concavity 54, 119, **124**, 141, 147, 151, 190
Conchae 282
Condyles 134–137, **129**, 211, 242/3
Constipation 53, 163, 185, 303
Contraindications 7, 17, 51, 54, 106, 122, 134, 171, 207
Contralateral 70, **113**, 158, 160, 175
Convexity 147, 149
Co-operation 135, 141
   Patient assistance 135, 153,

167, 211
   Practitioner assistance **112**, **113**, 113
Corpora Quadrigemina 79
Corpus Callosum 79
   Luteum 99
Cortisol 96
Cranial
   Academy 7
   Assessment 133
   Base (Basicranium) 5, 22, 62, 128–143, **136**, 153, 164, 242–3, 246, 248–259, **249**, **253**, **259**
   Behaviour 26
   Bones **see** Individual Names
   Concept xii, 3–13, 218
   C.R.I. 15–28, 119/121
   Fossa 64
   Hypothesis **212**, 212/3
   Landmarks **216**, 217/8
   Nerves **see** Nerves
   Osteopathy xi, xii, 5, 7, 8, 134
   Rhythms **see** Rhythms
   Sutural Motion **see** Sutures-motion
   'The Cranial Bowl' **see** Bowl
   Vault **see** Vault
Cranio-Sacral
   Balance 56–62, 69, 103
   Locking 158, 174
   Mechanism 5, 15–28, 30, 51, 62, 133, 187 **see also** C.R.I.
   Motion 19, 21, 56, **130**, 134
   System 8, 28, 77, 133, 139, 191, 242, 251
C.R.I. **see** Cranial
Crista Galli 39, 73, 277
'Cross-Over Point' **196**, 197
Crura 190
Cruveilhier's Joint **see** O-A Articulation
C.S.F. 7, 17, 23, **26**, 30–43, **36–7**, 45, 65, 79, **109**, 111, 156, 209, 238, 291
   Fluctuation 5, 77, 111
Cushing, Harvey William 76, 98
Cyclic A.M.P. 45, 79, 86, 96

Defence Mechanism 97
Deglutional Stress 123, 173, 256
Dentate Ligaments **see** Ligaments
Dentistry 147, 164, 256, 271
Depression 28, 81, 106, 133, 162, 173, 177, 207
   Manic 103
Descartes René 79
Detoxification 54

Diabetes 78, 96
Diagnosis 75, 175, **see also** Evaluation & Palpation
Evaluation 22, 116–126, **117**, 212
   Differential 22, **60**, 173
   Indications 15, **16**, 181
   Sketch **208**, 212
Diaphragms 6, 30, 49, 125, **184**, 190
   1st. Thoracic 155
   2nd. Respiratory 30, 49, 51, 185, 190
   3rd. Pelvic 185, 302
Diarrhoea 97, 163, 185, 199
Diencephalon **see** Brain
Dietary Considerations 173
Digestive Disturbances 59, 97
Diplopia 154
Direct Action Technique **see** Technique
Direction of Energy **see** Techniques
   V-Spread 158, 160, 175
Disease 38, 51, 131
   Addison's, Thomas 97
   Cushing's 98
   Hashimoto's 89
   Hodgkin's 49
   Menière's 168
   Parkinson's 204
   Quervain's, Fritz de 89
   Stoke's (Grave's) 87
   Willis's 96
Dizziness 162, 169, 205
Dolicephalic **see** Head
Dorsum Sellae 69, 161, 251
Drainage 50–52
Drugs 17, 163, 174, 186, 204, 207
Duct, Lacrimal 272
   Pharyngeal 272
Dura 19, 21, 23, **40**, 57, 139, 161 **see also** Meninges
   Extra 27
   Spinal 8, **18**
Dural 164, 280
   Attachments **18**, **24**, 73, 161, 243
   Fascia Relationships 23, 137, 158, 162, 303
   Tent 38, **57**, 73
   Tube 27, 39
Dysmenorrhoea 183
Dysplasia 173, 211
Dysrhythmia 204

Ear
   Examination 141, 164

INDEX

Ossicles 5, 255, 291–292, **293**
Otitus Media 164, 190
Problems 164–168
Pull **166**, 167
Tinnitus 164/5, 168
Eczema 125
E.C.F. 45, 85
Embryology 26, **32, 34**, 84, 98, 131, 264
Eminentia Cruciata 243
Eminence 269, 302
   Arcuate 256
   Thenar 107
Emmissary Veins **see** Veins
Endocrine 25, **76**, **see also** Glands
   Dysfunction 17, 131, 173, 177
   Orchestra 76
   'The Endocrine Umbrella' 75–105
   Trigger 30
Endorphines 23, 28
Enzymes 27, 45, 77
Epidural Injections 181
Epilepsy 23
Epinephrine **see** Adrenaline
Epithalamus **see** Brain
Ethmoid 154, 277–280, **279**
   Articulations 149, 222, 280
   Lesions 277/8
   Movements 27, 228
   Sinuses 277
   Treatments 278
E.T.T. **see** Techniques
Eustachion Tube 153, 165, 256
Evaluation **20**, 116–126, **117**, 158, 175, 204, 212
Exaggeration 28, 49
Examination 181
   Abdominal 183
   Pelvic 183
Exopthalmic Goitre 87
Extension 19, 21/3, 71, **58**, **110**, 111, 121, 254 **see also** Flexion
   Lesions 128, 141, **130**
Extracranial
   Considerations 190–197
Eye Conditions 73, 87, 128, 154, 162, 164, 269
   Movements 27, 254
   Treatments **150**, 151, 153/4

Face The 261–286
Facets 41, 246, 299, 302
Facial 262-3
   Assymetry 15, 119, 211, 271
   Bones 5, 261–286, **267, 274, 276, 279, 285**, 288

Complex 145–156
Fields 147, 149, 251
Foramina **120**, 273
Lesions 94, 148, 256
Treatment 149, 151, 153, 155
Fascia 23, 25, 46, 92, 185, 239
   -Dural 162, 255
   Extra-cranial 23, 174
   Mobility 123, 137
   Planes **184**, 185, 190
   Restrictions 59, 162, **184**, 185
   Treatment 185
Fallopian Tubes 179, 183
Falx
   Cerebri 27, 71, 125, 139, 161, **166**, 171, 234
   Cerebelli 27, 30, 33, 39, 161, 243
Fasting 96
Fatigue **see** Tiredness
Feet **see** Pedic
Femoral Triangle 196
Fever 17, 49, 93
Flexion **see also** Extension 19, 21/3, **58**, **110**, 121, 191, 254, 283
   Characteristics 39, 71
   Lesions **130**, 141
   Sacral **88**, 106, 205/6
Fibroids 181, 183
Flatulence 199
Fluid
   Balance 56–62
   Body 45–54, **48, 52**
   Bombardment 61
   Flow 13, 58, 89, 119
   Exchange 135
   Mechanics **36–7**, 48, 56–62, 106
   Patterns xii, 3
   Stasis 23, 49, 61, 106, 147, 163, 206, 210, 256
Foetal **32, 34**
   Behaviour 174
   Skull 129, 295/6, **129, 296**
Foetus 133
Folds
   Naso-labial 15, **16**, 119
   Supra-nasal **16**, 119
Fontanelles 234, 239, 242, **296**
Foramina 299
   Cranial 163, 234, 251, 256, 277
   Basal 23, 135, 251, 254, 256
   Facial **120**, 154, 264, 268/9, 273
   Internal 22, 246, 256, 277
   Miscellaneous 238
   Occasional 281

Orbital 251, 270
Sphenoidal 67/8, 251, 254
Luschka (Hubert von) 35
Magendie 35
Magnum 8, **11, 18**, 135, 175, 243
Monro (Alexander) 23, 79
Sacral 299
Stenson & Scarpa 270
Forceps 131, 133, 145
Fortification Figures 163
Fossae 191, 251, 256
   Incisive 146, 149, 264, 269
   Pterygopalatine 151, 265, 280
   Vermiform 243
Fourth (4th) Ventricle
   Compression 106–114, **107/8**, 141
   Application **107**, 141, 153/4, 164, 186, 204, 206
   Compression 106
   Contraindications 106, 207
   Effectiveness 106, 114
   Methods 107–114, **107/8**
   Summary 114
Frontal **16**, 133, 154, 234–8, **235, 237**
   Articulations 221, 238
   Lesions 238
   Lifts **138**, 139, 280
   Movements 26, 227
   Moulding 175
   Spread 140, 280
Frozen
   Shoulder 179
   Pelvis 179
Fryette H.H. 56, 63, 298
F.S.H. 98–100
Fulcrum 53, 77/8, 255
   Sutherland's 30

Gait Disturbances 78, 211, 190
Galen, Veins of, **see** veins
Ganglion 81, 163
   Gasserian 256, 265
   of Impar 21, 170
   Sphenopalatine 147, 151/3, 256, 276, 281
Gastritis 162, 173
Genetics 17, 94
Genitalia
   Female 99, 177, **180, 182**
   Male 70, 100, 103/4, 170, 185
Gladston Iago 188–9
Glands 46, 79, 94, 257, 264 **see also** individual names
Glaucoma 154
Glucagon 96

Glycogen 96, 100
Gonads 81, 84, 98–102, **101/2**
Gonadotrophin 79, 98, 185
Goitre 87, 89
Growth 81, 86
    Hormone 84, 186
Gynaecology 177–187
    Structure & Function 98–100, **180, 182**
    Disorders 100, 106, 133–135, 170, 181–7, 302
    P.P.P.D. 186–7
    Treatment 181–187

Haemorrhoids 22, 185
Hayfever 106, 145, 164, 277
Head 27, 106, 121, 139, 312
    -aches 28, 98, 106, 139, 152, 183
        Evaluation 256
        Migraine 106, 125, 139, 162/4
    Dimensions 41, 312
    Injuries 106, 164
    Shapes 131/2, 312
        'Banana' 22, 151
        Dolicephalic 22
Heamorrhage 51, 106, 207, 291
Heart **see** Cardia
Heredity 145, 162, 173
Hiatus Hernia 185
    Sacral 299
H.I.O.M.T. 79
Hippocrates xiv
Histamine 25, 79
Holds **see** Techniques
Homoeostasis 3, 6, 25, 30, 54, 56, 58, 62, 73, 79, 83, 86, 92, 103, 128, 133, 164, 193
Hormones 25, 30, 45, 77/8/9, 81, 84–86, 91–94, 97, 99, 100, 103
'Hot Spots' 158
Hunter John 55
Hydrocephalus 23, 78, 292
Hyoid 5, 91, 206, 256, 265, 288–291, **293**
    Articulations 288
    Muscles 206, 289–90
    Ligaments 206, 289–90
    Lesions 289
Hyper-
    -Activity 106, 205
    -Glycaemia 81, 85, 96
    -Hidrosis 87
    -Tension 57, 83, 97, 163–4
    -Tonicity 27, 51, 264, 268
Hypothalamus
    Hormonal Secretion 81, 137

Relations 75/6, 78, **82**, 84/5, 87, 104, 137
Structure & Function 75–78, **82**, 84/5

Ilia 6, 17, 65, 81, 170, 179, 196
Immune System 46, 93/4
Impotence 78, 98, 185, 209
Incontinence 209
Indigestion 61, 199
Infection 49, 93, 164
Inferior
    Maxilla **see** Mandible
    Nasal Conchae 282, **285**
        Articulations 222
        Lesions 285
        Movements 228
Infertility 99, 178
Inflammation 49, 89, 181, 257
Infundibulum 23, 83
Insomnia **see** Sleeplessness
Insulin 94, 96
Interstitial Fluids 45
Intracranial
    Membranes **see** Membranes
    Rhythms **see** Rhythms
'Irritable Bowel Syndrome' 185
Ischaemia 51

Jaw **see** Mandible
Jayasuriya Prof Dr Anton ix
Joints 3, 6, 288, 299
    'Universal' 286
Jugular 21
    Foramina 22, 246, 256
    Notch 255
    Veins 38, 165, 246, 256

Ketone Bodies 96
'Kettle-Lid' Method 71
Key Pairs 226
    Vertebrae 223–226
Kidney 46, 91, 97, 100, 191
'Kink' 23, 28, 191, 206
Kimberley Paul E 44
'Knock-On' Effect 151, 155
Kyphosis 51, 175

Labour 179, 181, 298
Lacrimals 272, **276**
    Articulations 222, 272
    Lesions 153
    Drainage **152**, 153
Lactation 85, 97
Lamina Papyracea 154, 277
Langerhan's Islets of 96
Leber's, Theodore
    Corpuscles 92

Lemniscate Action 77, 78, 92
Lesions 22
    Ascending/Descending 22, 62, 201
    Cranio-sacral 19, 56, 104, 128, 132, 163
        T.M.J. 154–6, 164, 257
        O-A 134
        O-M 106, 122, 135, 246
        Side-bending 22, **59**, 71, **130**, 164, 211, 243, 251, 281
        Vault & Base 62, 128–143, 238/9, 255, 283
    Differential Diagnosis 22, 123
    Facial 17, 151, 153, 265, 268, 271/2, 277/8, 281/3
    Gynaecological 100, 106, 133–5, 170, 181–7, 302
    Minimal 199–202, **200**
    Multiple 15, 17
    Orbital 123, 153
    Osteopathic 6, 199
    Pelvic 17, 107, 170, 211
    Psoas 194, 209
    Vertical Strain 141
Leucorrhea 181
L.H. 99
Lifts **see** Techniques
Ligaments 6, 98, 243, 256, 264
    Dentate **18**, 39
    Hyoidal 206, 288, 290
    Pelvic 39, 171, 181, 186, 191, 195, 299, 302
    Sphenoidal 67/8, 255
    Uterine 181
Little Kenneth E 74
Littlejohn John H **8**, 198
Lippincott Howard A & Rebecca C viii, 144, 147
Liver 46, 91, 96, 128
    & Spleen 53
Locus Ceruleus 23
Lordosis 41, 179
Low Back Problem **see** Backache
Lumbarization 299
Lymphatic 23, 92
    Structure & Function 16, 45, **47/48**
    Drainage 49, **50**, 51, 53
    Duct/Inlet **50**, 53
    Pump 45, **50**, 51, 77
Lymphocytes 92/3

Magoun Harold Ives viii, 5, 30, 33, 65, 106, 113, 147, 174/6, 298
Malar **see** Zygoma
Malignancy 49, 79, 84, 91, 93,

INDEX

177, 181, 183 **see also** Cancer
Mandible 264–7, **267**
   Articulation 221, 256, 265
   Lesions 265
   Movements 228
   Treatment **146**, 149, 154/5, 206
Manipulation 9, 19
   Soft Tissue 51, 54, 162, 207
Martindale Richard E
   Postulation **200**, 201
Maxilla 269–71, **274**, 280
   Articulations 221/2, 271
   Inferior **see** Mandible
   Lesions 271
   Movements 128, 228
   Treatment **146**, 147/9, 206
Meatus Auditory 256/7
Mechanism
   Cranio-sacral 5, 15–28
   Healing 49
   Protective 46
   Slack-tension 41
Medicine World of 5, 7
Medulla Oblongata **see** Brain
Melancholia 173, 206
Melatonin 79, 81
Membranes 7, 23, 33, 38, 41, 64, 123, 128, 165, 242, 254 **see also** Meninges
   Reciprocal Tension 13, 15, 21, 30
Membraneous
   activity 15, 158
   Tension 6, 21, **60**
   Tent 73, 175
Meninges **36–7**, 162/3
   Arachnoid 18
   Dura 18, 22, **24**, 27–39, **40, 57**, 73, 125, 162, 239, 242, 255/6
   Pia 18
Menstrual Cycle 98, 163, 186
   Disorders 163, 177
   Menopause 99, 177
Mental 191
   Disturbances 17, 103, 121, 133, 162, 164, 234
   Point 264
Metabolism 75, 78, 100
Mettrie Julien Offray de la 260
Migraine 106, 125, 139, 162–164
Minimal Lesion **see** Lesion
Miscarriages 179, 185
Mitchell Fred L 231
Motility 3, 33
Motion 33, 141
   Sensing the 8, 13, 139, 140, 149
   Still-point 25, 78, 113, 135,

158, 160
   Testing the **60**, 147
Movement 100, 161
   Articular 5, 13, 128, 219–222, 228
   Cessation of 155
   Cranio-sacral 19, 21, 56, **113**, 134
   Gliding 7
   Physiological 23, 30, 33, 227–230
Moulding 171–175, 211
   Infantile 131/2, 134, 173/4
   Sacral **172**, 174/5
   Vault **172**, 174/5
Muscles 23, 27, 93–94, 96, 165, 201
   Abdominal 193
   of Base 68/9
   Coccygeal 171, 302
   of Face 94, 264
   Gluteals 177, 302/3
   of Hyoid 206, 289–290
   Iliopsoas 41, 51, 190–197, **192**
   Pelvic 183, 195
   Piriformis 41, 62, 190, **192**, 194–7
   Sacral 219
   Sternocleidomastoid 51, 89, 264, 288
   Sphenoidal **66**, 67/8
   Stimulus 193
   Temporalis 239, 254, 255
   Tonus 65, 111, 264
   Vault 243, 239, 254/5
Musculo-Skeletal 17, 19, 78, 100, 179, 204
Myasthenia Gravis 93
Myopia 15, 73, 164
Myxoedema 87

Nasal 147, 238, **263**, 272/3, **276**
   Articulations 222, 273
   Distraint 151, **152**, 206
   Lesions 272
   Movements 27, 28/9
   Treatment **152**, 153
Negative Feed-Back 85
Nerves 243
   Cranial 71, 162, 163, 185, 246, 254, 256, 264, 281
   Sacral 195, 298
Nervous Disorders 173
   System 9, 33, 133
      Autonomic 23, 57, 75, 97, 137, 170, 177
      Parasympathetic 23, 79
      Sympathetic 79, 163

Neural Tube 33
Neuralgia 164
Neuro Endocrine Gangliform
   Contractions 51
Nor Adrenaline 81, 97
   Epinephrine 94
Nose 128, 271
Nuchal tissues 137, 158, 167
Nystagmus 154

O-A Joint 57, 221
O.A. Association 56
Obesity 173, 178
Observation 116, **117**, 119, 183
Occiput 8, **11–12**, 69, 167, 242–6, **245**
   Articulations **129**, 134, 220, 246
   Lesions 21, 59, 211, 243
   Movements 27, 141, 227
   O.M. Joint 106, 122, 135, 246
   -Sacral **26, 109**
   Supra- 106
   Treatment 106, 135–7, 109
Oedema 49, 53, 83, 106, 163, 181
Oestrogen 81, 99
Oligodendroglia 33
Optic Chiasma 83
   Groove 71
   Nerve 71
Orbit
   Structure & Function 27, 151/3, 234, 238, 251, **263**, 268–270, 280
   Lesions 73
   Treatment 27, **150**
Orbital Diameter 65, 73, 123, **150**, 153
Ossification 134, 234, 238, 242, 265, 270, 272/3, 280, 282, 288, 291, 298, 302
Ossicles **see** Ear
'Osteopathy in the Cranial
   Field' xi, 7
Osteopathic xi, 149, 199
   Armamentarium xii, 106
   Lesions 6, 199
   Methods 5, 149
   Principles 3, 116
Ovaries
   Structure & Function 98–99, **101**
   Hormonal Secretion 99
Overmoulding 174
Owen Dr Charles 17
Oxyphil 91
Oxytoxin 85, 163

Pacchionian Bodies 30
   Depressions 238

Page Leon E 127
Pain 15, 62, 94, 167, 181, 207
  Abdominal 97, 177, 190
  Headaches see Head
  High Threshold 163
  Migraine 162–4
  Period 177, 181, 183
  Referred 41, 183
Palate 128, 145–7, 269, 271, 280/1
  Cleft 270
Palatine 167, 280–282, **285**
  Articulations 64, 149, 222, 281
  Lesions 281
  Movements 27, 228
  Process 269
  Treatment 149, 151
Palpation 13, 17, **20, 60,** 71, 116–122, 147
Pancreas
  Structure & Function 94–96, **95**
  Hormonal Secretions 53, 94
  Islets of Langerhans 96
Paracelsus 247
Paralysis 94, 164, 181
Parathormone 86, 91
Parathyroids 86, **90,** 89, 91–2
Parietal **12,** 238–242, **241**
  Articulations 239, 242, 221
  Lesions 239
  Moulding 175
  Movements 140, 227
  Treatment **138,** 140, 164
Pars 85
  Distalis 84
  Tuberalis 84
Pascall Blaise Laws 35
Pathology 17, 92, 133, 164, 210
  Indications **16,** 104
  Osseous 173/4, 265
Patient 15, 106
  Behaviour 122, 158
  History 131, 164, 168, 173, **212**
  Signs & Symptoms 15, 117, 131, 201, **208**
Pedic
  Angle **118,** 119, 196
  Assistance 113, **110, 113**
Pelvis 17, 133, 177, 179, 211
Pelvic 298
  Diaphragm see Diaphragms
  Lesions 170, 211
Pendulum (Cranial) 19, 23, 211
Periods see Menstrual & Pain
Periosteum 270, 283
Petrous Portion see Temporal
Phaeochromocytoma 98
Pharnyx 91, 153, 243, 291
Phenomenon 25, 30, 39, 56, 65, 170, 174
Sleep-wake 23, 137
V-Spread 161
Phosphorus 46, 91
Photophobia 162
Physiology xi
Pia Mater see Meninges
Pineal Structure & Function 78–83, **82**
  & Pituitary 41, 76/7
  as 'third eye' 79, 81
  Secretions 79
  Treatment 25
Pinealocytes 79
Pioneers
  Osteopathic **6, 8**
  Cranial xi, **6**
Pituitary 27, 98
  & Hypothalamus 78, **82,** 104
  & Pineal 41, 76/7
  Hormonal secretions 46, 71, 84, 103
  Structure & Function 75, 83–86, 131
Placenta 174
Plato 297
Plexus 43, 91
  Hypogastric 21
Polarity 41, **77**
Poles of Attachment **24,** 73, 161
Polposis 195
Polyps 283
Position, Knee-chest 186
  Sim's semi-prone 186
Postural Balance 190
  disorders 137, 173, 179
Pouch of Douglas **180,** 183
P.P.P.D. 186/7
Practitioner xii
  Behaviour 161
  Stance 19, **117,** 120, 137
Pregnancy 86, 100, 106, 178, 298
  Ectopic 183
Pressure 22, 163, 175
  Intra-orbital 153
  Sub-atmospheric 163
Principles 3, 116
P.R.M. 5, 23, 25, 30–43, 65, 110–13, 125, 131, 170, 193, 204
Process, Clinoid 73, 251, 255
  Pterygoid 154
  Pyramidal 281
  Styloid 256
  Uncinate 277
  Zyphoid **88**
Prolactin 79, 84
Prolapse 177, 181, 183, 185, 302
Promontory 298

Proptosis 87
Prostaglandin 25, 30
Prostate 17, 170, 185
Proturberance see Eminentia Cruciata
Psoas 190–197, **192**
  Psoitis 194, 209
  Treatment 191, 193, **194**
Psyche 190
Psychosomatic Release 23
Ptosis 185
Pulsation 17, 116, 135, 139, 149
P.W.F. 81

Quadrant Analysis 113, 141/2, **142**
Raphe 243, 268, 270, 280
Rathke's Pouch 84
Record Keeping 183
Rectum 171, 185/6
Reflexes 25, 163, 209
  Chapman's 17, 54
  Coccygeal 170
  Genitourinary 185
  Stretch 25
  Visceral Somatic 185, 199
Research xii, xiii, 5
Respiratory Action 25, 39, **40,** 207, 269, 302
  Cooperation 135, 141, 167, 171, 211
  Diaphragmatic 6, 30, 125
  Distress 94, 106, 171, 179
  Coccygeal 170
  P.R.M. 25, 30–43, 65, 111, 113
Restrictions xii, 56
  Fascial 58, 162
  Intracranial 35, 119
  Osseous 147, 155
Rete Chords 100
Rhythms & Impulses xii, 8, 21, 33, 38, 62, 81, 119, 122, 140, 190
Ribs 89, 133, 190, 193
Rotation 78
  Axial 21
  Osseous **59**
R.T.M. see Membrane
Sacral
  Base 22, 41, 299
  Flexion **88,** 111, 205, 206
  Lesions 22
  Moulding **172,** 175
  -Occipital balancing **26, 109,** 113
Sacralization 299
Sacro-Iliac Joint 21, 181, 298
Sacrum **18,** 21, 39, 62, 111, 171, 174–178, 181, 185, 229, 251

INDEX

& Coccyx 298–304
& Ilia 5, 65, 170
Scars **see** Tissue
Schizophrenia 103
Schooley Dr Thomas xiii
School of Osteopathy, Kirksville, Missouri 5
Sciatica 195
Scoliosis 173/5, 195
Sella Turcica 161
  as Pituitary housing 71, 83, 251
  position 41, 65, 131
Selye Hans 38, 103
Septal Cartilage 147, 251, 273, 277, 282
Seratonin 25, 79, 94
Sex Glands **see** Gonads
Shoulder Conditions 156
Sinuses
  Air 238, 251, 256, 270, 277
  Cavernous 153, 186, 251
  Confluence of 27, 161/2, 243
  Petrosal 153, 246, 256
  Sphenoidal 153, 283
  Straight 23, 27, 30, **31**, 39, 78, 123, 206
  Sagittal 30, 35, 39, 140, 238
  Transverse 243
  Venous 27, **42–3**, 153, 163, 238
Sinusitis 145, 164, 190, 205, 238, 272, 277
Skull **4, 10–12**, 41, 65, 128, **129**, 134, **216**, 218, 239, 296 **see also** Head
  Shape 125, 131, 174, 312
  Size 133
Slackation 153/4, 186, 205
Sleeplessness 17, 98
  Insomnia 202
Somatostatin 96
Spasm **see** Psoas
Spheno-Basilar
  Flexion & Extension 26, **58**, 190
  Lesions 71, 113, 164
  Side-bending 22, **59**, 71, **130**, 164, 281
  Synchondrosis 65, 134, 243, 254
  Symphysis **58/9, 70, 72**, 123, 134, 141/2, 226, 234, 254, 299
  Techniques **110, 112/3**, 112/3
  Testing 121
  Torsion 22, **69**, 164, 167, 185, 281
Sphenoid 55, 64–73, 120, 251–55, **253**
  Articulations 64, 73, 220, 254, 256

Lesions 22, 251, 254
Movements 27, 134, 227
Muscles **66**, 67/8, 251
Processes 73, 154, 251, 254/5
Sinuses 251
Wings 25, 64, 140, 164, 254
Sphenopalatine 286
  Ganglia 151
  Notch 151, 281
Spine 39, 183, 196, 211 **see also** Vertebrae
Spinal **69**
  Canal 35
  Cord 35, 39, 41
Stasis **see** Fluid
Stefansson Vilhjalmur 287
Sterility 178
Sternum 88, 89
A.T. Still xiii, 5, **6**, 7, 17, 19, 25, 29, 75, 104, 154
Still-Point 25, 78, 113, 135, 139, 141, 158, 161
Strain & Stress xii, xiii, 81, 85, 87, 93, 162
Stretch Olive M xiii, 105
Struma Lymphomatoza **see** Disease – Hashimoto's
Sub-Arachnoid Space 35
Sudden Death Syndrome 94
Suicide 28, 81, 206
Surgery 163, 185
Sutherland William Garner xi, xiii, 3, **6**, 7, 8, 14, 15, 19, 30, 39, 64, 75, 104, 147, 251, 255/6
  His experiments 5
Sutural Behaviour xi, 121, 158
  Bevels 219–222, **233**
  Harmony 134
  Imbalance 158
  Irregularities/Anomalies 19
  Restrictions 51, 131, 158
Sutures 19, 219–222
  Cranial 3, 30, **148**
  Basal 220/221
  Coronal 140, 220, 239
  C.S.M. 220, 246
  Lambdoidal 125, 140, 220, 292
  Metopic 27, 139, 220, 234, 292
  O.M. 22, 41, 220, 246
  Sagittal 125, 140, **126**, 220
  Sphenoidal 64, 220
  Squamosal 140, 219/220, 256
  Temporal 154, 221, 256
Symphysis **70, 72**
  Menti 149, 153/4, 264/5
  Pubis 181
Synovial Fluid 45

System 163
  Cardio-vascular 17
  Circulatory 35–46, **42–3**, 58
  Lymphatic 46–49, 53

Tactile
  Capacity 158
  Finesse 19, 135, 171
Taylor, Best & 75
Taylor, Robert B 6
Techniques xii, 54, **110, 112–3**, 167
  Balancing **109**
  Bi-temporal rolling **80**, 83
  Cranial Base
    Decompression 134, **136**
    Decongestion 135, **136**
  Direct Action 28
  Direction of Energy
    E.T.T. 158–162, **159–60**, 206, 209
    V-Spread 158, 160, 174
  Exaggeration 28
  4 Finger **159, 160**, 160
  4 V.C. 106–114, **107–8**, 141
  'Kettle-Lid' 71
  Lifts **138**, 139, 280
  Moulding 171–5, **172**
  'Shot-gun' method 155, 193
  Special 158–177, **166, 169**
  Spread **126**, 139, 140, 280
  Spontaneous Release 135
  Thoracic Inlet **50**, 53
  Vault Holds 206
Teeth 91, 128, 145–7, 154, 164, 239, 244, 270–1
Temporal 17, 23, 25, 164, 255–259, **259**
  Articulations 221, 257
  Lesions 133–135, 255
  Movements 164, 227, 255
  Rotation 135
  Treatment 80, 83, 166/7
  'Wobbling Wheel' 256
Tendon
  Central 185
  Orbital 254
Tentorium Cerebelli 39, 162, 239, 255/6, **see also** Dural
Testes 99/100, **101**
Testosterone 99/100
Thalamus **82**
Thoracic
  Drainage 50, 51
  Duct 49, **50**
  Inlet 53
Thumb-Sucking 145, 147, 271
Thymosin 93

323

Thymus 79, **90**
  Secretion 93
  Structure & Function 92–94
Thyroxin 86/7, 97
Thyroid 17
  Hormonal secretion 79, 84, 86
  Structure & Function 86–91, **90**, 185
  Treatment **88**, 89, 204
Thyroiditis 89
Tic Douloureux 256
Tidy, Noel M 179
Tinnitus see Ear
Tiredness 93, 201, 204
Tissue 86, 89, 119, 242, 299
  Cerebral 128
  Connective 35, 91, 209
  Cervical 158
  Relaxation of 162
  Scar 162, 181
  Slack-tension 41
  T.M.J. 64, 154/6, 164, 239, 265
Tone 106, 116, 201
Tonus 65, 111, 264
Torsion 21, 41, **69, 70**, 141, 147, 195, **see also** Sphenobasilar
  Coccygeal 169
Torus Palatinus 147, 149, 205, 271, 281
Toxicity 28, 89, 93, 121, 145, 162, 168, 190
Traction 23
  Caudal 156
  Digital 155
  Induced 131
Transverse Functioning Muscle Stimulus 193
Trauma 14, 163, 170
  Birth 8, 17, 128–135, 174, 206
  Direct 135, 175, 239, 268, 271/2, 281
  Indirect 272
  Infantile 133
  Shock 25, 135, 164, 171
Treatment 15
  Coccygeal 169–171, **169**

Contraindications 7, 17, 51, 54, 134
Cranial 75, 100
Facial 145–156, **146, 152**, 206, 278
Frequency of 135, 149, 161, 171, 186
Gynaecological 181–187
Sacral **26, 88, 109–110**, 113, **172**, 175, 205/6
Tubercinereum 83
Tumours, Malignant 49, 79, 84, 92, 93, 181, 183
Uterine 178, 181, 183, 185

Uterus 99, 100, 177/8, **180**
  Displacements 170, 181–187
  Inertia 100, 106, 186
  Structure & Function 98–100, 106
  Treatment 181–187
Upledger, John E (& Jon D Vredevoogd) 147

Vagina 177, 181/2, 186
Vasoconstrictors 163
Vasopression 78, 85
Vault xii, 5, 41, 65, 218, 221, 227, 232–246, **233, 235, 237, 241, 245**
  Lesions 21, 59, 62, 128, 143, 153, 211, 239, 243, 283
  Structure & Function 221, **see also** individual bones
  Techniques 71, **126**, 128–143, **138**, 206, 280
Ventricles 33, **36–7**, 106
  1 & 2. Lateral 33–38
  3rd 38, 79, 83, 106
  4th 30, 35, 38, 57, 78, 100, 106–114, **107, 108, 109**, 141
Vertebrae 184, 201–2
  Cervical 22, 27, 39, 57, 86, 163, 167, 288
  Coccygeal 169–71, 302–4, **304**
  Dorsal 22, 177, 183, 185, 191–7, 201

Key 185, 223–226
Key Pairs 226
Lumbar 22, 41, 51, 111, 162, 170, 177–187, 191–197, **196**, 201, 299
Modified 69
Neutral 201
Sacral **18**, 21, 39, 111, 174–178, 181, 185, 298–301
Vertigo 162, 164, 168–9, 205
Veins 30, 39, 165
  Emissary 153, 239, 257
  Neck 163, 256
  of Galen 28, 149
  Opthalmic 153
Vital Capacity 170
Vomer 147, 151, 282, **285**
  Articulations 221, 283–6
  Lesions 283
  Movements 27, 228
  Treatment 28, **148**
  -vaginal canal 286
Vomitting 107, 162
'V' Spread 158–61, 175

Walton, Izaak 294
Waves 33
  C.S.F. 33, 35
Whitnall's Tubercle 268
'Wobbling Wheel' see Temporal
Willis Disease see Disease Circle of 28
Wilson, Perrin T 56
Wormian Bones see Bones

X-Rays 79, 116, 121, 197, 251

Yutang Lin 203

Zygoma 17, 65, **148, 274**
  Articulations 220/221, 256, 269
  Lesions 151, 268
  Movements 27, 228
  Structure & Function 153, 268–9